D0520202

ACP | MKSAP® 17

Medical Knowledge Self-Assessment Program®

Neurology

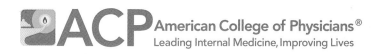

American College of Physicians®
Leading Internal Medicine, Improving Lives

Welcome to the Neurology Section of MKSAP 17!

In these pages, you will find updated information on headache and facial pain, head injury, epilepsy, stroke, cognitive disorders, movement disorders, multiple sclerosis, disorders of the spinal cord, neuromuscular disorders, and neuro-oncology. All of these topics are uniquely focused on the needs of generalists and subspecialists *outside* of neurology.

The publication of the 17th edition of Medical Knowledge Self-Assessment Program (MKSAP) represents nearly a half-century of serving as the gold-standard resource for internal medicine education. It also marks its evolution into an innovative learning system to better meet the changing educational needs and learning styles of all internists.

The core content of MKSAP has been developed as in previous editions—newly generated, essential information in 11 topic areas of internal medicine created by dozens of leading generalists and subspecialists and guided by certification and recertification requirements, emerging knowledge in the field, and user feedback. MKSAP 17 also contains 1200 all-new, psychometrically validated, and peer-reviewed multiple-choice questions (MCQs) for self-assessment and study, including 96 in Neurology. MKSAP 17 continues to include *High Value Care* (HVC) recommendations, based on the concept of balancing clinical benefit with costs and harms, with links to MCQs that illustrate these principles. In addition, HVC Key Points are highlighted in the text. Also highlighted, with blue text, are *Hospitalist*-focused content and MCQs that directly address the learning needs of internists who work in the hospital setting.

MKSAP 17 Digital provides access to additional tools allowing you to customize your learning experience, including regular text updates with practice-changing, new information and 200 new self-assessment questions; a board-style pretest to help direct your learning; and enhanced custom-quiz options. And, with MKSAP Complete, learners can access 1200 electronic flashcards for quick review of important concepts or review the updated and enhanced version of Virtual Dx, an image-based self-assessment tool.

As before, MKSAP 17 is optimized for use on your mobile devices, with iOS- and Android-based apps allowing you to sync your work between your apps and online account and submit for CME credits and MOC points online.

Please visit us at the MKSAP Resource Site (mksap.acponline.org) to find out how we can help you study, earn CME credit and MOC points, and stay up to date.

Whether you prefer to use the traditional print version or take advantage of the features available through the digital version, we hope you enjoy MKSAP 17 and that it meets and exceeds your personal learning needs.

On behalf of the many internists who have offered their time and expertise to create the content for MKSAP 17 and the editorial staff who work to bring this material to you in the best possible way, we are honored that you have chosen to use MKSAP 17 and appreciate any feedback about the program you may have. Please feel free to send us any comments to mksap_editors@acponline.org.

Sincerely,

Philip A. Masters, MD, FACP
Editor-in-Chief
Senior Physician Educator
Director, Content Development
Medical Education Division
American College of Physicians

Neurology

Committee

Robert Kaniecki, MD, Section Editor[2]
Director, The Headache Center
Chief, Headache Division
Assistant Professor of Neurology
University of Pittsburgh
Pittsburgh, Pennsylvania

Jack Ende, MD, MACP, Associate Editor[1]
The Schaeffer Professor of Medicine
Perelman School of Medicine at the University of
    Pennsylvania
Philadelphia, Pennsylvania

Anahita Adeli, MD[2]
Assistant Professor of Neurology
Department of Neurology
The Ohio State University Wexner Medical Center
Columbus, Ohio

Elizabeth E. Gerard, MD[2]
Assistant Professor of Neurology
Feinberg School of Medicine
Northwestern University
Chicago, Illinois

Daniel M. Harrison, MD[2]
Assistant Professor of Neurology
Johns Hopkins Multiple Sclerosis Center
Johns Hopkins University School of Medicine
Baltimore, Maryland

Houman Homayoun, MD[1]
Assistant Professor of Neurology
Department of Neurology
University of Pittsburgh Medical Center
Pittsburgh, Pennsylvania

Joshua Z. Willey, MD, MS[2]
Assistant Professor of Neurology
Columbia University Medical Center
New York, New York

Editor-in-Chief

Philip A. Masters, MD, FACP[1]
Director, Clinical Content Development
American College of Physicians
Philadelphia, Pennsylvania

Director, Clinical Program Development

Cynthia D. Smith, MD, FACP[2]
American College of Physicians
Philadelphia, Pennsylvania

Neurology Reviewers

Thomas E. Finucane, MD, FACP[1]
Lois Geist, MD[1]
Richard M. Hoffman, MD, MPH, FACP[1]
Bashar Katirji, MD, FACP[2]
Adrian Sequeira, MD, FACP[1]

Neurology Reviewer Representing the American Society for Clinical Pharmacology & Therapeutics

Linda A. Hershey, MD[2]

Neurology ACP Editorial Staff

Ellen McDonald, PhD[1], Senior Staff Editor
Margaret Wells[1], Director, Self-Assessment and Educational
    Programs
Becky Krumm[1], Managing Editor

ACP Principal Staff

Patrick C. Alguire, MD, FACP[2]
Senior Vice President, Medical Education

Sean McKinney[1]
Vice President, Medical Education

Margaret Wells[1]
Director, Self-Assessment and Educational Programs

Becky Krumm[1]
Managing Editor

Valerie A. Dangovetsky[1]
Administrator

Ellen McDonald, PhD[1]
Senior Staff Editor

Katie Idell[1]
Digital Content Associate/Editor

Megan Zborowski[1]
Senior Staff Editor

Randy Hendrickson[1]
Production Administrator/Editor

Linnea Donnarumma[1]
Staff Editor

Susan Galeone[1]
Staff Editor

Jackie Twomey[1]
Staff Editor

Kimberly Kerns[1]
Administrative Coordinator

---

1. Has no relationships with any entity producing, marketing, reselling, or distributing health care goods or services consumed by, or used on, patients.

2. Has disclosed relationship(s) with any entity producing, marketing, reselling, or distributing health care goods or services consumed by, or used on, patients.

Disclosure of Relationships with any entity producing, marketing, reselling, or distributing health care goods or services consumed by, or used on, patients:

Anahita Adeli, MD
Other
Eli-Lily, Lundbeck, Envivo, Merck, Pfizer

Patrick C. Alguire, MD, FACP
Board Member
Teva Pharmaceuticals
Consultantship
National Board of Medical Examiners
Royalties
UpToDate
Stock Options/Holdings
Amgen Inc, Bristol-Myers Squibb, GlaxoSmithKline, Covidien, Stryker Corporation, Zimmer Orthopedics, Teva Pharmaceuticals, Express Scripts, Medtronic

Elizabeth Gerard, MD
Research Grants/Contracts
Sage Pharmaceuticals, UCB

Daniel M. Harrison, MD
Research Grants/Contracts
Bayer Schering Pharmaceuticals, Sanofi Aventis, Avanir Pharmaceuticals, Biogen-IDEC, Merk-Serono
Consultantship
Questcor, MedImmune, Genzyme

Linda A. Hershey, MD
Employment
OU Health Science Center
Research Grants/Contracts
Baxter, NIH
Royalties
Med Link Co.

Robert Kaniecki, MD
Consultantship
Allergan
Honoraria
Zogenix

Bashar Katirji, MD, FACP
Royalties
Elsevier Publishers

Cynthia D. Smith, MD, FACP
Stock Options/Holdings
Merck and Co.; spousal employment at Merck

Joshua Z. Willey, MD, MS
Honoraria
Cardionet
Research Grants/Contracts
Genentech; AstraZeneca
Consultantship
Heartware Incorporated

Acknowledgments

The American College of Physicians (ACP) gratefully acknowledges the special contributions to the development and production of the 17th edition of the Medical Knowledge Self-Assessment Program® (MKSAP® 17) made by the following people:

Graphic Design: Michael Ripca (Graphics Technical Administrator) and WFGD Studio (Graphic Designers).

Production/Systems: Dan Hoffmann (Director, Web Services & Systems Development), Neil Kohl (Senior Architect), Chris Patterson (Senior Architect), and Scott Hurd (Manager, Web Projects & CMS Services).

MKSAP 17 Digital: Under the direction of Steven Spadt, Vice President, Digital Products & Services, the digital version of MKSAP 17 was developed within the ACP's Digital Product Development Department, led by Brian Sweigard (Director). Other members of the team included Dan Barron (Senior Web Application Developer/Architect), Chris Forrest (Senior Software Developer/Design Lead), Kara Kronenwetter (Senior Web Developer), Brad Lord (Senior Web Application Developer), John McKnight (Senior Web Developer), and Nate Pershall (Senior Web Developer).

The College also wishes to acknowledge that many other persons, too numerous to mention, have contributed to the production of this program. Without their dedicated efforts, this program would not have been possible.

MKSAP Resource Site (mksap.acponline.org)

The MKSAP Resource Site (mksap.acponline.org) is a continually updated site that provides links to MKSAP 17 online answer sheets for print subscribers; the latest details on Continuing Medical Education (CME) and Maintenance of Certification (MOC) in the United States, Canada, and Australia; errata; and other new information.

ABIM Maintenance of Certification

Check the MKSAP Resource Site (mksap.acponline.org) for the latest information on how MKSAP tests can be used to apply to the American Board of Internal Medicine for Maintenance of Certification (MOC) points.

Royal College Maintenance of Certification

In Canada, MKSAP 17 is an Accredited Self-Assessment Program (Section 3) as defined by the Maintenance of Certification (MOC) Program of The Royal College of Physicians and Surgeons of Canada and approved by the Canadian Society of Internal Medicine on December 9, 2014. Approval extends from July 31, 2015 until July 31, 2018 for the Part A sections. Approval extends from December 31, 2015 to December 31, 2018 for the Part B sections.

Fellows of the Royal College may earn three credits per hour for participating in MKSAP 17 under Section 3. MKSAP 17 also meets multiple CanMEDS Roles, including that of Medical Expert, Communicator, Collaborator, Manager, Health Advocate, Scholar, and Professional. For information on how to apply MKSAP 17 Continuing Medical Education (CME) credits to the Royal College MOC Program, visit the MKSAP Resource Site at mksap.acponline.org.

The Royal Australasian College of Physicians CPD Program

In Australia, MKSAP 17 is a Category 3 program that may be used by Fellows of The Royal Australasian College of Physicians (RACP) to meet mandatory Continuing Professional Development (CPD) points. Two CPD credits are awarded for each of the 200 *AMA PRA Category 1 Credits*™ available in MKSAP 17. More information about using MKSAP 17 for this purpose is available at the MKSAP Resource Site at mksap.acponline.org and at www.racp.edu.au. CPD credits earned through MKSAP 17 should be reported at the MyCPD site at www.racp.edu.au/mycpd.

Continuing Medical Education

The American College of Physicians (ACP) is accredited by the Accreditation Council for Continuing Medical Education (ACCME) to provide continuing medical education for physicians.

The ACP designates this enduring material, MKSAP 17, for a maximum of 200 *AMA PRA Category 1 Credits*™. Physicians should claim only the credit commensurate with the extent of their participation in the activity.

Up to 16 *AMA PRA Category 1 Credits*™ are available from July 31, 2015, to July 31, 2018, for the MKSAP 17 Neurology section.

Learning Objectives

The learning objectives of MKSAP 17 are to:
- Close gaps between actual care in your practice and preferred standards of care, based on best evidence
- Diagnose disease states that are less common and sometimes overlooked or confusing
- Improve management of comorbid conditions that can complicate patient care
- Determine when to refer patients for surgery or care by subspecialists
- Pass the ABIM Certification Examination
- Pass the ABIM Maintenance of Certification Examination

Target Audience

- General internists and primary care physicians
- Subspecialists who need to remain up-to-date in internal medicine and in areas outside of their own subspecialty area
- Residents preparing for the certification examination in internal medicine
- Physicians preparing for maintenance of certification in internal medicine (recertification)

Earn "Instantaneous" CME Credits Online

Print subscribers can enter their answers online to earn instantaneous Continuing Medical Education (CME) credits. You can submit your answers using online answer sheets that are provided at mksap.acponline.org, where a record of your MKSAP 17 credits will be available. To earn CME credits, you need to answer all of the questions in a test and earn a score of at least 50% correct (number of correct answers divided by the total number of questions). Take any of the following approaches:

1. Use the printed answer sheet at the back of this book to record your answers. Go to mksap.acponline.org, access the appropriate online answer sheet, transcribe your answers, and submit your test for instantaneous CME credits. There is no additional fee for this service.

2. Go to mksap.acponline.org, access the appropriate online answer sheet, directly enter your answers, and submit your test for instantaneous CME credits. There is no additional fee for this service.

3. Pay a $15 processing fee per answer sheet and submit the printed answer sheet at the back of this book by mail or fax, as instructed on the answer sheet. Make sure you calculate your score and fax the answer sheet to 215-351-2799 or mail the answer sheet to Member and Customer Service, American College of Physicians, 190 N. Independence Mall West, Philadelphia, PA 19106-1572, using the courtesy envelope provided in your MKSAP 17 slipcase. You will need your 10-digit order number and 8-digit ACP ID number, which are printed on your packing slip. Please allow 4 to 6 weeks for your score report to be emailed back to you. Be sure to include your email address for a response.

If you do not have a 10-digit order number and 8-digit ACP ID number or if you need help creating a user name and password to access the MKSAP 17 online answer sheets, go to mksap.acponline.org or email custserv@acponline.org.

Disclosure Policy

It is the policy of the American College of Physicians (ACP) to ensure balance, independence, objectivity, and scientific rigor in all of its educational activities. To this end, and consistent with the policies of the ACP and the Accreditation Council for Continuing Medical Education (ACCME), contributors to all ACP continuing medical education activities are required to disclose all relevant financial relationships with any entity producing, marketing, re-selling, or distributing health care goods or services consumed by, or used on, patients. Contributors are required to use generic names in the discussion of therapeutic options and are required to identify any unapproved, off-label, or investigative use of commercial products or devices. Where a trade name is used, all available trade names for the same product type are also included. If trade-name products manufactured by companies with whom contributors have relationships are discussed, contributors are asked to provide evidence-based citations in support of the discussion. The information is reviewed by the committee responsible for producing this text. If necessary, adjustments to topics or contributors' roles in content development are made to balance the discussion. Further, all readers of this text are asked to evaluate the content for evidence of commercial bias and send any relevant comments to mksap_editors@acponline.org so that future decisions about content and contributors can be made in light of this information.

Resolution of Conflicts

To resolve all conflicts of interest and influences of vested interests, the American College of Physicians (ACP) precluded members of the content-creation committee from deciding on any content issues that involved generic or trade-name products associated with proprietary entities with which these committee members had relationships. In addition, content was based on best evidence and updated clinical care guidelines, when such evidence and guidelines were available. Contributors' disclosure information can be found with the list of contributors' names and those of ACP principal staff listed in the beginning of this book.

Hospital-Based Medicine

For the convenience of subscribers who provide care in hospital settings, content that is specific to the hospital setting has been highlighted in blue. Hospital icons (H) highlight where the hospital-based content begins, continues over more than one page, and ends.

High Value Care Key Points

Key Points in the text that relate to High Value Care concepts (that is, concepts that discuss balancing clinical benefit with costs and harms) are designated by the HVC icon (HVC).

Educational Disclaimer

The editors and publisher of MKSAP 17 recognize that the development of new material offers many opportunities for error. Despite our best efforts, some errors may persist in print. Drug dosage schedules are, we believe, accurate and in accordance with current standards. Readers are advised, however, to ensure that the recommended dosages in MKSAP 17 concur with the information provided in the product information material. This is especially important in cases of new, infrequently used, or highly toxic drugs. Application of the information in MKSAP 17 remains the professional responsibility of the practitioner.

The primary purpose of MKSAP 17 is educational. Information presented, as well as publications, technologies, products, and/or services discussed, is intended to inform subscribers about the knowledge, techniques, and experiences of the contributors. A diversity of professional opinion exists, and the views of the contributors are their own and not those of the American College of Physicians (ACP). Inclusion of any material in the program does not constitute endorsement or recommendation by the ACP. The ACP does not warrant the safety, reliability, accuracy, completeness, or usefulness of and disclaims any and all liability for damages and claims that may result from the use of information, publications, technologies, products, and/or services discussed in this program.

Publisher's Information

Copyright © 2015 American College of Physicians. All rights reserved.

This publication is protected by copyright. No part of this publication may be reproduced, stored in a retrieval system, or transmitted in any form or by any means, electronic or mechanical, including photocopy, without the express consent of the American College of Physicians. MKSAP 17 is for individual use only. Only one account per subscription will be permitted for the purpose of earning Continuing Medical Education (CME) credits and Maintenance of Certification (MOC) points/credits and for other authorized uses of MKSAP 17.

Unauthorized Use of This Book Is Against the Law

Unauthorized reproduction of this publication is unlawful. The American College of Physicians (ACP) prohibits reproduction of this publication or any of its parts in any form either for individual use or for distribution.

The ACP will consider granting an individual permission to reproduce only limited portions of this publication for his or her own exclusive use. Send requests in writing to MKSAP® Permissions, American College of Physicians, 190 N. Independence Mall West, Philadelphia, PA 19106-1572, or email your request to mksap_editors@acponline.org.

MKSAP 17 ISBN: 978-1-938245-18-3
(Neurology) ISBN: 978-1-938245-23-7

Printed in the United States of America.

For order information in the United States or Canada call 800-523-1546, extension 2600. All other countries call 215-351-2600, (M-F, 9 AM – 5 PM ET). Fax inquiries to 215-351-2799 or email to custserv@acponline.org.

Errata

Errata for MKSAP 17 will be available through the MKSAP Resource Site at mksap.acponline.org as new information becomes known to the editors.

Table of Contents

Movement Disorders

Multiple Sclerosis

Disorders of the Spinal Cord

Neuromuscular Disorders

Neuro-oncology

Bibliography

Self-Assessment Test

Index

Neurology High Value Care Recommendations

The American College of Physicians, in collaboration with multiple other organizations, is engaged in a worldwide initiative to promote the practice of High Value Care (HVC). The goals of the HVC initiative are to improve health care outcomes by providing care of proven benefit and reducing costs by avoiding unnecessary and even harmful interventions. The initiative comprises several programs that integrate the important concept of health care value (balancing clinical benefit with costs and harms) for a given intervention into a broad range of educational materials to address the needs of trainees, practicing physicians, and patients.

HVC content has been integrated into MKSAP 17 in several important ways. MKSAP 17 now includes HVC-identified key points in the text, HVC-focused multiple choice questions, and, for subscribers to MKSAP Digital, an HVC custom quiz. From the text and questions, we have generated the following list of HVC recommendations that meet the definition below of high value care and bring us closer to our goal of improving patient outcomes while conserving finite resources.

High Value Care Recommendation: A recommendation to choose diagnostic and management strategies for patients in specific clinical situations that balance clinical benefit with cost and harms with the goal of improving patient outcomes.

Below are the High Value Care Recommendations for the Neurology section of MKSAP 17.

- Guidelines specifically recommend against neuroimaging studies in patients with stable headaches that meet criteria for migraine or uncomplicated headache (see Item 48).
- No evidence supports the superiority of anticoagulation over antiplatelet therapy in prevention of stroke after carotid and vertebral artery dissections, and most patients are initially managed with aspirin.
- Patients with unruptured intracranial aneurysms should be counseled to stop smoking because of the increased risk of aneurysmal rupture (see Item 72).
- Because of the documented significantly higher rates of medication overuse headache in patients exposed to butalbital compounds and opioid analgesics, these agents should be avoided in headache management.
- One way of remedying the high rate of misdiagnosis of migraine is to use the POUND mnemonic, which includes the following criteria: headache that is Pulsatile, is One-day in duration (with episodes lasting 4-72 hours if untreated), is Unilateral, is accompanied by Nausea/ vomiting, and is Disabling; patients with greater than three of these criteria can be diagnosed with migraine without further evaluation.
- Evidence-based guidelines suggest that NSAIDs, triptans, and dihydroergotamine are effective treatments for acute migraine without aura and that NSAIDs are preferred as initial treatment because of their greater cost-effectiveness (see Item 69).
- No good evidence supports the superior efficacy of any oral NSAID or triptan choice; cost, formulary availability, and results of previous medication trials are all considerations in the selection of acute migraine medication.
- In order to improve health outcomes, such as attack frequency, intensity, disability, and cost, the use of preventive agents should be considered in patients with eight or more total days or four or more disabling days of migraine per month.
- In persons who sustain mild traumatic brain injury, neuroimaging is only recommended if symptoms of worsening headache, repeated vomiting, drowsiness, persistent confusion, dysarthria, or focal neurologic findings are present; head CT is preferable to brain MRI for initial neuroimaging because of its wider availability, lower cost, and greater sensitivity for identifying skull fractures.
- Contact sports should be prohibited in patients who are symptomatic after sustaining a mild traumatic brain injury (see Item 51).
- Because patients older than 75 years have the highest rates of morbidity, hospitalization, and mortality after traumatic brain injury, prevention is key; preventive measures include avoiding overmedication and encouraging regular physical activity and living area modifications.
- Single seizures that are provoked usually do not require treatment with an antiepileptic drug and instead should be addressed by correcting the underlying condition or removing the offending agent; further diagnostic evaluation, such as neuroimaging and electroencephalography, may not be needed if a clear reversible cause of the seizure is identified and the patient has normal findings on neurologic examination.
- In a patient with a single unprovoked seizure and a normal electroencephalogram and MRI, the 2-year recurrence risk is 30% to 40%; because seizure medications reduce this risk by only approximately 50%, antiepileptic drug therapy is not typically recommended.

- Choosing an AED for an individual patient depends on several factors, including his or her epilepsy syndrome, age, sex, and comorbid medical conditions and the drug's adverse-effect profile and cost.
- The use of generic antiepileptic drugs (AEDs) is a way to control costs for patients with epilepsy, and the major consideration in using a generic AED is its bioavailability, which may differ by as much as 20% between manufacturers; because drug level maintenance is critical to maintaining seizure threshold, patients taking generic AEDs should try to use the same drug manufacturer from month to month.
- Most patients with asymptomatic extracranial internal carotid artery stenosis should be treated with aggressive risk factor control and not stenting or elective endarterectomy, which should only be considered in patients with a greater than 80% stenosis and low cardiovascular risk (as long as the operative complication rate is less than 3%).
- Using a statin to treat patients with asymptomatic internal carotid artery stenosis is associated with a stroke risk of less than 2% per year (see Item 35) and may prevent the need for endarterectomy.
- No reliable clinical markers or diagnostic tests can predict the likelihood that an individual patient with mild cognitive impairment will develop dementia, and no intervention has been shown to delay the onset of dementia in such a patient.
- For older patients with suspected cognitive impairment who are asymptomatic, insufficient evidence supports routine cognitive testing.
- Currently, the use of Alzheimer disease biomarkers in the clinical setting has no role because of the absence of disease-modifying therapies and the cost of advanced neuroimaging techniques and laboratory testing.
- Cholinesterase inhibitors have not been approved to treat frontotemporal dementia and vascular neurocognitive disorder or to delay progression from mild cognitive impairment to dementia.
- Nonpharmacologic interventions are often effective in treating the behavioral symptoms experienced by patients with dementia and should be the first-line treatment.
- No pharmacologic therapy is currently FDA approved for the prevention or treatment of delirium.
- Neurologic examination, particularly assessments of motor function and gait, is a low risk, high value means to distinguish the various movement disorders.
- The diagnosis of Parkinson disease can be made on the basis of clinical findings and requires the presence of bradykinesia and at least one of the other cardinal features of resting tremor, rigidity, or postural instability (see Item 73).
- Single photon emission CT of the brain should be reserved for differentiating Parkinson disease from drug-induced parkinsonism in patients with an atypical clinical picture.
- Recent studies have shown the beneficial role of rigorous daily exercise in improving motor fitness and gait in patients with Parkinson disease, and thus physical activity or physical therapy should be encouraged in all patients with the disease.
- Cerebrospinal fluid testing can be helpful when the diagnosis of MS is not clear but is not required for diagnosis if the full McDonald criteria have been met and other causes have been excluded.
- Maintenance of an active healthy lifestyle and strengthening, stretching, and aerobic exercise are recommended for all patients with multiple sclerosis to mitigate disability and preserve appropriate muscle tone.
- Routine vaccinations, such as an annual influenza vaccination, are recommended for patients with multiple sclerosis (MS) to prevent infections leading to a heightened immune state and potential MS relapse (see Item 68).
- Smoking cessation is strongly advised for all patients with multiple sclerosis because of the threefold increased risk of conversion to secondary progression associated with cigarette smoking.
- Treatment of a pseudorelapse of multiple sclerosis, which is worsening of baseline neurologic symptoms or recurrence of previous symptoms in the setting of physiologic stressors, should consist of observation and supportive therapy and not include increased immunosuppressive therapy (see Item 74).
- Although newer medications, such as pregabalin and duloxetine, have been used successfully to treat neuropathic pain in multiple sclerosis, less expensive generic alternatives, such as tricyclic antidepressants and gabapentin, are as effective and well tolerated.
- Low doses of tricyclic antidepressants, such as amitriptyline and nortriptyline, are a cost-effective, first-line treatment option for patients with painful peripheral neuropathy.
- Nerve biopsy is indicated only in a small subset of neuropathies when concern for vasculitic, infectious, or infiltrative neuropathy exists.
- Meralgia paresthetica, a compressive neuropathy of the lateral femoral cutaneous nerve that causes isolated anterolateral thigh numbness without weakness, can be clinically diagnosed and treated conservatively.
- Carpal tunnel syndrome can be diagnosed clinically by the presence of hypalgesia in the distribution of the median nerve; initial treatment involves wrist bracing, occupational therapy, and anti-inflammatory medications; electromyographic studies are not necessary.
- Bell palsy is idiopathic paralysis of the facial nerve that leads to complete unilateral facial paralysis; patients with a classic presentation and no other neurologic deficits can be diagnosed without brain imaging and laboratory testing.

- Early treatment of Bell Palsy with oral prednisone (within 72 hours of symptom onset) improves outcomes; antiviral therapy does not affect prognosis.
- Diagnosis of diabetic peripheral neuropathy is clinical, and electromyographic studies are not necessary for patients with classic symptoms.
- Amyotrophic lateral sclerosis (ALS) is a fatal disease involving the motoneurons that is associated with progressive weakness and muscle wasting for which treatment is supportive; it is essential to discuss prognosis and establish goals of care with patients and families, thereby avoiding unnecessary diagnostic and therapeutic measures.
- Small asymptomatic meningiomas can be followed conservatively with an initial repeat MRI at 3 to 6 months.
- Prophylactic use of antiepileptic drugs is not recommended in most patients with brain tumors.

Neurology

Headache and Facial Pain

Approach to the Patient with Headache

Headache is one of the most common reasons for presentation to an internist or emergency department. The diagnostic classification outlined in the third edition of the International Classification of Headache Disorders (ICHD-3) categorizes headache as primary, secondary, or related to a cranial neuralgia. Primary headaches are biologic disorders of the brain that are differentiated on the basis of clinical criteria (**Table 1**). Secondary headache disorders are defined by identifiable organic causation (**Table 2**) and typically display one of the following clinical "red flags."

- First or worst headache
- Abrupt-onset or thunderclap attack
- Progression or fundamental change in headache pattern
- Abnormal physical examination findings
- Neurologic symptoms lasting greater than 1 hour
- New headache in persons younger than 5 years or older than 50 years
- New headache in patients with cancer or immunosuppression or in pregnant women
- Association with alteration in or loss of consciousness
- Headache triggered by exertion, sexual activity, or Valsalva maneuver

The neurologic examination must involve thorough cranial nerve assessments, including funduscopic and visual field testing; additional examination of the cervical spine, carotid and temporal vessels, and temporomandibular joint may be helpful. Neuroimaging is indicated for suspected secondary headaches that exhibit one of the clinical red flags but is rarely appropriate in the evaluation of primary headache disorders; guidelines specifically recommend against neuroimaging studies in patients with stable headaches that meet criteria for migraine. When neuroimaging is necessary, MRI is preferred over CT (except in emergency settings, such as trauma-related headache or suspected acute intracerebral hemorrhage) because of its greater sensitivity and lack of radiation exposure. Suspected giant cell (temporal) arteritis should provoke measurement of erythrocyte sedimentation rate and C-reactive protein level. Lumbar puncture may be helpful in patients with suspected infectious or neoplastic meningitis or disorders of

TABLE 1. Primary Headache Syndromes
Migraine
Migraine without aura
Migraine with aura
Migraine with typical aura
Migraine with brainstem aura
Hemiplegic migraine
Retinal migraine
Chronic migraine
Complicated migraine
Probable migraine
Episodic syndromes possibly associated with migraine
Tension-Type Headache
Infrequent episodic tension-type headache
Frequent episodic tension-type headache
Chronic tension-type headache
Trigeminal Autonomic Cephalalgias
Cluster headache
Chronic paroxysmal hemicrania
Short-lasting unilateral neuralgiform headache attacks
With conjunctival injection and tearing (SUNCT)
With cranial autonomic symptoms (SUNA)
Hemicrania continua
Other Primary Headache Disorders
Primary cough headache
Primary exercise headache
Primary headache associated with sexual activity
Primary thunderclap headache
Cold-stimulus headache
External-pressure headache
Primary stabbing headache
Nummular headache
Hypnic headache
New daily persistent headache

Adapted with permission of SAGE Publications Ltd., London, Los Angeles, New Delhi, Singapore and Washington DC, from Headache Classification Committee of the International Headache Society (IHS). The International Classification of Headache Disorders, 3rd edition (beta version). Cephalalgia. 2013 Jul;33(9): 636–7. [PMID: 23771276]. Copyright SAGE Publications Ltd., 2013.

TABLE 2.	Secondary Headache Syndromes

Posttraumatic headache

    Head injury

    Whiplash injury

Headache attributed to cranial or cervical vascular disorder

    Ischemic stroke or transient ischemic attack

    Parenchymal or subarachnoid hemorrhage

    Unruptured vascular malformation or aneurysm

    Intracranial or extracranial arteritis

    Arterial dissection

    Venous or sinus thrombosis

Headache attributed to nonvascular intracranial disorders

    Intracranial hypotension or hypertension

    Brain neoplasia

    Noninfectious inflammatory disorders (sarcoidosis)

    Chiari malformation

Headache attributed to substance use or withdrawal

    Medication adverse event (nitrates)

    Alcohol

    Caffeine withdrawal

    Medication overuse headache

Headache attributed to infection

    Intracranial infection (meningitis, encephalitis, brain abscess)

    Extracranial infection (systemic bacterial infection, viral syndrome)

Headache attributed to disorder of homeostasis

    Hypertensive crisis, dialysis, hypoxia, hypercapnia, hypothyroidism

Headache attributed to disorder of the neck, eyes, ears, nose, sinuses, teeth, or mouth

Cranial neuralgias

Adapted with permission of SAGE Publications Ltd., London, Los Angeles, New Delhi, Singapore and Washington DC, from Headache Classification Committee of the International Headache Society (IHS). The International Classification of Headache Disorders, 3rd edition (beta version). Cephalalgia. 2013 Jul;33(9): 637-41. [PMID: 23771276]. Copyright SAGE Publications Ltd., 2013.

intracranial pressure. Electroencephalography has no role in the assessment of headache disorders.

After exclusion of secondary headache, primary headaches are best classified by evaluation of headache frequency, duration, and phenotypic expression, including pain descriptors and any associated neurologic, sensory, gastrointestinal, or autonomic components. The term episodic is used when headache-free days outnumber headache days over a defined period of time, and the term chronic when the number of days with headache is greater than the number of days without headache. Quantification of acute headache medication use is critical to identify those at risk for medication overuse headache. Greater than 90% of primary headaches involve a variant of migraine. Other primary disorders, such as tension-type

and cluster headache, should be considered only after both secondary headache and migraine have been excluded. An algorithmic approach to headache assessment is provided in **Figure 1**.

KEY POINTS

- Primary headaches are biologic disorders of the brain, whereas secondary headaches have an identifiable organic causation and typically display a clinical red flag.
- Guidelines specifically recommend against neuroimaging studies in patients with stable headaches that meet criteria for migraine.

HVC

Secondary Headache

Thunderclap Headache

The term thunderclap headache is applied to severe headaches that reach maximum intensity within 1 minute. The patient characteristically describes an attack as "the worst headache of my life." Although many benign primary headache syndromes can present with severe pain, the abrupt onset and rapid escalation of thunderclap headache signal the potential for serious intracranial disorders, most commonly subarachnoid hemorrhage (SAH). The headache can present as an isolated symptom and be global or localized. Associated features can vary depending on the underlying pathology and may include neck stiffness, nausea, vomiting, photophobia, phonophobia, or focal neurologic symptoms. Examination findings can be normal but can include nuchal rigidity, focal deficits, or alteration in consciousness.

Affected patients require emergent evaluation with head CT, and if CT scans are normal, lumbar puncture is mandatory. Neurovascular imaging with catheter magnetic resonance or CT angiography may be necessary to diagnose cerebral aneurysm, vascular malformation, arterial dissection, venous thrombosis, or reversible cerebral vasoconstriction syndrome (RCVS; also known as Call-Fleming syndrome).

Approximately 25% of thunderclap headaches result from SAH, with most of these (85%) involving rupture of previously unidentified saccular aneurysms. Risk of rupture is highest for cerebral aneurysms greater than 5 mm in diameter and those located in the posterior circulation. SAH-associated thunderclap headache can be spontaneous or associated with physical exertion. Many patients experience warning sentinel leaks, manifested as transient headaches, in the days or weeks before aneurysmal rupture. Head CT identifies 98% of SAHs within the first 12 hours, but sensitivity drops to 50% after 7 days. Lumbar puncture typically reveals an elevated opening pressure, high protein levels, and an erythrocyte count usually greater than $10,000/\mu L$ ($10,000 \times 10^6/L$). Xanthochromia, or yellowing of the cerebrospinal fluid (CSF) due to breakdown of heme into bilirubin, is 100% sensitive for SAH between 12 hours and 7 days but may take 4 hours or more to develop. Because SAH has a 50% mortality rate and 25% serious morbidity rate, urgent neurosurgical evaluation is warranted.

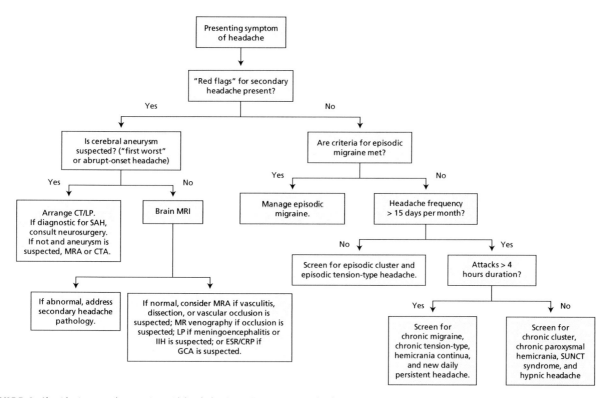

FIGURE 1. Algorithmic approach to a patient with headache. CRP = C-reactive protein level; CTA = CT angiography; ESR = erythrocyte sedimentation rate; GCA = giant cell (temporal) arteritis; IIH = idiopathic intracranial hypertension; LP = lumbar puncture; MRA = magnetic resonance angiography; SAH = subarachnoid hemorrhage; SUNCT = short-lasting unilateral neuralgiform headache with conjunctive injection and tearing syndrome.

Thunderclap headache occurs in two thirds of patients with cervical (carotid or vertebral) artery dissection but is rarely the only symptom. Dissections of the cranial vessels may occur spontaneously or as a result of either trivial or serious trauma. More than 90% of patients will have additional neck pain or associated neurologic features related to ischemic events within the territory of the affected artery. The headache may be diffuse but commonly is ipsilateral to the dissected vessel, with frontotemporal locations more common in carotid artery dissection and occipital locations more frequent in vertebral artery dissection. Visual amaurosis fugax, diplopia, or Horner syndrome can indicate carotid artery involvement, whereas dissections of the vertebral artery sometimes present with ataxia, vertigo, nausea and vomiting, and brainstem findings. Pulsatile tinnitus or audible bruits can be present with either type of dissection. No evidence supports the superiority of anticoagulation over antiplatelet therapy in prevention of stroke after carotid and vertebral artery dissections, and most patients are initially managed with aspirin.

Thrombosis of the cerebral veins or dural sinuses can present with abrupt-onset headache. Clinical symptoms may be related to the resulting increase in intracranial pressure and include pain exacerbation with the Valsalva maneuver, pulsatile tinnitus, and diplopia. Papilledema and focal findings, such as sixth nerve palsy, can be present, and some patients develop altered mentation and seizures. Suspicion of

venous thrombosis should increase in the presence of hypercoagulable states, pregnancy and the puerperium, oral contraceptive use, infections of the ears or sinuses, or dehydration. Treatment with low-molecular-weight heparin results in lower hospital mortality than treatment with unfractionated heparin. Anticoagulation with warfarin is generally continued for 3 to 6 months.

Recurrent thunderclap headaches occur in patients with RCVS. This disorder is more common in women, particularly before menopause. RCVS appears to arise from transient failure of cerebrovascular autoregulation and is often triggered by exposure to adrenergic or serotonergic drugs. Headaches occur over the span of several days or weeks. Episodes can be triggered by exertion, the Valsalva maneuver, or abrupt head movements. Some patients have focal neurologic deficits, and neuroimaging may show evidence of parenchymal strokes, hemorrhages, or cerebral edema. A subset of patients have clinical and imaging features of posterior reversible encephalopathy syndrome, including seizures, confusion, visual loss, and cerebral edema, particularly of the parietal and occipital lobes. The CSF in RCVS is normal or near normal, and angiographic studies reveal multifocal areas of cerebral vasoconstriction. Management includes normalization of blood pressure and elimination of any triggering drug or substance. Nimodipine and verapamil have shown benefit in headache control. Although RCVS is sometimes complicated by stroke, seizures, or (rarely) death, most outcomes are benign.

Posterior reversible encephalopathy syndrome (PRES) is a disorder of cerebrovascular regulation frequently showing clinical and neuroimaging overlap with RCVS. Headaches are common but not necessarily thunderclap in type. Nausea, vomiting alterations in mental status, seizures, and visual compromise are all frequently noted. Brain MRI reveals areas of white matter edema in posterior brain regions (occipital and parietal cortex), and vasoconstriction may not be present. Causes include malignant hypertension, eclampsia, and various drugs, such as sympathomimetic agents and immunosuppressive drugs.

KEY POINTS

- Thunderclap headache requires emergent evaluation with head CT; if CT scans are normal, lumbar puncture is mandatory.
- Most (85%) thunderclap headaches resulting from subarachnoid hemorrhage involve rupture of previously unidentified saccular aneurysms.
- **HVC** No evidence supports the superiority of anticoagulation over antiplatelet therapy in prevention of stroke after carotid and vertebral artery dissections, and most patients are initially managed with aspirin.

Idiopathic Intracranial Hypertension (Pseudotumor Cerebri)

Idiopathic intracranial hypertension (IIH), also called pseudotumor cerebri, is characterized by increased intracranial pressure without identifiable structural pathology. This disorder may arise from elevated venous pressure and secondarily increased resistance to CSF absorption. More than 90% of affected patients are female, obese, and of child-bearing age. Other risk factors include hypervitaminosis A, tetracycline antibiotics, isotretinoin, pregnancy, and glucocorticoid use or withdrawal. Headaches are typically diffuse, steady or throbbing, and worse in the mornings or with the Valsalva maneuvers. Brief episodes of bilateral dimming of vision lasting seconds ("visual obscurations") are classically reported, but blurring, scotomas, and diplopia also are noted. Pulsatile tinnitus, dizziness, and neck pain are common. Papilledema is almost always present on examination. Diagnosis is confirmed by a CSF opening pressure greater than 250 mm H_2O with normal fluid composition. Brain MRI may either be normal or show small ventricles, a partially empty sella turcica, widening of the optic nerve sleeves, or flattening of the optic globes. Visual field testing is crucial in the initial and follow-up evaluations of IIH. Enlargement of the blind spot and reduction in peripheral fields are commonly seen, and patients who do not improve with standard treatment may require surgical methods that reduce CSF pressure along the optic nerve to preserve vision.

The carbonic anhydrase inhibitor acetazolamide is considered the drug of choice to treat this disorder. Topiramate possesses a weak carbonic anhydrase effect but may provide the added benefit of weight loss. In patients with an elevated BMI, a weight-reduction program is necessary, with some requiring bariatric procedures. Repeated lumbar punctures may be helpful in the early stages of the disorder as medication takes effect and in the settings of pregnancy or poor surgical risk. CSF decompressive procedures (such as optic nerve fenestration) or lumboperitoneal shunting should be considered when medical options are ineffective.

KEY POINT

- Carbonic anhydrase inhibitors, such as acetazolamide or topiramate, are generally used to treat idiopathic intracranial hypertension.

Headaches from Intracranial Hypotension

Headaches from intracranial hypotension are characteristically postural, worsening in the upright and improving in the supine position. Some affected patients may report dull interval head pain, neck pain or stiffness, diplopia, nausea, vertigo, tinnitus, or hyperacusis. Physical examination findings are usually normal, although sixth nerve palsy or other abnormalities are possible. CSF hypotension may arise as a result of lumbar puncture, surgery, or trauma or may occur spontaneously. Risk factors for postdural puncture headaches include young age, female sex, low BMI, and the use of larger gauge or conventional cutting (traumatic) needles. Contrary to previous reports, a migraine history does not appear to increase the risk.

Evaluation of patients with spontaneous intracranial hypotension is initiated with contrast-enhanced MRI scans of the brain and spinal cord. Brain MRI can be normal or reveal diffuse pachymeningeal thickening and enhancement, subdural fluid collections, or caudal cerebellar tonsillar descent suggestive of a Chiari malformation. If the spinal MRI does not reveal the site of leak, CT myelography should then be performed.

Conservative treatment measures for all forms of intracranial hypotension include bed rest, analgesia, and fluid resuscitation. In patients who do not respond to conservative measures, 10 to 15 mL of homologous blood can be injected into the epidural space. The resultant blood patch is associated with resolution of symptoms in 80% to 90% of patients. Alternative treatments include intravenous caffeine and epidural saline infusions, local injections of fibrin glue, and surgical correction of the dural tear or diverticula.

KEY POINT

- Epidural blood patching is highly effective in resolving headaches from cerebrospinal fluid leaks that failed to respond to conservative management.

Trigeminal Neuralgia

Trigeminal neuralgia involves paroxysms of severe facial pain isolated to the territory of the trigeminal nerve. More common in older patients, this disorder also can affect younger adults, particularly those with multiple sclerosis. Patients describe electric, lancinating pain that can be repetitive at short intervals and typically involves the second or third divisions of the trigeminal nerve on one side, occasionally occurring bilaterally. Patients with multiple sclerosis are more likely to have bilateral pain. Paroxysms typically last seconds but may build in duration over time. Episodes can be spontaneous or triggered by sensory stimulation to the face or teeth, seriously affecting nutrition and facial and oral hygiene. Interictal pain of lower intensity may be noted. Neurologic examination may be impaired by reluctance of the patient to allow examination of the face, but results of facial sensory and motor examinations are generally normal. Brain MRI with contrast should be used to identify potential compressive or demyelinating causes.

Carbamazepine is the drug of choice for initial management, with a greater than 50% response rate. Dizziness and drowsiness are common adverse effects. Serum carbamazepine drug levels, complete blood counts (to check for potential agranulocytosis), and serum electrolyte levels (to check for potential hyponatremia) should be intermittently monitored. Oxcarbazepine, a structural derivative of carbamazepine, is a more expensive choice that has fewer adverse effects and drug interactions. Second-line agents, such as gabapentin, baclofen, clonazepam, lamotrigine and other antiepileptic drugs, may be considered as adjunctive therapies. Approximately 30% of patients do not respond to drug treatment, even after two or three trials of single or multiple agents, at which point surgical procedures should be considered. Noninvasive options include percutaneous radiofrequency coagulation, glycerol injection, or focused stereotactic (gamma knife) radiation. These techniques are generally effective in greater than 50% of patients. Posterior fossa microvascular decompression of a vessel adjacent to the trigeminal nerve root is more invasive but typically more than 90% effective and is recommended in settings of low surgical risk.

KEY POINT

- Carbamazepine is the drug of choice for initial management of trigeminal neuralgia, with a greater than 50% response rate; for the 30% of patients not responding to drug therapy, surgical procedures should be considered.

Medication-Induced Headache

Medication may provoke headache directly or aggravate an underlying headache disorder. The most common drugs directly provoking headache include nitrates, phosphodiesterase inhibitors, and hormones. This type of headache can occur in patients without a history of previous headache. Medication overuse headache (or rebound headache) requires both a patient susceptible to headache (someone, for example, with repeated migraine or tension-type headaches) and exposure to an offending agent. These patients develop either a marked worsening of their underlying headache or a new milder nonspecific headache associated with the overuse of the acute headache medication. Medication overuse headache must be considered in all patients taking simple or combination analgesics, ergotamine products, or triptans for more than 10 days per month. In light of evidence documenting significantly higher rates of medication overuse headache in patients exposed to butalbital compounds and opioid analgesics, these agents should be avoided in headache management.

KEY POINTS

- Medication overuse headache must be considered in all patients taking simple or combination analgesics, ergotamine products, or triptans for more than 10 days per month.
- Because of the documented significantly higher rates of medication overuse headache in patients exposed to butalbital compounds and opioid analgesics, these agents should be avoided in headache management.

HVC

Primary Headache

Migraine

Clinical Features and Diagnosis

The diagnosis of migraine is made if several specific clinical criteria are present, as outlined by the International Headache Society (**Table 3**). Because some symptoms overlap with those of secondary headache disorders, the criteria for migraine also include the stipulation that potentially causative conditions be excluded. Phenotypic expression of migraine attacks varies widely among patients and among attacks experienced by an individual patient. In addition to severe or disabling attacks, most patients experience milder episodes of headache that frequently represent milder migraine. This phenotypic variability, combined with the misperception that any single clinical feature (aura, nausea, throbbing discomfort) is a requirement for migraine, may be responsible for misdiagnosis in as many as 50% of affected patients. One way of remedying this high rate of misdiagnosis is to use the POUND mnemonic, which includes the following criteria: headache that is Pulsatile, is One-day in duration (with episodes lasting 4-72 hours if untreated), is Unilateral, is accompanied by Nausea/vomiting, and is Disabling. Patients with greater than three of these criteria can be diagnosed with migraine without further evaluation. Unidentified migraine is usually mislabeled as either a tension-type or sinus headache, even though the latter is now felt to be exceedingly uncommon outside the context of acute sinusitis.

The aura of migraine is present in as many as 30% of migraine episodes and may precede, occur concurrently with, or occur outside the context of a headache attack. Migraine auras without headache are often referred to as silent or

TABLE 3. International Headache Society Criteria for Migraine Headache

Without Aura

A. At least five attacks fulfilling criteria B-D

B. Headache attacks lasting 4-72 hours (untreated or unsuccessfully treated)

C. Headache with at least two of the following four characteristics:

1. Unilateral location

2. Pulsating quality

3. Moderate or severe pain intensity that inhibits or prohibits daily activities

4. Aggravation by walking up or down stairs or similar routine physical activity

D. During headache, occurrence of at least one of following symptoms:

1. Nausea/vomiting

2. Photophobia/phonophobia

E. Not better accounted for by another ICHD-3 diagnosis

With Aura

A. At least two attacks fulfilling criteria B and C

B. One or more of the following fully reversible aura symptoms:

1. Visual

2. Sensory

3. Speech and/or language

4. Motor

5. Brainstem

6. Retinal

C. At least two of the following four characteristics:

1. At least one aura symptom spreads gradually over >5 minutes, and/or two or more symptoms occur in succession.

2. Each individual aura symptom lasts 5-60 minutes.

3. At least one aura symptom is unilateral.

4. The aura is accompanied, or followed within 60 minutes, by headache.

D. Headache not better accounted for by another ICHD-3 diagnosis, and transient ischemic attack has been excluded.

ICHD-3 = International Classification of Headache Disorders, 3rd edition.

Adapted with permission of SAGE Publications Ltd., London, Los Angeles, New Delhi, Singapore and Washington DC, from Headache Classification Committee of the International Headache Society (IHS). The International Classification of Headache Disorders, 3rd edition (beta version). Cephalalgia. 2013 Jul;33(9):645-6. [PMID: 23771276]. Copyright SAGE Publications Ltd., 2013.

homonymous visual, hemisensory, or language symptoms. Purely monocular aura falls into the retinal migraine category. Previously known as basilar migraine, migraine with brainstem aura is defined by the presence of vertigo, ataxia, dysarthria, diplopia, tinnitus, hyperacusis, or alteration in consciousness. Any aura complex that involves some degree of motor weakness is categorized as hemiplegic migraine. Both migraine with brainstem aura and hemiplegic migraine must be recognized because triptan therapy is contraindicated for both.

Migraine with aura is a strong contributor to stroke risk in women, comparable to systolic hypertension, obesity, and diabetes mellitus. Strokes usually occur outside the context of acute migraine, but when infarction is noted during the course of a typical migraine with aura attack, it is termed migrainous infarction. These strokes typically occur in the posterior circulation (occipital-parietal cortex, cerebellum) and in young women. Estrogen-containing oral contraceptives must be avoided in women experiencing migraine with aura because of the already increased risk of stroke. The risk of stroke also is slightly elevated in men who have migraine with aura. However, most studies have shown no association between stroke and migraine without aura. Management of stroke does not differ in those with migraine, although an adjustment in acute migraine therapy may be necessary because cerebrovascular disease is a contraindication for triptan use. Clinical stroke must be differentiated from MRI-identified subclinical deep white matter hyperintensities, which tend to be smaller than lesions associated with cerebrovascular or demyelinating disease and are clinically insignificant in most patients with migraine. In the absence of vascular risk factors, further investigation or management adjustments are unnecessary.

Episodic migraine occurs less than 15 days per month. Mean migraine frequency is nearly three episodes per month, with an average duration of less than 24 hours. Chronic migraine describes headache occurring on 15 or more days per month for more than 3 months, with headache possessing the features of migraine on at least 8 days per month. Chronic migraine affects 2% of the adult population and imposes substantial burdens on patients, their families, and their workplaces. Most cases arise from gradual transformation of episodic to chronic migraine, but the transition can occur abruptly, particularly with significant life events, trauma, or (in female patients) hormonal changes. Patients whose baseline frequency of headache or acute medication use is greater than 10 days per month are 20 times more likely to experience transformation. Additional factors, some potentially modifiable, also have been shown to increase the risk of transformation, such as older age, female sex, obesity, excessive intake of caffeine or nicotine, trauma, low socioeconomic status, and the presence of comorbid pain, sleep, or psychiatric conditions.

Acute Migraine Management

The goal of acute migraine management is to resolve the entire symptom complex of migraine and return the patient to

acephalgic migraine. Aura symptoms generally develop gradually and last between 5 and 60 minutes. Both positive (visual lights, paresthesias) and negative (visual loss, numbness) symptoms are typically described. Aura that occurs for the first time after age 40 years usually involves solely negative symptoms or is either very short or prolonged; other causes, such as transient ischemic attack, should be excluded. Aura is considered typical if it involves any combination of normal function. Ideally, pain, nausea, and sensory sensitivities are resolved completely within 1 to 2 hours of treatment, and the patient remains free of symptoms for at least 24 hours. Evidence-based guidelines suggest the medications that are most effective as acute migraine therapy are NSAIDs, triptans, and dihydroergotamine (DHE) (**Table 4**). Trials of NSAIDs are preferred initially because of their cost-effectiveness. Guidelines recommend against the use of opioid- or butalbital-containing compounds as first-line treatments for headache. Because these drugs have been linked to lowered responsiveness to other acute and preventive migraine therapies, to increased rates of emergency department utilization, and to increased risk of transformation into chronic migraine, they should be reserved for those with medical conditions that preclude the use of NSAIDs or triptans.

Most patients manage the majority of migraine attacks with an oral medication. NSAIDs are often effective in the management of mild to moderate migraine. Triptans are used in patients not responding to one or more NSAID. No good evidence supports the superior efficacy of any oral NSAID or triptan choice. Cost, formulary availability, and results of

previous medication trials are all considerations in the selection of acute migraine medication. Each drug is best evaluated after three episodes to assess efficacy and consistency, and it is reasonable to try several different drugs in any class. Evidence indicates that outcomes are more favorable when acute medication is administered within the first hour of the attack. Unless medication overuse headache is a concern, patients should be advised to treat at the first sign of pain. Because migraine intensity is highly variable, occasional attacks that are less responsive to medication are to be expected. Certain patients may benefit from coadministration of an antiemetic agent or from combination treatment with NSAIDs and triptans.

Nonoral routes of administration may be necessary in certain settings when early administration of an oral agent is impossible or ineffective. Migraine with severe nausea or vomiting, migraine that occurs on awakening, and migraine that escalates rapidly within minutes may be best treated by nasal triptans, subcutaneous sumatriptan, or nasal or subcutaneous DHE (see Table 4).

Refractory migraine may require management in emergency department or inpatient settings. Data also support the use of intravenous antidopaminergic agents, such as prochlorperazine, in the treatment of severe migraine. These are often combined with intravenous fluids and diphenhydramine, with the latter drug aimed at preventing potential dystonic reactions from the antidopaminergic drugs. Ketorolac is frequently administered for pain. Parenteral opioids should be avoided if possible. Status migrainosus, defined as an attack duration greater than 72 hours, is the most common complication of acute migraine. A short course of glucocorticoids may be helpful for outpatients, and repetitive intravenous DHE is effective in inpatient settings. The latter is typically delivered over 3 days and is combined with fluid resuscitation and parenteral antidopaminergic agents. H

TABLE 4. Acute Migraine Therapies	
Drug	**Recommended Dose**
NSAIDs[a]	
Aspirin	325-900 mg
Ibuprofen	400-800 mg
Naproxen	250-1000 mg
Combination of acetaminophen/aspirin/caffeine	2 tablets
Diclofenac (oral solution)	50 mg
Migraine-Specific Oral Agents[a]	
Almotriptan	6.25-12.5 mg
Eletriptan	20-40 mg
Frovatriptan	2.5 mg
Naratriptan	1-2.5 mg
Rizatriptan	5-10 mg
Sumatriptan	25-100 mg
Sumatriptan-naproxen	85-500 mg
Zolmitriptan	2.5-5 mg
Nonoral Therapies[a]	
Dihydroergotamine	1 mg nasally
Dihydroergotamine	1 mg subcutaneously
Prochlorperazine	10 mg intravenously
Sumatriptan	5-20 mg nasally
Sumatriptan	4-6 mg subcutaneously
Zolmitriptan	5 mg nasally

[a]Doses listed may be administered once or twice daily.

Migraine Prevention

Reduction in migraine frequency and intensity may be accomplished initially through lifestyle modification. Triggers should be identified and avoided when possible. The patient should be advised to sleep regular hours, eat small but frequent meals, hydrate appropriately, and exercise regularly. Although evidence supporting these recommendations is limited, hunger, dehydration, and changes in sleep schedule are common aggravating factors in migraine. Valuable stress management techniques include relaxation therapy, biofeedback, and cognitive behavioral therapy. Caffeine may be helpful in the acute management of migraine, but chronic excessive exposure may exacerbate the condition. Daily caffeine intake should be limited to less than 100 mg. Good evidence supports the use of *Petasites hybridus* (butterbur), magnesium, riboflavin, and feverfew for migraine prevention.

In order to improve health outcomes, such as attack frequency, intensity, disability, and cost, the use of preventive agents should be considered in patients with eight or more total days or four or more disabling days of migraine per month. However, research has shown that most patients with migraine who might benefit from preventive medications do not receive them. Additional indications for using preventive medications include the use of acute medications (over-the-counter or prescription) more frequently than 8 days per month and persistent disability despite aggressive management of migraine attacks. Evidence-based guidelines for selecting an effective agent for episodic migraine prevention are available (**Table 5**). Only topiramate and injectable onabotulinumtoxinA have good evidence in the setting of chronic migraine, but both are marginally effective. Given the potential for medication overuse headache, long-term opioids are not recommended for migraine prevention except in extremely limited circumstances. The selection of a preventive agent additionally should be guided by patient age, sex, and medical history; by the presence of comorbid conditions; and the results of previous treatments. The goal is to reduce headache frequency and intensity by 50%. A titration phase, which can take 2 to 3 months to achieve benefit, is followed by a maintenance phase of 6 to 12 months. Many patients then tolerate a slow taper of the drug, with future reinstitution possible if headache frequency escalates.

KEY POINTS

HVC

- One way of remedying the high rate of misdiagnosis of migraine is to use the POUND mnemonic, which includes the following criteria: headache that is Pulsatile, is One-day in duration (with episodes lasting 4-72 hours if untreated), is Unilateral, is accompanied by Nausea/vomiting, and is Disabling; patients with greater than three of these criteria can be diagnosed with migraine without further evaluation.

(Continued)

TABLE 5.	Episodic Migraine Preventive Therapies
Drug	**Recommended Daily Dose**
Level A: Effective	
Divalproex sodium/ valproic acid	500-1000 mg
Metoprolol	50-200 mg
Propranolol	40-240 mg
Timolol	10-30 mg
Topiramate	50-200 mg
Level B: Probably Effective	
Amitriptyline	25-150 mg
Atenolol	50-100 mg
Fenoprofen	600-1800 mg
Ibuprofen	400 mg
Ketoprofen	150 mg
Naproxen	500-1100 mg
Venlafaxine	150 mg

KEY POINTS *(continued)*

- Evidence-based guidelines suggest that the most effective medications for acute migraine therapy are NSAIDs, triptans, and dihydroergotamine; trials of NSAIDs are preferred initially because of their cost-effectiveness.   HVC

- No good evidence supports the superior efficacy of any oral NSAID or triptan choice; cost, formulary availability, and results of previous medication trials are all considerations in the selection of acute migraine medication.   HVC

- In order to improve health outcomes, such as attack frequency, intensity, disability, and cost, the use of preventive agents should be considered in patients with eight or more total days or four or more disabling days of migraine per month.   HVC

Tension-Type Headache

Tension-type headache is the most prevalent primary headache disorder. Despite its common occurrence, tension-type headache is an uncommon reason for medical consultation. The clinical classification identifies tension-type headache largely by the absence of disabling features (**Table 6**). By definition, pain is never severe, nausea is absent (or possibly mild, with the chronic form), and photophobia and phonophobia are never present together. Neurologic and autonomic features are lacking. Basically, tension-type headache is defined by the absence of migraine. Subclassification based on attack frequency has been found to be clinically helpful.

TABLE 6. International Headache Society Criteria for Tension-Type Headache
A. At least 10 attacks fulfilling criteria B-D
B. Headache attacks (untreated or unsuccessfully treated) lasting from 30 minutes to 7 days

C. Headache with at least two of the following four characteristics:
  1. Bilateral location
  2. Pressing/tightening (nonpulsating) quality
  3. Mild or moderate intensity
  4. Not aggravated by walking or climbing stairs or similar routine physical activity

D. Headache characterized by both of the following:
  1. No nausea/vomiting
  2. No more than one episode of photophobia or phonophobia

E. Not better accounted for by another ICHD-3 diagnosis

ICHD-3 = International Classification of Headache Disorders, 3rd edition.

Adapted with permission of SAGE Publications Ltd., London, Los Angeles, New Delhi, Singapore and Washington DC, from Headache Classification Committee of the International Headache Society (IHS). The International Classification of Headache Disorders, 3rd edition (beta version). Cephalalgia. 2013 Jul;33(9):660. [PMID: 23771276]. Copyright SAGE Publications Ltd., 2013.

Infrequent episodic tension-type headache (<1 day/month) is benign and requires no medical attention. Frequent episodic tension-type headache (1-14 days/month) may occasionally cause disability warranting the use of prescription medication. Chronic tension-type headache (>14 days/month) is a serious disorder with significant morbidity that requires acute and preventive medications. Brain MRI is also required to exclude organic pathology.

Acetaminophen, aspirin, and NSAIDs are often successful in the acute treatment of tension-type headache. Caffeine-containing compounds may help those not responding to simple analgesics. Preventive medication may be necessary for those with headache frequency greater than 8 days/month. Amitriptyline is considered the drug of choice for prevention of tension-type headache, and efficacy may be enhanced by the addition of stress management techniques. Venlafaxine and mirtazapine may be useful alternatives. Muscle relaxants, benzodiazepines, and onabotulinumtoxinA have no role in the acute or preventive treatment of tension-type headache.

KEY POINT

- Acetaminophen, aspirin, and NSAIDs are often successful in the acute treatment of tension-type headache; amitriptyline is considered the drug of choice for prevention of this type of headache.

Cluster Headache

Cluster headache is considered the most severe of the primary headache syndromes and is the most common of the headaches classified as trigeminal autonomic cephalgias. These disorders are characterized by severe unilateral pain, typically in the first division of the trigeminal nerve (periorbital, frontal, temporal), and are accompanied by ipsilateral cranial autonomic symptoms (**Table 7**). Although episodes of migraine and other primary headaches may occur repeatedly over the course of several days or weeks, the term "cluster" is derived from this disorder's characteristic short cycles of headache activity (weeks) interrupted by long periods of complete remission (month or years). Attacks of cluster headache can best be differentiated from migraine on the basis of their shorter duration. Whereas untreated migraine typically lasts between 4 and 72 hours, most cluster attacks have a duration of less than 3 hours. Male sex and cigarette smoking are risk factors for the development of cluster headache, and most affected patients are young or middle aged. Alcohol is a commonly reported trigger during an active cycle. Cluster periods can occur at specific times of year, most often in the spring or fall. Nocturnal attacks are the norm. Frequency may vary from attacks every other day to eight attacks per day. Approximately 10% of affected patients develop a chronic form notable for absent or brief remissions. Brain MRI should be performed initially to exclude structural lesions mimicking cluster headache. Oxygen inhalation and subcutaneous sumatriptan are first-line therapies for acute cluster headache. Transitional prophylaxis with 2 to 3 weeks

TABLE 7. International Headache Society Criteria for Cluster Headache

A. At least five attacks fulfilling criteria B-D

B. Severe or very severe unilateral orbital, supraorbital, and/or temporal pain lasting 15-180 minutes (when untreated)

C. Either or both of the following:

1. At least one of the following symptoms or signs, ipsilateral to the headache:

    a) conjunctival injection and/or lacrimation

    b) nasal congestion and/or rhinorrhea

    c) eyelid edema

    d) forehead and facial sweating

    e) forehead and facial flushing

    f) sensation of fullness in the ear

    g) miosis and/or ptosis

2. A sense of restlessness or agitation

D. Attack frequency from 1 every other day to 8 per day when the disorder is active

E. Not better accounted for by another ICHD-3 diagnosis

ICHD-3 = International Classification of Headache Disorders, 3rd edition.

Adapted with permission of SAGE Publications Ltd., London, Los Angeles, New Delhi, Singapore and Washington DC, from Headache Classification Committee of the International Headache Society (IHS). The International Classification of Headache Disorders, 3rd edition (beta version). Cephalalgia. 2013 Jul;33(9):665-6. [PMID: 23771276]. Copyright SAGE Publications Ltd., 2013.

of glucocorticoid administration may help reduce attacks at the onset of the cycle. Verapamil is the drug of choice for prevention of cluster headache. Refractory headaches may require trials of lithium carbonate, anticonvulsant agents, or pericranial nerve blockade.

Chronic paroxysmal hemicrania (CPH) and short-lasting unilateral neuralgiform headaches with conjunctival injection and tearing (SUNCT) have phenotypic features identical to cluster headache but differ in attack frequency and duration. CPH attacks occur at least five times daily and last between 3 and 20 minutes. Diagnosis of CPH is confirmed by absolute response to indomethacin, which is unhelpful in cluster headache. SUNCT typically recurs dozens or even hundreds of times per day, with durations of 1 second to 10 minutes. Although lamotrigine has been recommended, SUNCT is often refractory to treatment. The presence of ipsilateral autonomic features and the typical distribution of pain in the first division of the trigeminal nerve help distinguish these syndromes from trigeminal neuralgia.

KEY POINTS

- In patients with suspected cluster headache, brain MRI should be performed initially to exclude structural lesions mimicking cluster headache.

- Oxygen inhalation and subcutaneous sumatriptan are first-line therapies for acute cluster headache.

Other Primary Headache Syndromes

Primary stabbing headaches ("ice-pick headaches") are characterized by brief episodes of stabbing head pain typically lasting a few seconds but occasionally extending to a few minutes. They have no associated autonomic features. Although the eye may be affected ("needle in the eye" sensation), the face is typically spared. The location of pain is fixed in one third of patients, and brain MRI may be justified in some of these patients. Primary stabbing headache may be seen in isolation or in those with migraine. Indomethacin can be helpful during cycles of more frequent attacks.

Primary cough headache develops abruptly after a cough, remains severe for seconds to minutes, and then fades. The pain is typically bilateral and described as an intense pressure. Mild headache may then linger for several hours. A significant correlation exists between cough frequency and headache intensity. Primary cough headache is most common in older adults, and response to indomethacin is typical. Secondary cough headaches have a structural cause, such as a Chiari malformation, and constitute up to half of cough headaches. If this diagnosis is suspected, brain MRI is mandatory.

KEY POINT

- Primary cough headache develops abruptly after a cough, remains severe for seconds to minutes, and then fades; response to indomethacin is typical.

Head Injury
Traumatic Brain Injury

Traumatic brain injury (TBI) arises from the exposure of the brain to external physical forces that cause either temporary dysfunction or permanent damage to brain tissue from blunt or penetrating trauma. **Table 8** outlines the classification of mild, moderate, and severe brain injury.

TABLE 8.	Classification of Brain Injury Severity		
	Mild	**Moderate**	**Severe**
Neuroimaging findings	Normal	Normal or abnormal	Normal or abnormal
Duration of loss of consciousness	0-30 minutes	>30 minutes and <24 hours	>24 hours
Duration of alteration in consciousness	Momentary-24 hours	>24 hours	>24 hours
Duration of posttraumatic amnesia	0-1 day	1-7 days	>7 days
Glasgow Coma Scale score	13-15	9-12	3-8

Skull fracture, intracranial (epidural, subdural) hematomas, parenchymal hemorrhages, and contusions may be complications of TBI.

Mild Traumatic Brain Injury

Mild TBI, also known as concussion, is the most common form of TBI. Initial manifestations include any loss of consciousness or alteration in awareness (such as feeling "dazed" after a head injury), amnesia near the time of the event, or focal neurologic deficit. Symptoms, which may persist, can be divided into physical, cognitive, psychological, and sleep-related domains (**Table 9**). A thorough neurologic examination is necessary, with findings of hemotympanum (blood in the middle ear), orbital ecchymoses ("raccoon eyes"), or mastoid ecchymoses (Battle sign) suggesting a basilar skull fracture. Neuroimaging and, possibly, hospital admission are recommended for persons with worsening headache, repeated vomiting, drowsiness, persistent confusion, dysarthria, or focal neurologic findings. In the emergent setting, head CT is preferable to brain MRI because of its wider availability, lower cost, and greater sensitivity for identifying skull fractures.

TABLE 9.	Symptoms of Mild Traumatic Brain Injury
Physical	
Headache	
Nausea/vomiting	
Dizziness/vertigo	
Gait disturbance	
Photophobia or phonophobia	
Visual blurring	
Dysarthria	
Seizures	
Cognitive	
Poor concentration	
Mental "fogginess" or confusion	
Poor memory	
Learning impairment	
Slowed reaction times	
Psychological	
Irritability	
Depression	
Anxiety	
Sleep	
Fatigue	
Insomnia	
Hypersomnia	
Drowsiness	
Vivid dreams	

KEY POINT

HVC
- In persons who sustain mild traumatic brain injury, neuroimaging is only recommended if symptoms of worsening headache, repeated vomiting, drowsiness, persistent confusion, dysarthria, or focal neurologic findings are present; head CT is preferable to brain MRI for initial neuroimaging because of its wider availability, lower cost, and greater sensitivity for identifying skull fractures.

Head Injury in Special Populations

Athletes

Any athlete suspected of sustaining a mild TBI should be immediately removed from play and undergo sideline assessment through administration of standardized tools, such as the Graded Symptom Checklist and the Standardized Assessment of Concussion. Neuropsychological testing may be helpful in identifying and tracking those with cognitive dysfunction. Future participation in contact sports must be prohibited until the patient returns to cognitive baseline and is asymptomatic without taking any medication to treat trauma-related symptoms.

KEY POINT

- Any athlete suspected of sustaining mild traumatic brain injury should be immediately removed from play and prohibited from participating in contact sports until he or she returns to cognitive baseline and is asymptomatic without taking any medication to treat trauma-related symptoms.

Military Personnel

Blast injuries from weaponry, especially improvised explosive devices, now account for most TBIs in members of the armed services returning from combat. Guidelines recommend that these military personnel undergo mandatory screening for TBI if involved in a vehicular accident, exposed to an explosive blast, struck by a direct blow to the head, or instructed to by a superior officer. Specifically, a Military Acute Concussion Evaluation and a mandatory 24-hour rest period are required, with full recovery necessary before return to duty. Because the manifestations of TBI may vary widely, treatment programs should be individualized. Headaches and sleep dysfunction should be managed with appropriate medications. Emotional disorders, such as depression and posttraumatic stress disorder, must be identified early and managed with counseling and medication, when necessary. The addition of pain medicine or mental health providers to the health care team is highly recommended.

Older Patients

Adults older than 75 years have the highest rates of morbidity, hospitalization, and death from TBI. Falls, motor vehicle accidents, and accidental blows to the head are the leading causes of TBI in this population. Older age also is associated with less rapid and less complete recovery. Therefore, TBI prevention is key. Prevention involves decreasing the risk of falls by avoiding overmedication and encouraging regular physical activity and living area modifications, such as removal of trip hazards and installation of appropriate lighting, nonslip mats in the bathroom, and handrails in the bathroom and along stairways.

KEY POINT

- Because patients older than 75 years have the highest **HVC** rates of morbidity, hospitalization, and mortality after traumatic brain injury, prevention is key; preventive measures include avoiding overmedication and encouraging regular physical activity and living area modifications.

Postconcussion Syndrome

The term postconcussion syndrome (PCS) is applied to those persons who continue to report symptoms of mild TBI beyond a typical recovery period of several weeks. Risk factors predictive of PCS include female sex, low socioeconomic status, headaches, unsettled court cases, severe bodily injury from the TBI, or previous TBI. Management of PCS is largely supportive and rehabilitative, with medical treatments directed at specific symptoms. NSAIDs and triptans may be useful in treating posttraumatic headache. Opioids should be avoided. Tricyclic antidepressants, selective serotonin reuptake inhibitors, and serotonin-norepinephrine reuptake inhibitors can be effective in managing posttraumatic headache, mood, and anxiety disorders. Although data are inconclusive, those with visual accommodation issues may benefit from visual therapy, and those with balance disorders from vestibular rehabilitation. Similarly, those with cognitive impairment may benefit from a rest period followed by gradual reintroduction of cognitive activities.

KEY POINT

- Management of postconcussion syndrome is largely supportive and rehabilitative, with medical treatments directed at specific symptoms.

Epidural and Subdural Hematomas

Epidural hematomas involve the collection of blood from an arterial source between the inner table of the skull and the dura (**Figure 2**). Most of these hematomas result from blunt head injury causing fracture of the temporal bone and laceration of the middle meningeal artery, with blood accumulation under arterial pressure. Headache, mental status abnormalities, and rapid neurologic decline with ipsilateral pupillary dilatation and brain herniation can occur. Some patients exhibit a brief "lucid interval" before subsequent precipitous decline. Prognosis is often excellent with emergent evacuation

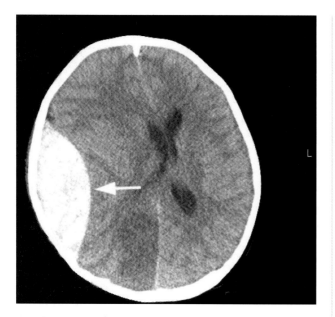

FIGURE 2. CT scan of an epidural hematoma. Note the biconvex lens appearance as blood under arterial pressure collects between the skull and outer margin of the dura (*arrow*).

of the hematoma because the underlying brain tissue is frequently uninjured. Without immediate surgical evacuation, however, death can occur within a matter of hours.

Subdural hematomas (**Figure 3**) arise from injury to the small bridging veins between the cortex and the dura. Because the collection of blood is under venous pressure, the clinical course is often more indolent than with epidural hematomas. Acute subdural hematomas can develop over hours to days,

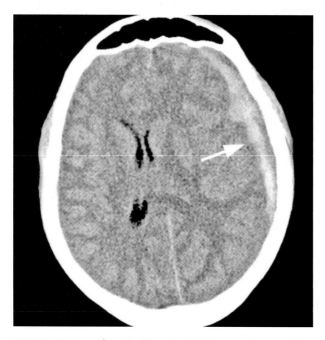

FIGURE 3. CT scan of a subdural hematoma. Note the crescent shape as blood under venous pressure separates the dura from the arachnoid membrane (*arrow*).

and chronic subdural hematomas over weeks to months. The latter can occur in the absence of significant trauma, particularly among older patients and those taking anticoagulant drugs. Patients may warrant either observation or surgical evacuation, depending on their specific presentation.

KEY POINTS

- The prognosis of epidural hematomas is often excellent after emergent surgical evacuation because the underlying brain tissue is frequently uninjured; without immediate evacuation, however, death can occur within a matter of hours.

- Subdural hematomas can occur in the absence of significant trauma, particularly among older persons and those taking anticoagulant drugs; observation or surgical evacuation is appropriate treatment, depending on the specific presentation.

Seizures and Epilepsy
Clinical Presentation of Seizures

Seizures are stereotyped paroxysmal events caused by hypersynchronization of neurons. Approximately 10% of the population will experience isolated seizures in their lifetimes. Epilepsy, which occurs in 1% to 3% if the population, is diagnosed after two unprovoked seizures have occurred. Tonic-clonic seizures (often referred to as convulsions) are the most commonly recognized seizures; they are characterized by loss of consciousness associated with tonic stiffening and clonic jerking of all extremities. However, seizures can have many different manifestations depending not only on where in the brain they begin, but also on the extent of their spread throughout the brain. Tonic-clonic seizures can be focal or generalized in onset. Properly labeling the seizure type helps identify the potential cause of a seizure, the associated epilepsy syndrome (if any), and the appropriate therapy.

Partial (Focal) Seizures

Most seizures occurring in adults are partial seizures, or seizures caused by abnormal electrical activity beginning in a single region of the brain. Determining whether an isolated tonic-clonic seizure was partial or generalized at onset can be difficult. Clinical clues to identifying a partial seizure that has progressed to a generalized tonic-clonic seizure (also known as a secondarily generalized seizure) include unilateral shaking, head turning to one side (versive head turning), or a subjective aura before the onset of convulsion. Focal weakness after a convulsion (Todd paralysis) may occur. The absence of one of these focal features does not exclude a partial onset. It is generally helpful to inquire if the patient has had other types of seizures in the past.

Simple partial seizures and complex partial seizures are two types of partial seizures; although more common than convulsions, they may be subtle and often are not recognized as seizures. Simple partial seizures do not impair consciousness. Their symptoms depend on the area of the brain involved. Whereas simple partial seizures in the motor cortex can cause rhythmic jerking in one body part, in other areas of the brain they may cause subjective phenomena known as auras. For example, the most common temporal lobe aura is a difficult-to-describe epigastric rising sensation; patients sometimes describe this sensation as nausea or simply motion towards their chest with an upward gesture. Temporal lobe auras also can cause paroxysmal feelings of fear or déjà vu. These temporal lobe seizures are often misdiagnosed as panic attacks, although the stereotyped features, paroxysmal onset, and short duration (usually less than 1 minute) are distinguishing features. Complex partial seizures are associated with a disturbance of awareness. During these seizures, patients may exhibit semipurposeful behaviors known as automatisms, such as lip smacking or fumbling of the fingers. Patients with complex partial seizures may recognize a typical aura before losing consciousness, but they often are unaware that they have become impaired and may have no recollection of the seizure. This makes interviewing family and friends imperative in patients with a suspected seizure disorder.

KEY POINTS

- Simple partial seizures are partial-onset seizures that do not impair consciousness, whereas complex partial seizures are partial seizures associated with a disturbance of awareness.

- During complex partial seizures, patients may exhibit semipurposeful behaviors (automatisms), such as lip smacking or fumbling of the fingers.

Generalized Seizures

Generalized seizures involve both hemispheres of the brain at onset. Primary generalized seizures are tonic-clonic seizures without a focal onset. Absence seizures, which typically develop in childhood or adolescence, are another type of generalized seizure characterized by a brief behavioral arrest and impairment of awareness. The term absence seizure is often incorrectly used to describe a complex partial seizure; as with complex partial seizures, patients may be unaware they have experienced absence seizures, noting at most "missed time," but absence seizures are usually much shorter (<5 seconds versus 30-90 seconds) and are not associated with postictal confusion. Myoclonic seizures are characterized by quick, nonrhythmic, shock-like muscular contractions that can occur in rapid succession and usually are not associated with impaired consciousness. These seizures are typical of juvenile myoclonic epilepsy.

KEY POINT

- Absence seizures are shorter than complex partial seizures (<5 seconds versus 30-90 seconds) and are not associated with postictal confusion.

Epilepsy Syndromes

Epilepsy syndromes also are classified as partial or generalized. The diagnosis of an epilepsy syndrome depends on the seizure type(s) a patient experiences and can be supported by electroencephalographic and MRI findings.

Focal (Partial) Epilepsy

Temporal lobe epilepsy is the most common type of focal epilepsy and the most common epilepsy syndrome presenting in adulthood. Patients with this type of epilepsy typically experience complex partial seizures, which often begin with auras (an epigastric rising sensation or a feeling of déjà vu). These patients also may have simple partial or secondarily generalized seizures. Mesial temporal sclerosis (neuronal loss and gliosis in the hippocampus) is a characteristic finding in patients with temporal lobe epilepsy (**Figure 4**). Frontal lobe epilepsy is the second most common type of focal epilepsy and is often characterized by nocturnal complex partial seizures that awaken patients from sleep because of chaotic movements. Structural causes of focal epilepsy syndromes include brain tumors, vascular malformations (**Figure 5**), malformations of cortical development (**Figure 6**), chronic strokes, and head trauma. An increasing number of genetic focal epilepsy syndromes are being recognized. Most of the time, however, the cause of focal epilepsy remains unknown.

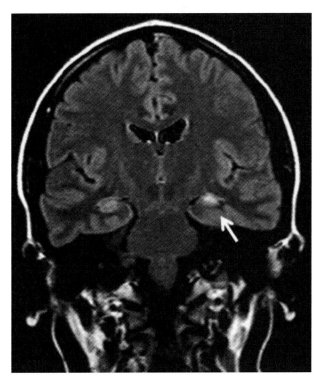

FIGURE 4. Mesial temporal sclerosis. Coronal flair MRI shows increased signal intensity and atrophy of the left mesial temporal lobe (*arrow*).

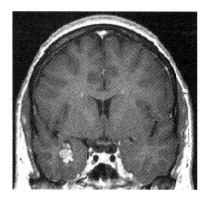

FIGURE 5. Cavernous malformation. Coronal T1-weighted MRI shows an intra-axial mass (cavernous hemangioma) in the right temporal lobe with a surrounding hemosiderin ring.

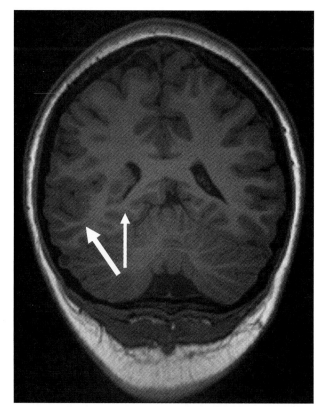

FIGURE 6. Focal cortical dysplasia with periventricular nodular heterotopia. Coronal MRI showing a focal area of thickened cortex in the right temporal region (*thick arrow*) and nodules of abnormal neuronal tissue along the ventricular surface (*thin arrow*).

KEY POINT

- Temporal lobe epilepsy is the most common type of focal epilepsy; in most patients, the cause of focal epilepsy remains unknown.

Idiopathic Generalized Epilepsy

Idiopathic generalized epilepsy (IGE) accounts for approximately one third of all epilepsy syndromes. IGE is typically diagnosed in patients before age 20 years and is presumed to be genetic in origin, although a close relative with the disorder often cannot be identified. Patients with IGE may have any combination of tonic-clonic seizures, absence seizures, and myoclonic seizures. Juvenile myoclonic epilepsy (JME) is one of the most common types of IGE. Typically beginning in adolescence, JME is characterized by morning myoclonus, which is often perceived as tremors or "jitteriness." Patients with JME often also have primary generalized seizures and may or may not have absence seizures. IGE syndromes are presumed to be genetic; a family history of epilepsy is common but not always present.

Although all patients with epilepsy are sensitive to the effects of alcohol and sleep deprivation, patients with IGE are particularly susceptible to these triggers. MRI findings are typically normal, and an EEG may show generalized spike-wave activity (**Figure 7**).

KEY POINTS

- Idiopathic generalized epilepsy is genetic, accounts for one third of all epilepsy syndromes, and may manifest as tonic-clonic seizures, absence seizures, or myoclonic seizures.

- Juvenile myoclonic epilepsy, one of the most common types of idiopathic generalized epilepsy, is characterized by morning myoclonus; affected patients often also have tonic-clonic seizures and sometimes absence seizures.

Initial Approach to the Patient with a First Seizure

General Comments

The appropriate immediate management of a seizure focuses on stabilization of the patient, with attention paid to the airway and vital signs, and on rapid identification of any reversible causes. If a serum glucose level cannot be obtained quickly, thiamine followed by glucose should be administered. Basic metabolic function and liver chemistry panels should be ordered, as should an electrocardiogram; if appropriate, urine toxicology and serum alcohol and antiepileptic drug (AED) levels also should be obtained.

The clinical history and evaluation of a potential seizure should focus on answering the following questions:

- Was the event a seizure?

- Was the seizure provoked?

- Was this a first seizure?

- Does the patient have risk factors for subsequent seizures?

There are several paroxysmal events that can mimic a seizure (**Table 10**). For example, syncope is associated with tonic-clonic activity in 5% to 15% of patients. The distinction between seizures and similar events relies heavily on a careful clinical history, which usually requires interviewing observers. The patient and his or her friends and family members also should be asked about more subtle events in the past that may

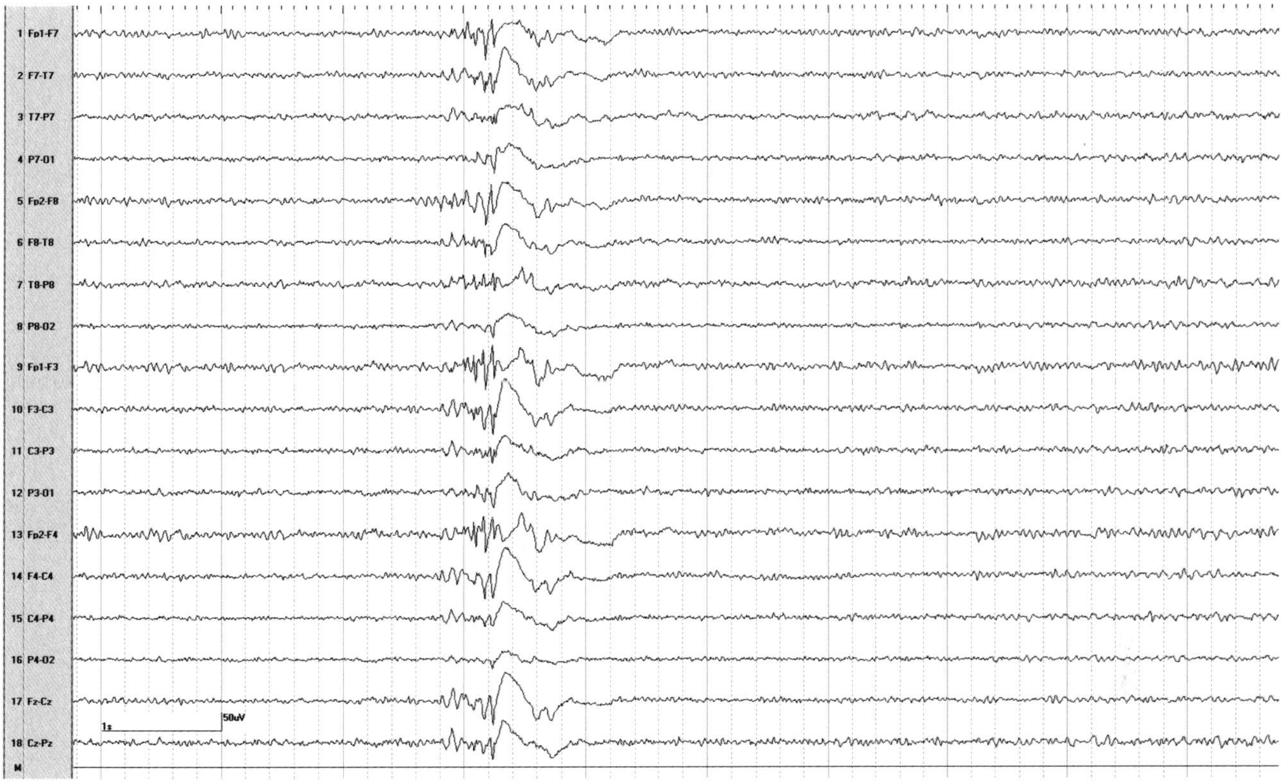

FIGURE 7. Characteristic electroencephalogram of a patient with idiopathic generalized epilepsy shows a generalized interictal epileptiform discharge during sleep.

TABLE 10.	Characteristics of Seizures and Common Mimics in Adults					
Characteristic	**Epileptic Seizure**	**Psychogenic Nonepileptic Seizure**	**Syncope**	**TIA**	**Migraine**	**Vertigo**
Warning/aura	Variable (<1 min)	Variable	Lightheaded feeling, sweating	None	Variable (15-30 min)	None
Duration	1-2 min	5-15 min	Seconds to minutes	5-30 min	Hours	Minutes to days
Position dependent	No	No	Typically, but not always	No	No	Often on standing or moving head, but not always
Symptoms during episode	Variable: automatisms, confusion, aphasia, tonic-clonic movements	Pelvic thrusting, jerking that waxes and wanes, forced eye closure	Loss of tone, brief tonic extension or clonic jerks	Hemiparesis, hemisensory loss, visual loss, aphasia	Visual disturbance, vertigo, paresthesias, aphasia, dysarthria	Nausea, ataxia
Altered consciousness	Common	Common	Common	Rare	Rare	No
Incontinence	Variable	Variable	Variable	None	None	None
Heart rate	Increased	Variable	Irregular and decreased	Variable	No effect	Variable
Symptoms after episode	Confusion, fatigue	Variable	Alert	Alert	Fatigue	Alert
EEG during event	Epileptiform pattern	Unaltered	Diffuse slowing	Focal slowing	Rare slowing	Unaltered

EEG = electroencephalogram; TIA = transient ischemic attack.

CONT.

not have been recognized as seizures (such as auras and periods of inattention) and about precipitating factors (such as sleep deprivation and toxic exposures [alcohol, illicit drugs, and certain medications]) and the presence of epilepsy risk factors, including:

- Family history of epilepsy
- Childhood febrile convulsions
- History of head trauma with loss of consciousness
- History of central nervous system infection
- Central nervous system lesion (brain tumor, vascular malformation, stroke)
- Prenatal or birth injury

Neuroimaging is indicated in most patients with a first unprovoked seizure. An urgent noncontrast head CT is recommended to exclude hemorrhage in patients with focal neurologic deficits, impaired mental status, or head trauma. An MRI is preferred in otherwise clinically stable patients and should be performed at, or very soon after, presentation. EEG also is recommended for all patients with an unprovoked seizure. If the patient is not returning toward baseline mental status by 15 minutes after a first seizure, continuous EEG monitoring (to rule out nonconvulsive seizures) is indicated. Lumbar puncture should be considered in patients with a seizure in the setting of suspected meningitis or encephalitis or in the setting of immunosuppression.

Because seizures are unpredictable, all patients who have had a seizure should be counseled to avoid situations in which a momentary loss of consciousness could be hazardous; avoiding heights, heavy lifting, and swimming or bathing alone are recommended. Additionally, it is the physician's obligation to counsel any patient who has had a seizure about the risks of driving. Driving restrictions apply in patients with an unexplained loss of consciousness even if the diagnosis is unclear. Some states require the reporting of a patient's seizures to the department of motor vehicles (state driving laws can be found at www.epilepsy.com/driving-laws). Although laws vary from state to state, most require that patients abstain from driving for a period of 3 to 12 months after any event causing an impairment of consciousness, including complex partial and absence seizures and convulsions. The laws apply to patients who have had a single seizure (provoked or unprovoked) and to patients with diagnosed epilepsy.

KEY POINTS

- The appropriate immediate management of a seizure focuses on stabilization of the patient with attention paid to the airways and vital signs and on rapid identification of any reversible causes.
- Brain imaging is recommended in any patient with an unprovoked seizure; an urgent noncontrast head CT is recommended to exclude hemorrhage in patients with focal neurologic deficits, impaired mental status, or head trauma.

Provoked Seizures

Several medical conditions and treatments can provoke seizures (**Table 11**). Single seizures that are provoked should be addressed by correcting the underlying condition or removing the causative agent; they usually do not require treatment with an AED. Further diagnostic evaluation, such as neuroimaging and EEG, may not be needed if a clear reversible cause of the seizure is identified and the patient has normal findings on neurologic examination. In patients with recurrent provoked seizures, AED treatment occasionally is needed on a short-term basis, but long-term therapy usually is not indicated. Similarly, patients with acute symptomatic seizures that occur within 1 week of head trauma or acute brain injury, such as intracerebral hemorrhage, may benefit from a short course of an AED but do not necessarily require long-term treatment.

KEY POINT

- Single seizures that are provoked usually do not require treatment with an antiepileptic drug and instead should be addressed by correcting the underlying condition or removing the offending agent; further diagnostic evaluation, such as neuroimaging and electroencephalography, may not be needed if a clear reversible cause of the seizure is identified and the patient has normal findings on neurologic examination.

HVC

Psychogenic Nonepileptic Seizures

At least 20% of patients evaluated at epilepsy referral centers receive a diagnosis of psychogenic nonepileptic seizures (PNES). Although some patients with PNES may be malingering, PNES typically is a type of conversion disorder, with affected patients remaining unaware of why they have these

TABLE 11.	Medical Conditions and Treatments Provoking Seizures
Condition	**Specific Cause**
Metabolic disturbance	Hyponatremia, hypo- or hypercalcemia, hypo- or hyperglycemia, uremia
Drug intoxication	Cocaine, phencyclidine, methamphetamines
Drug withdrawal	Alcohol withdrawal, benzodiazepine withdrawal, barbiturate withdrawal, baclofen withdrawal
Medication-induced lowered seizure threshold[a]	Bupropion, cefepime, ciprofloxacin, clozapine, cyclosporine, imipenem, isoniazid, tacrolimus, theophylline, tricyclic antidepressants, tramadol
Infection	Encephalitis, meningitis
Vasculopathy	Eclampsia, hypertensive encephalopathy, posterior reversible leukoencephalopathy syndrome

[a]The medications listed are those most commonly associated with lowered seizure threshold, particularly at supratherapeutic levels or in association with chronic kidney disease. Note that both cyclosporine and tacrolimus have been associated with posterior reversible leukoencephalopathy syndrome; therefore, patients taking these medications should be evaluated with MRI.

events. A history of trauma or abuse is common in patients with PNES but is not always present. Some of the characteristic features of PNES are summarized in Table 10 and include forced eye closure, long duration, and hypermotor activity that starts and stops.

Inpatient video EEG monitoring is required to make this diagnosis because of the difficulty in distinguishing between PNES and epileptic seizures, particularly frontal lobe seizures. A high index of suspicion is critical for making a diagnosis of nonepileptic events, particularly in patients who do not respond to AED therapy. Early diagnosis by video EEG and referral to appropriate psychological resources provide the best chance of a good outcome. Limiting or eliminating unnecessary AEDs is critical, particularly in women of childbearing age. Approximately 10% to 30% of patients with PNES also have epileptic seizures, which underscores the need for a careful and complete assessment.

KEY POINT

- Inpatient video electroencephalographic monitoring is required to make the diagnosis of psychogenic nonepileptic seizure.

Diagnostic Evaluation of Seizures and Epilepsy

Imaging Studies

All patients with unprovoked seizures should have brain MRI to identify structural lesions that increase the risk of recurrent seizure, such as tumors and small vascular lesions (see Figure 5), malformations of cortical development (see Figure 6), and

mesial temporal sclerosis (see Figure 4). Most centers have seizure or epilepsy MRI protocols that include a coronal flair sequence (see Figures 4 and 5), which is critical in identifying lesions in the mesial temporal region (common in epilepsy). MRI results are normal in most patients with generalized epilepsy and in many patients with focal epilepsy. The older the patient, the more likely a structural cause will be detected.

Electroencephalography

A routine EEG is a 30- to 60-minute recording of brain activity. Under ideal circumstances, the recording captures both the awake and sleep states because sleep is more sensitive for revealing epileptiform abnormalities. Seizures are rarely recorded on routine EEG, but the presence of interictal epileptiform discharges is highly correlated with an increased risk of recurrent seizures. Interictal epileptiform abnormalities also can help characterize the epilepsy syndrome as focal (**Figure 8**) or generalized (see Figure 7). An EEG can help confirm the presence of epilepsy but cannot be used to exclude the diagnosis. The likelihood that a single 30-minute EEG will record interictal epileptiform discharges in a patient with epilepsy is approximately 25% to 50%, varying by the type of epilepsy. Performing a second EEG increases the sensitivity for detecting epileptiform abnormalities, as does performing an EEG shortly after a seizure.

Epilepsy Monitoring Units

Epilepsy monitoring units are inpatient units designed for continuous simultaneous video and EEG monitoring. Patients are admitted electively to the hospital for 2 to 7 days, during which time their AED(s) may be withdrawn. Inpatient

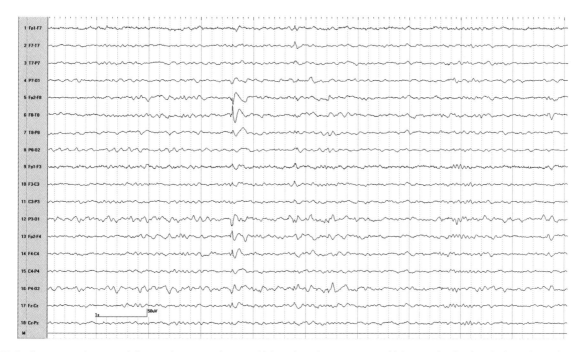

FIGURE 8. Characteristic electroencephalogram of a patient with temporal lobe epilepsy showing an interictal left temporal epileptiform discharge during sleep.

epilepsy monitoring is recommended for most patients who have not responded to two or more AEDs to determine their candidacy for epilepsy surgery and to exclude PNES. It may be reasonable to admit patients sooner if their epilepsy diagnosis is uncertain or if they are women of childbearing age.

Continuous Electroencephalographic Monitoring

Continuous EEG monitoring, which typically includes video monitoring, has become increasingly more available outside of epilepsy monitoring units. This type of monitoring is useful in detecting nonconvulsive seizures and nonconvulsive status epilepticus (NCSE) in patients who are comatose or have an altered mental state. Approximately 8% to 37% of patients with coma will be found to have nonconvulsive seizures on continuous EEG. Risk factors for nonconvulsive seizures and NCSE include intracerebral hemorrhage, traumatic brain injury (TBI), and central nervous system infections. The greatest risk for nonconvulsive seizures and NCSE occurs in patients with persistent altered mental status after apparently successful treatment of convulsive status epilepticus (CSE), with 48% of these patients showing evidence of seizures on EEG. Notably, only 50% of nonconvulsive seizures and NCSE will be detected on a 1-hour EEG, but continuous EEG monitoring for 12 to 24 hours increases the sensitivity for nonconvulsive seizures to 80%, and sensitivity approaches 96% after 48 hours of monitoring.

Treatment of Epilepsy

Antiepileptic Drug Therapy

Treatment with an AED is recommended for all patients who have had two or more unprovoked seizures. In a patient with a single unprovoked seizure and a normal EEG and brain MRI, the 2-year recurrence risk is 30% to 40%. Because seizure medications reduce this risk by only approximately 50%, AED therapy is not typically recommended. The risk of seizure recurrence is higher in patients older than 65 years and in those with a history of significant head trauma or partial seizure, postictal Todd paralysis, and focal findings on an EEG or brain MRI. The presence of one or more of these risk factors argues for the institution of AED treatment after a single seizure.

Selection of Antiepileptic Drugs

No single AED is recommended for the initial treatment of epilepsy. Approximately 50% of patients with this disorder will respond to the first AED administered. Choosing an AED for an individual patient depends on several factors, including his or her epilepsy syndrome, age, sex, and comorbid medical conditions and the drug's adverse-effect profile and cost. Only a few AEDs (lamotrigine, levetiracetam, topiramate, valproic acid, and zonisamide) are considered broad-spectrum agents and can be used to treat both generalized and partial epilepsy syndromes. Other narrow-spectrum AEDs (carbamazepine, gabapentin, oxcarbazepine, phenobarbital, phenytoin, and pregabalin) have the potential to exacerbate seizures in patients with generalized epilepsy. Phenytoin may control the tonic-clonic seizures in generalized epilepsy and is indicated in the treatment of convulsive status epilepticus but also can worsen other seizure types when used for chronic treatment of generalized epilepsy.

Because only a few randomized placebo-controlled trials of various epilepsy treatments exist and little evidence suggests a significant difference in efficacy between different AED monotherapy regimens, most experts recommend choosing an AED based on tolerability and the adverse-effect profile that is most appropriate for a particular patient. Treatment options and considerations are summarized in **Table 12**. Levetiracetam is a common first-line drug because it can be used for both generalized and partial epilepsy and for patients in whom the specific epilepsy syndrome is not yet apparent (for example, a patient with two convulsive seizures and no history of other seizures or focal features). Levetiracetam also can be started quickly, has few drug-drug interactions, and is typically well tolerated; however, it has the common adverse effect of irritability and also has been associated in some patients with anxiety, depression, and psychosis. In a patient with a clear focal epilepsy syndrome at presentation, carbamazepine provides a relatively cost-effective option, although its common adverse effects of fatigue and dizziness make it not well tolerated by some (particularly older) patients.

Carbamazepine and other enzyme-inducing AEDs (such as felbamate, oxcarbazepine, phenobarbital, and phenytoin)

TABLE 12.	Initial Treatment of Epilepsy and Considerations in Special Populations							
Epilepsy Syndrome	Best Evidence	Commonly Used Drugs	Least Expensive Drugs	Women of Childbearing Age	Older Patients	Liver Failure	Chronic Kidney Disease	Mood Disorder
Partial epilepsy	Carbamazepine, levetiracetam, phenytoin, zonisamide	Lacosamide, lamotrigine, oxcarbazepine, topiramate, valproic acid	Carbamazepine, phenobarbital, phenytoin	Lamotrigine, levetiracetam (avoid valproic acid and topiramate)	Lamotrigine, levetiracetam, gabapentin	Levetiracetam, gabapentin (avoid valproic acid)	Lamotrigine, levetiracetam	Carbamazepine, lamotrigine, oxcarbazepine, valproic acid (avoid levetiracetam)
Generalized epilepsy	No high-quality evidence available	Lamotrigine, levetiracetam, topiramate, valproic acid, zonisamide	Valproic acid	Lamotrigine, levetiracetam (avoid valproic acid and topiramate)	Lamotrigine, levetiracetam	Levetiracetam (avoid valproic acid)	Lamotrigine, levetiracetam	Lamotrigine, valproic acid (avoid levetiracetam)

can have significant interactions with other hepatically metabolized drugs and also are associated with an increased risk for osteoporosis and hypercholesterolemia. Phenobarbital is another inexpensive option for treating partial epilepsy but is rarely used because of its significant adverse effects, including sedation and the risk of a severe withdrawal syndrome. Valproic acid has been shown in one trial to be superior to other AEDs for treating generalized epilepsy, but its associated adverse effects include sedation, weight gain, and hypercholesterolemia; in young women, it has the additional adverse effect of polycystic ovary syndrome. It should never be used as a first-line drug in women of childbearing age because of the significantly elevated risk of congenital and cognitive abnormalities in exposed offspring (see Epilepsy and Pregnancy section and Table 12). Lamotrigine is commonly prescribed in women of childbearing age and is also a good option for older patients or those who have depression or other mood disorders. Topiramate and zonisamide can be used for both generalized and partial epilepsy and are associated with weight loss; however, both drugs have been associated with an increased risk of kidney stones and should be avoided in patients with a history of nephrolithiasis.

Common adverse effects of AEDs and less common but more serious adverse reactions to AEDs are summarized in **Table 13**. The most common serious adverse reactions associated with AEDs are hypersensitivity syndromes, such as Stevens-Johnson syndrome and drug reaction with eosinophilia and systemic symptoms (DRESS) syndrome (see MKSAP 17 Dermatology); systemic findings include facial edema, widespread erythema, fever, lymphadenopathy, skin necrosis, purpura, eosinophilia, hepatitis, and nephritis. Hypersensitivity reactions are most common in the weeks following initiation of the drug but can occur at any time during therapy. The AEDs most commonly associated with rashes and hypersensitivity reactions are carbamazepine, lamotrigine, oxcarbazepine, phenobarbital, and phenytoin. Lamotrigine needs to be titrated

TABLE 13. Adverse Effects of Antiepileptic Drugs

Drug	Common Adverse Effects	Serious Adverse Reactions
Carbamazepine	Sedation, fatigue, dizziness, ataxia, mild leukopenia, hyponatremia	Aplastic anemia, agranulocytosis, acute liver failure, rash, severe hyponatremia, Stevens-Johnson syndrome, DRESS
Clobazam	Sedation, dizziness, constipation	Tolerance, pyrexia, Stevens-Johnson syndrome; abrupt or excessively rapid discontinuation of therapy associated with benzodiazepine withdrawal syndrome
Ezogabine	Sedation, dizziness	Blue skin discoloration and retinal pigment changes, QT prolongation, urinary retention, confusion, psychosis, hallucinations
Felbamate	Insomnia, weight loss, nausea, headache	Aplastic anemia, acute liver failure
Gabapentin	Sedation, lower extremity edema, weight gain	—
Lacosamide	Sedation, dizziness, ataxia, diplopia, nausea, prolonged PR interval	Cardiac conduction abnormalities (bradyarrhythmias, AV block), rash
Lamotrigine	Insomnia, headache, acne, dizziness, double vision	Rash, Stevens-Johnson syndrome, DRESS, acute liver failure, blood dyscrasias
Levetiracetam	Irritability, sedation	Depression, psychosis, blood dyscrasias
Oxcarbazepine	Sedation, dizziness, ataxia, mild leukopenia, hyponatremia	Rash, Stevens-Johnson syndrome, DRESS, severe hyponatremia
Phenobarbital	Sedation, nausea, ataxia	Rash, Stevens-Johnson syndrome, acute liver failure, blood dyscrasias, barbiturate withdrawal
Phenytoin	Sedation, dizziness, ataxia	Rash, Stevens-Johnson syndrome, DRESS, blood dyscrasias, gingival hyperplasia, acute liver failure, drug-induced lupus, cardiac conduction abnormalities
Pregabalin	Sedation, weight gain, lower extremity edema	—
Topiramate	Word-finding difficulty, anorexia	Kidney stones, acute angle-closure glaucoma, heatstroke, metabolic acidosis
Valproic acid	Weight gain, tremor, hirsutism, hair loss, hyperammonemia, menstrual irregularity	Acute liver failure, pancreatitis, aplastic anemia, thrombocytopenia, platelet dysfunction
Vigabatrin	Sedation, headache, dizziness	Peripheral vision loss (irreversible), peripheral neuropathy, rash
Zonisamide	Sedation, anorexia	Kidney stones, rash

[a]AV = atrioventricular; DRESS = drug reaction with eosinophilia and systemic symptoms.

CONT.

slowly because the risk of rash has been specifically related to rapid titration; this dose escalation needs to be even slower in patients also taking valproic acid because valproic acid inhibits lamotrigine metabolism and increases the risk of a hypersensitivity syndrome. Asian patients who have the HLA-B*1502 allele are at an increased risk for hypersensitivity reactions to the aromatic AEDs (carbamazepine, lamotrigine, oxcarbazepine, and phenytoin). Therefore, genotype testing is recommended before starting one of these drugs in patients of Asian heritage; alternatively, other AEDs can be used as first-line therapy. **H**

Monitoring and Discontinuing Medications

The target dose for an AED is the dose that controls a patient's seizures without significant adverse effects. Therapeutic drug ranges published by many laboratories are useful guides, but the patient's response defines his or her own therapeutic drug level. For example, if a patient requires a drug level above the recommended range for seizure control and has no adverse effects to this higher level, the dose does not need to be adjusted; a notable exception to this is phenytoin, for which supratherapeutic levels are associated with an increased risk of cardiac arrhythmias. In general, AED levels do not need to be monitored routinely in a patient who is doing well. A baseline level (ideally, a trough level) should be established once the target dose has been reached and the patient's seizures are well-controlled. Further AED monitoring is indicated in pregnancy, kidney or liver disease, menopause, change from a brand name to a generic medication, or around the time of initiating a new medication that may affect metabolism or protein binding. In these situations, doses should be adjusted to maintain the patient's personal therapeutic drug level.

The use of generic medications is a major way to control costs for patients with epilepsy. The major consideration in using a generic drug is its bioavailability, which may differ by as much as 20% between manufacturers. Because drug level maintenance is critical to maintaining seizure threshold, patients taking generic AEDs should try to use the same drug manufacturer from month to month.

Certain AEDs are associated with adverse effects that require additional monitoring. For example, both carbamazepine and oxcarbazepine can cause hyponatremia. Evaluation of the serum sodium level after initiating the drug and at 3 months is recommended. Because many AEDs are associated with liver abnormalities and/or blood dyscrasias, obtaining a complete blood count and comprehensive metabolic profile at 6 and 12 months in the first year of therapy is advisable; if no abnormalities are detected, yearly monitoring is reasonable.

Patients taking AEDs should be regularly screened for suicidal thoughts. All AEDs carry a black box warning indicating a potentially increased risk of suicidal ideation, which is based on a pooled analysis of clinical trials. Mood disorders also are prevalent in patients with epilepsy.

Epilepsy can go into remission, and many childhood epilepsy syndromes often resolve in adulthood. A major exception is JME, which typically is regarded as a life-long condition requiring continuous treatment. Many patients who have been seizure free for 2 to 4 years can choose to be weaned from AEDs; seizure recurrence after AED withdrawal in these patients is 30% to 40% over 5 years. Those with normal EEG and MRI results who have no other risks factors for epilepsy are more likely to remain seizure free after stopping their medications. Discontinuing medications is a difficult decision that requires careful counseling about the risks of recurrent seizures, including a discussion of sudden unexplained death in epilepsy (SUDEP; see later discussion) and the implications for driving.

KEY POINTS

- In a patient with a single unprovoked seizure and a normal electroencephalogram and MRI, the 2-year recurrence risk is 30% to 40%; because seizure medications reduce this risk by only approximately 50%, antiepileptic drug therapy is not typically recommended. **HVC**

- Choosing an AED for an individual patient depends on several factors, including his or her epilepsy syndrome, age, sex, and comorbid medical conditions and the drug's adverse-effect profile and cost. **HVC**

- The antiepileptic drugs (AEDs) lamotrigine, levetiracetam, topiramate, valproic acid, and zonisamide are considered broad-spectrum agents and can be used to treat both generalized and partial epilepsy syndromes; some narrow-spectrum AEDs (such as carbamazepine, gabapentin, oxcarbazepine, phenobarbital, phenytoin, and pregabalin) have the potential to exacerbate seizures in patients with generalized epilepsy.

- The use of generic antiepileptic drugs (AEDs) is a way to control costs for patients with epilepsy, and the major consideration in using a generic AED is its bioavailability, which may differ by as much as 20% between manufacturers; because drug level maintenance is critical to maintaining seizure threshold, patients taking generic AEDs should try to use the same drug manufacturer from month to month. **HVC**

Counseling and Lifestyle Adjustments

Alcohol, stress, and sleep deprivation can reduce a patient's seizure threshold. Therefore, counseling patients to minimize exposure to these triggers is an important part of epilepsy treatment. Likewise, use of interventions to optimize adherence to AED regimens (such as the use of pill boxes) should be encouraged. Several medications, including antibiotics, antihistamines, and psychiatric and pain medications, can lower seizure threshold and interact negatively with AEDs. Patients and their physicians should discuss any new medications, and alternatives should be used when appropriate. Testing for and treating sleep apnea when appropriate also may improve seizure control. All patients must be counseled about driving restrictions.

KEY POINT

- Alcohol, stress, sleep deprivation, and certain drugs—including antibiotics, antihistamines, and psychiatric and pain medications—can lower a patient's seizure threshold; these agents also can interact negatively with antiepileptic drugs.

Comorbidities and Complications of Epilepsy

Common comorbidities of epilepsy include mood disorders, sleep disorders, metabolic bone disease, and hyperlipidemia. Screening for these conditions is a vital part of caring for a patient with epilepsy.

Sudden Unexplained Death in Epilepsy

Sudden unexplained death in epilepsy (SUDEP) is nonaccidental death in otherwise healthy patients with epilepsy. SUDEP is a significant cause of mortality in epilepsy, with approximately 1 in 1000 patients with epilepsy dying of it each year. The mechanism of SUDEP is poorly understood, but it is likely related to a disturbance in cardiac or respiratory autoregulation. Death often occurs during sleep. Risk factors include refractory epilepsy, cognitive impairment, generalized tonic-clonic seizures, and poor medication adherence.

Intractable Epilepsy

Epilepsy Surgery

Patients who do not respond to either their first or their second AED (in sequence or combination) have a less than 10% chance of experiencing seizure remission with pharmacotherapy. These patients are considered to have refractory epilepsy and should be referred to a comprehensive epilepsy center to confirm the diagnosis of epilepsy and determine their candidacy for epilepsy surgery.

KEY POINT

- Patients with epilepsy who do not respond to either their first or their second antiepileptic drug are considered to have refractory epilepsy and should be referred to a comprehensive epilepsy center to confirm the diagnosis and determine their candidacy for epilepsy surgery.

Seizures and Epilepsy in Specific Populations

Older Patients

Patients age 65 or greater who have a first unprovoked seizure at presentation are much more likely to have underlying brain disease (such as a tumor, previous stroke, or dementia) and a higher risk for recurrent seizures. Morbidity related to seizures in this population also is higher. For these reasons, it may be reasonable to start AED treatment after an initial seizure in older patients. Medication tolerability may be problematic in this age group. Lamotrigine, levetiracetam, and gabapentin are generally well-tolerated in older patients and have few drug-drug interactions. One study showed that lamotrigine was the most effective, followed by levetiracetam. Titration of the drug dosage may need to be slower, and the ultimate dosage should account for decreased glomerular filtration rate, when present.

KEY POINT

- Antiepileptic drugs (preferably lamotrigine, levetiracetam, and gabapentin) are sometimes given to older patients after a first seizure because their risks of recurrent seizure and seizure-related morbidity are higher.

Patients with Organ Failure

The management of AEDs in patients with liver failure or chronic kidney disease depends on the metabolism of the drug and the degree to which the drug is protein bound. **Table 14** summarizes dosing considerations for specific AEDs in organ failure. Levetiracetam is a good option in patients with either liver failure or chronic kidney disease, although dose adjustment is required in patients with chronic kidney disease.

Returning Combat Veterans

TBI, with or without evidence of intracranial abnormalities, is a risk factor for epilepsy. Therefore, it is reasonable to consider AED treatment in a combat veteran with a history of TBI and a single unprovoked seizure. Inpatient monitoring should be considered early in veterans whose seizures do not respond to AEDs because these patients are at risk not only for epileptic seizures, but also for nonepileptic seizures. The diagnosis of PNES is often delayed in veterans, most often because these patients often report a history of TBI. Early monitoring and diagnosis is critical, as are interventions to minimize disability. Posttraumatic stress disorder is strongly associated with PNES in veterans.

Women and Epilepsy

Women of childbearing age who have epilepsy require special consideration regarding AED treatment and management. Valproic acid in particular should be avoided in this population because the risk of teratogenesis is much higher with this drug than with other AEDs. Other adverse effects in a female population are weight gain, hair loss, and polycystic ovary syndrome. Contraception can be a particular challenge in women with epilepsy because AEDs have complex interactions with oral contraceptives and other forms of hormonal contraception.

Epilepsy and Pregnancy

Most women with epilepsy have healthy pregnancies and children. In most women with active epilepsy, AED therapy during pregnancy is required to control seizures, which can adversely affect the pregnancy. Early planning (well before a patient

TABLE 14. Dose Adjustment of Antiepileptic Drugs in Organ Failure

Drug	Requires Dose Adjustment in Chronic Kidney Disease	Requires Supplemental Dose After Dialysis	Requires Dose Adjustment in Liver Failure
Carbamazepine	No	No	Avoid
Clobazam	No	No	Yes
Felbamate	Yes	Possibly[a]	Avoid
Gabapentin	Yes	Yes	No
Lacosamide	Only with a glomerular filtration rate < 30 mL/min/1.73 m^2	Yes	Yes; avoid drug in patients with severe impairment
Levetiracetam	Yes	Yes	Yes, in severe disease
Oxcarbazepine	Yes	Possibly[a]	No, but avoid in patients with severe liver failure
Phenobarbital	No	Possibly[a]	Yes
Phenytoin	No, but monitoring free phenytoin levels recommended	Possibly[a]	Yes
Pregabalin	Yes	Yes	No
Topiramate	Yes	Yes	Possibly
Valproic acid	No	Possibly[a]	Avoid if possible
Vigabatrin	Yes	Probably	No
Zonisamide	No[b]	Possibly[a]	Possibly

[a]Filtration of these drugs during dialysis depends on the pore size of the dialyzer. Supplementation is needed with many of the new high-efficiency dialyzers. Checking antiepileptic drug levels pre- and postdialysis can help determine the need for supplemental dosing.

[b]Insufficient evidence for dose adjustment even with a glomerular filtration rate < 30 mL/min/1.73 m^2.

attempts pregnancy) can optimize the outcome of any future pregnancy. The initial drug choice in young women with seizures should keep a potential pregnancy in mind. Supplemental folic acid (1-4 mg) is recommended for all women of childbearing age who are taking AEDs.

Valproic acid is associated not only with an increased risk (6%-17%) of major congenital malformations (MCMs) compared with other AEDs, but also with decreased intelligence quotients (IQs) and autism in exposed children. Other drugs that are associated with a high risk of MCMs are phenobarbital and phenytoin; topiramate has recently been categorized as a class D drug in pregnancy (evidence of human fetal risk) because of a specifically increased risk of cleft lip and cleft palate; this drug should be avoided (if possible) in patients who are pregnant or may become pregnant.

Lamotrigine is a good option for women with epilepsy and has been associated with a relatively low risk of MCM (2%-6%) compared with a baseline risk of 2% to 3% in the general population. Levetiracetam also appears to have a low risk of birth defects, although the number of published exposures is still small. Carbamazepine has been associated with an overall low risk of MCMs in several studies but may have a specific association with spina bifida, one of the more severe MCMs.

AED levels must be followed closely during pregnancy. Lamotrigine and oxcarbazepine are particularly sensitive to the effect of estrogen on glucuronidation, which leads to an increase in liver metabolism. The levels of these AEDs can decrease precipitously during pregnancy and result in increased seizure frequency. Increasing the dosage of these drugs during pregnancy is thus recommended.

KEY POINT

- In most women with active epilepsy, antiepileptic drug (AED) therapy during pregnancy is required to control seizures, which can adversely affect the pregnancy; because of its association with major congenital malformations, decreased intelligence, and autism in exposed children (compared with other AEDs), valproic acid should be avoided.

Contraception

Enzyme-inducing AEDs, including carbamazepine, phenytoin, and phenobarbital, decrease both estrogen and progestin levels and thus inactivate many forms of hormonal contraception. Topiramate, oxcarbazepine, clobazam, and felbamate can have a similar effect. Because lamotrigine is metabolized by glucuronidation, a process induced by estrogens, estrogen-containing contraceptive agents can reduce lamotrigine levels and lead to more seizures if a patient's dosage is not increased.

KEY POINT

- Estrogen-containing contraceptive agents can reduce lamotrigine levels in women with epilepsy and lead to more seizures if the lamotrigine dosage is not increased.

Status Epilepticus

Convulsive Status Epilepticus

CSE is a medical emergency that can lead to significant morbidity and mortality. Prompt intervention is critical. CSE is defined as persistent tonic-clonic activity with impaired mental status that lasts longer than 5 minutes. Initial management of CSE requires rapidly assessing airways, breathing, and circulation; checking the blood glucose level; and administering thiamine with glucose, if needed. These steps should be performed simultaneously with initiating drug treatment. First-line pharmacologic treatment (**Figure 9**) is intravenous lorazepam followed by phenytoin. Intramuscular midazolam (or lorazepam) or rectal diazepam can be used as an alternative to lorazepam if intravenous access is not possible. If available, fosphenytoin, a prodrug of phenytoin, is preferable to phenytoin for initial treatment of CSE because it can be administered faster and does not carry the risk of thrombophlebitis or skin necrosis (purple glove syndrome) that is associated with phenytoin extravasation. Fosphenytoin can be given intramuscularly, if needed. Both fosphenytoin and phenytoin can cause hypotension and cardiac conduction abnormalities. Valproic acid is an alternative to phenytoin or

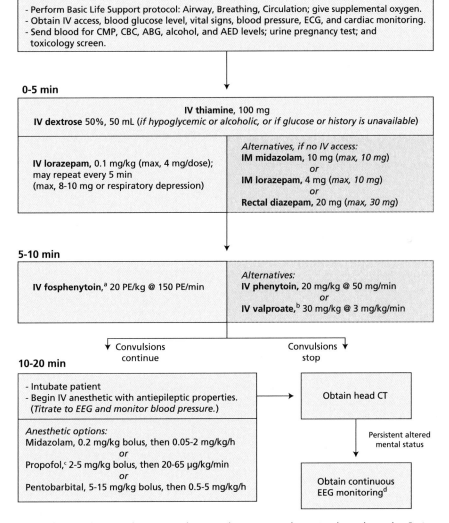

FIGURE 9. Management algorithm for generalized convulsive status epilepticus with ongoing convulsive activity lasting longer than 5 minutes *or* recurrent convulsive seizures without a regaining of consciousness. ABG = arterial blood gases; AED = antiepileptic drug; CBC = complete blood count; CMP = comprehensive metabolic panel; ECG = electrocardiogram; EEG = electroencephalogram; IM = intramuscular; IV = intravenous; max, maximum; PE = phenytoin equivalent.

[a]Monitor ECG and blood pressure with fosphenytoin and phenytoin use; monitor for drug extravasation with phenytoin use.

[b]Consider valproic acid (valproate) as first-line therapy in those with known idiopathic generalized epilepsy; avoid when possible in women of childbearing age.

[c]Note that propofol infusion is dosed in µg/kg/min unlike other infusions. Caution is advised with prolonged use and high doses of propofol because of an increased risk of propofol infusion syndrome, particularly with rates greater than 65 µg/kg/min.

[d]Should be obtained in all patients not recovering baseline mental status, including those receiving IV anesthesia.

CONT.

fosphenytoin, particularly in patients with an allergy to phenytoin or with IGE. No other AED is recommended as first-line treatment of CSE.

If a patient continues to convulse after receiving lorazepam, is medically unstable, or has an unprotected airway, intubation and intravenous anesthesia are typically required. Consensus about which anesthetic agent should be used first is lacking. Propofol is effective in stopping seizures but needs to be monitored closely because prolonged infusions of high-dose propofol can lead to rhabdomyolysis and multiorgan failure. All options are listed in Figure 9.

Patients with CSE who have stopped having clinical seizures are at high risk for NCSE. Thus, all patients with CSE who do not return to baseline within 15 minutes of pharmacologic treatment should be monitored with continuous EEG monitoring. **H**

KEY POINT

- First-line pharmacologic treatment for convulsive status epilepticus, defined as persistent convulsive activity with impaired mental status lasting longer than 5 minutes, is intravenous lorazepam followed by intravenous phenytoin (or, if available, fosphenytoin).

Nonconvulsive Status Epilepticus

NCSE is defined as persistent clinical or electrographic seizure activity without convulsive motor manifestations. The implications and treatment of NCSE depend greatly on the clinical context in which it occurs. Arguably, the most critical patients with NCSE are those in whom CSE is followed by NCSE. Although management of the electrographic pattern in these patients is controversial, it is usually aggressive and uses either additional AEDs or increasing amounts of anesthesia to control seizures or induce burst-suppression.

On the other end of the spectrum, NCSE can occur in ambulatory patients with complex partial status epilepticus or absence status epilepticus; these patients are sometimes referred to as "the walking confused." This situation most often involves patients with established epilepsy and sometimes can present de novo in older persons. Affected patients occasionally respond to treatment with a benzodiazepine or initiation of a new AED; an initial aggressive approach involving intubation can cause unnecessary morbidity and is not recommended.

NCSE also is increasingly diagnosed in critically ill comatose or stuporous patients with acute neurologic or medical conditions who have not had a convulsive seizure. Similar to NCSE following CSE, NCSE in these populations also is associated with increased morbidity and mortality and requires prompt attention and intervention. The definition of NCSE in these patients, however, is controversial, and scant evidenced-based data exist on treatment of this population.

In all patients with NCSE and CSE, the underlying cause determines outcome, and early attempts to identify and correct the underlying cause are critical. **H**

KEY POINT

- Although management of the electrographic pattern in patients with nonconvulsive status epilepticus is controversial, it usually is directed at controlling seizures.

Stroke

Definition of Stroke

Stroke is characterized by the sudden onset a focal neurologic impairment that can be ascribed to a specific location in the brain, retina, or spinal cord. The fourth leading cause of death in the United States and the leading cause of significant disability, stroke can be further subdivided into ischemic and hemorrhagic stroke, with the relative proportion of each varying by age and geographic location. Hemorrhagic stroke has two further subtypes: subarachnoid hemorrhage (SAH), which is usually caused by rupture of an intracranial aneurysm, and nontraumatic intracerebral hemorrhage (ICH). Ischemic stroke can be further classified as lacunar (a small subcortical infarct), large artery atherosclerotic (either intra- or extracranial), cardioembolic, or cryptogenic. One of the principal goals of hospitalization for stroke is the determination of stroke subtype, which has important implications for acute treatment, secondary prevention strategies, and prognosis. **H**

KEY POINT

- A principal goal of hospitalization in patients with stroke is to determine the stroke subtype, which has important implications for acute treatment, secondary prevention strategies, and prognosis.

Diagnosis of Stroke

A complete neurologic examination is warranted in all patients with suspected stroke to localize the deficit to the central nervous system and inform prognosis. In the acute stroke setting, when time is of the essence, validated scales for measuring neurologic impairment can be rapidly performed by any health care provider. The National Institutes of Health Stroke Scale (**Table 15**) is the most commonly used scale, and training is available online through several organizations for certification.

Because the predictive value of any specific finding from the history or physical examination is insufficient to distinguish ischemic from hemorrhagic stroke, prompt neuroimaging also is required. A noncontrast CT scan of the head will readily identify ICH and SAH (**Figure 10**) and is the initial test of choice. Any patient with suspected SAH

TABLE 15. National Institutes of Health Stroke Scale

Parameter (Testing Method)	Scores[a]
1a. LOC	0 = normal 1 = not alert but arousable by minor stimulation 2 = not alert and requires constant verbal or painful stimuli to remain interactive 3 = unresponsive or responds with only reflexive movements
1b. LOC, questions (state month and age)	0 = answers both correctly 1 = answers one correctly 2 = answers neither correctly
1c. LOC, commands (close and open eyes; make fist or close one hand)	0 = performs both tasks correctly 1 = performs one task correctly 2 = performs neither task correctly
2. Gaze (track a finger in a horizontal plane)	0 = normal 1 = partial gaze palsy or isolated cranial nerve paresis 2 = forced gaze deviation or total gaze paresis
3. Visual fields (each eye tested individually)	0 = no visual loss 1 = partial hemianopia 2 = complete hemianopia 3 = bilateral hemianopia
4. Facial strength (show teeth, raise eyebrows, close eyes)	0 = normal 1 = minor paralysis (flattening of the nasolabial fold or asymmetry on smiling) 2 = partial paralysis (paralysis of the lower face only) 3 = complete paralysis (upper and lower face)
5. Arm strength (hold arm with palms down or lift arm for 10 s; each arm scored separately)	0 = no drift 1 = some drift but does not hit bed 2 = drifts down to bed 3 = no effort against gravity 4 = no movement
6. Leg strength (hold leg at 30 degrees for 5 s; each leg scored separately)	0 = no drift 1 = some drift but does not hit bed 2 = drifts down to bed 3 = no effort against gravity 4 = no movement
7. Limb ataxia (finger-nose-finger test, heel-knee-shin slide)	0 = absent 1 = present in one limb 2 = present in two limbs
8. Sensation (pinch/pinprick tested in face, arm, and leg)	0 = normal 1 = mild to moderate sensory loss or loss of sensation in only one limb 2 = complete sensory loss
9. Language (describe a picture, name six objects, and read five sentences)	0 = no aphasia 1 = mild to moderate aphasia (difficulty with fluency and comprehension; meaning can be identified) 2 = severe aphasia (fragmentary language; meaning cannot be clearly identified) 3 = global aphasia or mute
10. Dysarthria (repeat or read words)	0 = normal 1 = mild to moderate 2 = severe (speech not understandable)
11. Extinction/inattention (visual and tactile stimuli applied on right and left sides)	0 = normal 1 = visual or tactile extinction or mild hemispatial neglect 2 = profound hemi-inattention or extinction to more than one modality

LOC = level of consciousness.

[a]Score interpretation: 0 = no stoke; 1-4 = minor stroke; 5-15 = moderate stroke; 16-20 = moderate to severe stroke; 21-42 = severe stroke (maximum score, 42).

Adapted from www.ninds.nih.gov/doctors/NIH_Stroke_Scale.pdf. Accessed February 9, 2015. Certification available at www.stroke.org/we-can-help/healthcare-professionals/improve-your-skills/tools-training-and-resources/training/nih?gclid=CJWx_IDO08MCFcnm7AodZloACA.

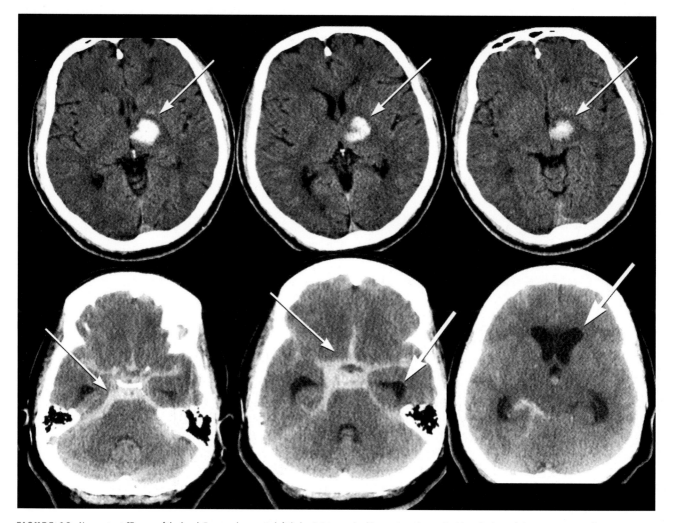

FIGURE 10. Noncontrast CT scans of the head. *Top panel*, an acute left thalamic intracerebral hemorrhage (*arrows*) without hydrocephalus or intraventricular extension is shown. *Bottom panel*, an acute subarachnoid hemorrhage is shown that involves the basal cisterns (*thinner arrows*) with associated enlargement of the lateral horn of the lateral ventricles, consistent with obstructive hydrocephalus and elevated intracranial pressure (*thicker arrows*).

whose head CT scan is normal should have a lumbar puncture to evaluate for blood or xanthochromia in the cerebrospinal fluid to rule out aneurysmal bleeding. A noncontrast CT scan of the head also can identify the early changes seen in the acute setting in some patients with cerebral infarction (**Figure 11**). In many instances, the initial noncontrast CT will not show any appreciable changes for as long as 24 hours after ischemic stroke, and small infarcts, particularly in the thalamus and brainstem, may not be visible with CT beyond that time window. After an initial evaluation with noncontrast head CT, other neuroimaging studies may provide information regarding stroke location and allow for evaluation of the cerebral vasculature. MRI (**Figure 12**) can help determine the presence of cerebral infarction when the CT scan is not informative and provide additional information about previous strokes or other intracranial pathology. However, because of its greater cost, less widespread availability, and generally longer duration, MRI is rarely the initial imaging technique of choice to evaluate for hemorrhage or suitability for systemic thrombolysis. Similarly, CT of the head with contrast is rarely helpful in the evaluation of brain parenchyma in patients with stroke unless it is being used to exclude other intracranial pathology (such as metastasis) that may mimic stroke in a patient who cannot receive an MRI.

The neurologic examination provides useful information about the specific neuroanatomic localization of stroke, which in itself can suggest the stroke subtype. For example, the absence of cortical features, such as aphasia and visuospatial neglect, can point to a small subcortical infarct, whereas monocular visual loss and a carotid bruit can suggest extracranial large artery atherosclerotic disease. The examination, however, is not sufficiently sensitive or specific to further identify the subtype of ischemic stroke, and vessel imaging and cardiac evaluation are required in most patients with ischemic stroke. ∎

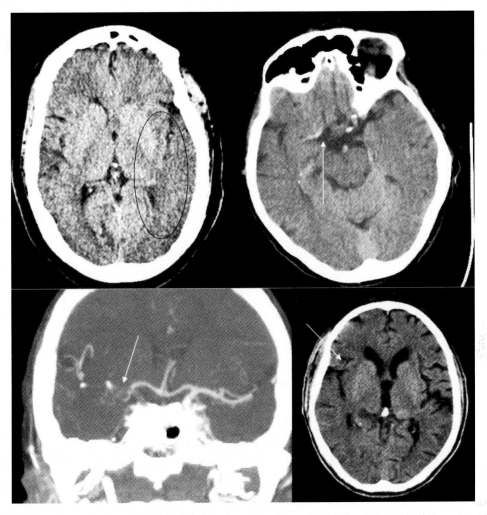

FIGURE 11. Head CT findings in acute ischemic stroke. *Top left,* sulcal effacement and loss of the gray-white differentiation (*oval circle*) in a patient 1.5 hours after the witnessed onset of global aphasia. *Top right,* hyperdensity (*arrow*) in the proximal right middle cerebral artery in a patient with left hemiparesis and left hemi-inattention 60 minutes after last being seen well. *Bottom left,* CT angiogram of the same patient that shows absent contrast in the right internal carotid and proximal middle cerebral arteries (*arrow*), consistent with a thrombus in the artery. *Bottom right,* loss of gray-white matter differentiation in the insula ("loss of the insular ribbon") on the right (*arrow*) compared with the left where the gray-white matter differentiation is clearly seen in a patient 2 hours after onset of left hemiparesis.

KEY POINT

- In patients with stroke, neuroimaging (usually a non-contrast CT scan of the head) is required to distinguish ischemic from hemorrhagic stroke; when subarachnoid hemorrhage is suspected but neuroimaging findings are normal, lumbar puncture is necessary to evaluate for blood or xanthochromia in the cerebrospinal fluid.

H Stroke Subtypes

Transient Ischemic Attack

Transient ischemic attack (TIA) is defined by transient focal neurologic symptoms resulting from brain, retinal, or spinal cord ischemia and was initially defined as lasting less than 24 hours. A more recently adopted definition recognizes the high prevalence of acute infarcts on neuroimaging and emphasizes that TIA is defined by the absence of infarction on neuroimaging, independent of symptom duration. TIA symptoms typically are short lasting, usually 5 minutes to 1 hour, and include sudden-onset hemiparesis, hemisensory loss, change in speech function (either aphasia or dysarthria), loss of vision, or inability to walk. Patients with a suspected TIA should thus undergo neuroimaging with either noncontrast MRI or CT within 24 hours of the onset of neurologic deficits.

TIA is considered a neurologic emergency given the subsequent 48-hour and 90-day risk of ischemic stroke. Several clinical scales have been developed for risk stratification of patients with a TIA (or stroke); the most widely accepted is the ABCD^2 score, which is based on a patient's Age, Blood pressure, Clinical presentation, Duration of symptoms, and the presence of Diabetes mellitus (**Table 16**). The risk of stroke increases as the ABCD^2 score increases, and hospital admission is recommended for all patients with an ABCD^2 score of 3 or

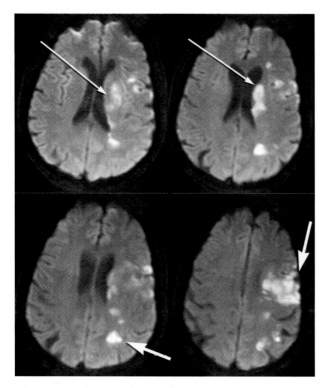

FIGURE 12. Diffusion-weighted MRIs from a patient with symptomatic left middle cerebral artery atherosclerosis reveal an acute infarction in deep (*thinner arrows*) and superficial (*thicker arrows*) structures in the left cerebral hemisphere.

TABLE 16.	ABCD Scoring System[a]
Patient Characteristics	**Score[b]**
Age ≥60 y	1
Blood pressure ≥140/90 mm Hg	1
Clinical symptoms	
Focal weakness with the TIA	2
Speech impairment without weakness	1
Duration of TIA	
≥60 min	2
10-59 min	1
Diabetes mellitus present	1

TIA = transient ischemic attack.

[a]Based on Age, Blood pressure, Clinical presentation, Duration of symptoms, and the presence of Diabetes mellitus.

[b]The 48-hour stroke risk based on score: 0-1 = 0%; 2-3 = 1.3%; 4-5 = 4.1%; 6-7 = 8.1%.

CONT.

greater so that rapid evaluation and treatment can occur. A noncontrast head CT is required to rule out hemorrhagic stroke. Hospital admission also can be considered in patients with a score of 0 to 2 if suspicion of infarction is high or if rapid outpatient evaluation cannot be completed within 48 hours. All patients with suspected TIA require an expedited evaluation within 48 hours with both cerebrovascular imaging and cardiac examination. Cerebrovascular imaging is necessary to exclude extracranial internal carotid artery disease, which is associated with a high risk of subsequent stroke, and can be performed with carotid ultrasonography; magnetic resonance and CT angiography are other options, but cost and risk from contrast and radiation should be considered. The cardiac examination is primarily focused on identifying patients who could be candidates for anticoagulation for stroke prevention; electrocardiography or cardiac event monitoring is performed to detect any atrial fibrillation, and echocardiography is needed to evaluate for ventricular thrombus or other high-risk embolic sources (for further discussion, see MKSAP 17 Cardiovascular Medicine).

KEY POINT

- In patients who have had a transient ischemic attack, the risk of stroke increases as the ABCD[2] score (based on a patient's Age, Blood pressure, Clinical presentation, Duration of symptoms, and the presence of Diabetes mellitus) increases; hospital admission is recommended for all patients with an ABCD[2] score of 3 or greater so that rapid evaluation and treatment can occur.

Ischemic Stroke

Cardioembolic Stroke

The most common cause of cardioembolic stroke is atrial fibrillation. Other potential cardioembolic sources can be identified during the diagnostic evaluation, including reduced left ventricular ejection fraction, severe calcific mitral stenosis, ventricular thrombus or apical aneurysm, or congenital abnormalities (such as a patent foramen ovale [PFO]). For further details on risk stratification with cardioembolic sources and anticoagulation criteria, see MKSAP 17 Cardiovascular Medicine.

Several findings on neuroimaging suggest a cardioembolic cause, such as involvement of the cortical surface in the absence of cerebral artery atherosclerosis; presence of more than one infarct, especially if bilateral or involving the territory of both the internal carotid and vertebrobasilar arteries; and involvement of the entire territory of a large intracranial artery. Cardiac rhythm evaluation is advisable for all patients with ischemic stroke, including electrocardiography and in-hospital telemetry, to evaluate for atrial fibrillation. Transthoracic echocardiography should be considered in patients with stroke who have a suspected embolic stroke or underlying heart disease without another identified cause to identify candidates for anticoagulation. Transesophageal echocardiography can be considered on a case-by-case basis to identify rare causes of stroke, such as valvular endocarditis or intracardiac tumors.

Large Artery Atherosclerosis

Stroke due to large artery atherosclerosis commonly occurs after local thrombus formation in the area of plaque rupture with subsequent distal embolization. Of the common causes of stroke, extracranial internal carotid artery atherosclerosis has the highest risk of recurrent stroke in the first 2 weeks. Suggestive clinical history and examination findings include recent monocular visual loss and the presence of a carotid bruit, both on the side of the affected hemisphere. The risk of recurrent stroke is highest when the stenosis is greater than 70%; stenosis in the 50% to 70% range has a more modest risk of recurrence. Prompt vascular imaging is therefore recommended for patients with a TIA or a carotid territory infarction seen on neuroimaging. Several imaging modalities are available for quantifying the degree of stenosis, including ultrasonography, magnetic resonance angiography

(MRA), and CT or catheter digital subtraction angiography. Carotid ultrasonography is a useful initial, noninvasive test, particularly because of its high sensitivity for hemodynamically significant stenosis and its low risk. If the carotid ultrasound shows significant stenosis, the percentage of narrowing and the anatomic location should be confirmed with either CT angiography or MRA without contrast before recommending stenting procedures or other surgery (see **Figure 13** for a comparison of different imaging modalities). Unless carotid artery angioplasty with stenting is planned, catheter angiography is not routinely necessary.

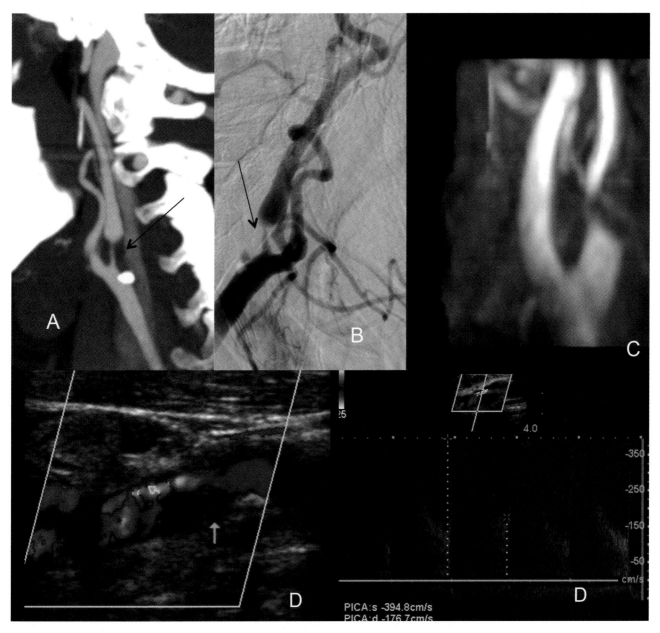

FIGURE 13. Diagnostic imaging modalities in a patient with a symptomatic extracranial internal carotid artery atherosclerotic plaque and associated 90% stenosis. *Top panels*: a CT angiogram (*A*), a digital subtraction angiogram (*B*), and a magnetic resonance angiogram (*C*) all show high-grade stenosis at the area of the origin of the internal carotid artery (*arrows*). *Bottom panel*: ultrasounds (*D*) of the extracranial proximal internal carotid artery show a large plaque at the origin (*arrow*) of the artery, with associated elevated systolic (−394.8 cm/s) and diastolic (−176.7 cm/s) velocities consistent with 80% to 99% stenosis. PICA = proximal internal carotid artery.

CONT.

Stroke arising from atherosclerosis of the intracranial arteries typically occurs with stenosis greater than 70% in the vertebrobasilar, intracranial internal carotid, and middle cerebral arteries. Intracranial atherosclerosis also is associated with a high long-term risk of recurrent stroke; its presence can be detected with either CT or MRA. Transcranial Doppler ultrasonography can detect accelerated velocities consistent with significant stenosis and can be used in patients unable to undergo CT or MRA; diagnostic cerebral angiography is rarely necessary in these patients.

Small Subcortical Infarcts (Lacunes)

Small subcortical infarcts (lacunes) are commonly less than 1.5 cm in size and arise from occlusion of small perforating arteries emanating from the large intracranial vessels. This stroke subtype typically presents with only motor or sensory findings on examination; cortical hemispheric symptoms, such as visual field cuts, aphasia, or hemispatial neglect, are lacking. The main risk factor for lacunar stroke is hypertension, leading to associated pathologic changes at the origin of the perforating arteries. Because these infarcts may still arise from atherothrombotic lesions in large cerebral arteries, vascular imaging is required in affected patients to initiate appropriate secondary stroke prevention.

Cryptogenic and Rare Causes of Stroke

A sizeable proportion of patients will have a cerebral infarction with no definitive cause identified on cardiac or vascular diagnostic testing. In these patients, prolonged cardiac rhythm monitoring or interrogation of a pacemaker, if present, may reveal undiagnosed paroxysmal atrial fibrillation that could change secondary prevention strategies. Other diagnostic testing can be considered on a case by case basis, depending on the specific circumstances. Headache preceding stroke in younger patients without cardiovascular disease risk factors, particularly those with recent head/neck trauma, suggests cervicocephalic arterial dissection and can be ruled out with head and neck vascular imaging. Testing for autoimmune and hypercoagulable disorders can be considered in young patients with otherwise unexplained stroke. Echocardiography may reveal a PFO, which is present in up to 25% of the general population. In younger patients, a PFO is likely to be causally related to the stroke, although these patients generally are at a low risk of subsequent stroke in the absence of a hypercoagulable disorder. Recently completed clinical trials, however, have failed to show the benefit of percutaneous closure compared with best medical therapy. For further details see MKSAP 17 Cardiovascular Medicine. **H**

KEY POINTS

- Cardiac rhythm evaluation, including electrocardiography and in-hospital telemetry, is advisable for all patients with ischemic stroke to evaluate for atrial fibrillation. *(Continued)*

KEY POINTS *(continued)*

- Stroke is commonly caused by large artery atherosclerosis, and the risk of stroke recurrence is highest when any associated stenosis is greater than 70%.

Hemorrhagic Stroke
Subarachnoid Hemorrhage

Nontraumatic SAH presents with the sudden onset of a severe headache, described by patients as the worst headache of their life or "thunderclap" in origin (see Headache and Facial Pain). The most common examination finding in patients with SAH is impairment in consciousness due to elevated intracranial pressure that manifests as a spectrum ranging from mild somnolence to coma or brain death. The initial clinical examination is often summarized by using clinical scales that correlate well with mortality (**Table 17**). Other early localizing findings include subhyaloid hemorrhages on funduscopy (**Figure 14**) and oculomotor nerve palsies with pupillary dilation from direct compression. In patients with elevated intracranial pressure from either

TABLE 17. Clinical Grading Scale for Subarachnoid Hemorrhage

Hunt-Hess Grade	Clinical Description
1	Asymptomatic or mild headache
2	Moderate to severe headache, cranial nerve palsies
3	Somnolence, confusion, or minor focal neurologic deficits
4	Significant impairment in consciousness, significant focal neurologic deficits
5	Coma, posturing

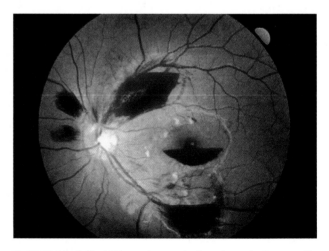

FIGURE 14. Subhyaloid hemorrhages on funduscopic examination suggesting an aneurysmal subarachnoid hemorrhage.

Adapted with permission from Laforest C, Selva D, Crompton J, Leibovitch I. Entopic phenomenon as initial presentation of acute myelogenous leukemia. Ann Intern Med. 2005 Dec 6;143(11):847. [PMID: 16330805]

cerebral edema or obstructive hydrocephalus, loss of brainstem reflexes, posturing in response to painful stimuli, and impairments in consciousness can occur. Any patient with sudden unexplained coma requires neuroimaging to exclude SAH and hydrocephalus. The principal cause of SAH is a ruptured cerebral saccular aneurysm, which often can be identified by CT angiography. Catheter angiography still is required in all patients to confirm the presence of a symptomatic aneurysm and to detect other pathology that may be

beyond the resolution of CT angiography, such as intracranial arterial dissection, intracranial vascular malformation, or small distal aneurysms. Catheter angiography has the additional benefit of being a treatment modality for ruptured intracranial aneurysms (**Figure 15**). Besides intracranial arterial dissections and intracranial vascular malformations, other conditions that can lead to SAH include reversible cerebral vasoconstriction syndrome and dural sinus thrombosis.

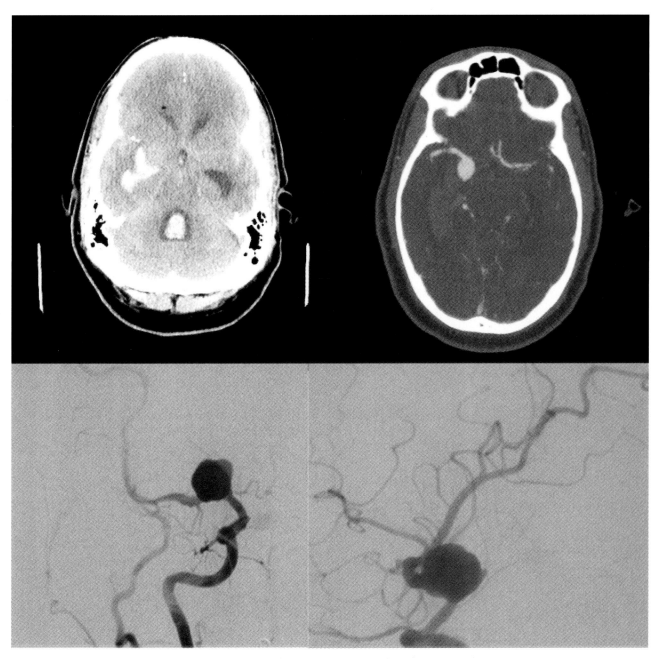

FIGURE 15. Angiograms showing an internal carotid artery aneurysm in a patient with a subarachnoid hemorrhage (SAH). *Top left*, noncontrast head CT scan showing an extensive SAH with intraventricular extension. *Top right*, CT angiogram showing a large right internal carotid artery aneurysm. *Bottom left*, anteroposterior view of a digital subtraction angiogram of the right intracranial internal carotid artery showing the same large aneurysm. *Bottom right*, lateral view of the digital subtraction angiogram showing the same large aneurysm.

Intracerebral Hemorrhage

ICH should be suspected in any patient with focal neurologic symptoms with associated headache, nausea, or impairment in consciousness. Other predictive features of ICH include hypertension at onset, use of oral anticoagulants, and sudden unexplained loss of consciousness. However, no reliable history or examination findings can reliably confirm or rule out hemorrhagic stroke, and the diagnosis of ICH requires a prompt CT scan of the head without contrast, which can readily identify the presence of blood. This procedure can be completed quickly and allows for the identification of associated pathology that can have a significant negative effect on prognosis, including cerebral edema and hydrocephalus. Repeat neuroimaging often is required in patients with ICH to detect hematoma expansion, worsening cerebral edema, or other causes of changes in neurologic status.

The location of the ICH correlates with different underlying pathologies, which can further dictate long-term prognosis and secondary prevention strategies. ICH originating from deep structures of the brain, such as the basal ganglia, pons, and cerebellum, is typically due to hypertension. With adequate control of the blood pressure, patients with deep hemorrhages may still be candidates for anticoagulation, if needed, in the future. Lobar hemorrhages in older patients without hypertension that originate near the cortical surface can be caused by amyloid angiopathy stemming from amyloid-β deposits in distal cerebral arterioles; this process is similar to what occurs in Alzheimer disease, in which amyloid-β deposits are found in the parenchyma. Amyloid angiopathy is associated with a high risk of recurrent lobar hemorrhage, and anticoagulation and statins should be avoided in these patients. Vascular imaging or MRI may be required in patients with atypical presentations or otherwise unexplained ICH. H

KEY POINTS

- The principal cause of subarachnoid hemorrhage is a ruptured cerebral saccular aneurysm, which can be identified by CT angiography; catheter angiography is required for confirmation of the diagnosis and potential treatment of the aneurysm.

- Repeat neuroimaging often is required in patients with intracerebral hemorrhages to detect hematoma expansion, worsening cerebral edema, or other causes of changes in neurologic status.

Acute Stroke Therapy

The initial therapy in acute stroke depends on whether the stroke is ischemic or hemorrhagic. Regardless of stroke etiology, a primary goal of hospitalizing all affected patients is the prevention and treatment of associated medical and neurologic complications.

Ischemic Stroke Treatment

Thrombolysis

The initial goal in the evaluation of a patient with acute ischemic stroke is to establish eligibility for intravenous thrombolysis. The primary determinant of eligibility is the time since stroke onset, which is determined by either self-report or the time when the patient was last witnessed at a prestroke baseline. Thrombolysis in stroke aims to restore cerebral blood flow to the ischemic penumbra where cerebral tissue has sustained ischemic injury but has not yet progressed to infarction. Intravenous thrombolysis in ischemic stroke is indicated within 3 hours of onset in patients with a measurable deficit who do not meet any of the exclusion criteria and is most effective the earlier it is administered. A focused history and physical examination and a fingerstick measurement of blood glucose level can determine any of the exclusion criteria; rapid imaging with noncontrast head CT is required to exclude ICH. Laboratory testing, including a complete blood count, coagulation profile, and basic metabolic profile, also should be obtained in all patients with acute ischemic stroke, although the results are not necessary to initiate thrombolysis unless a suspicion of coagulopathy or thrombocytopenia exists. The optimal time from hospital arrival to treatment with thrombolysis is 60 minutes or less, which is considered a marker of high-quality care. Additional testing is not indicated in most patients because it leads to unnecessary delays in treatment. Vascular imaging in the acute ischemic stroke setting also is not necessary and can lead to treatment time delays.

Treatment with intravenous thrombolysis between 3 to 4.5 hours from stroke onset can be considered in a select group of patients who meet strict inclusion/exclusion criteria, although this therapy lacks FDA approval. The efficacy of endovascular stroke therapy in lieu of, or after, intravenous thrombolysis has not been established by several recently completed clinical trials. Endovascular acute stroke therapy with intra-arterial thrombolytic or thrombectomy devices can be considered on a case by case basis for patients within 6 hours of stroke onset who are otherwise ineligible for intravenous thrombolysis. A proposed pathway for the evaluation and treatment of acute ischemic stroke is provided in **Figure 16**.

The main complication from intravenous thrombolysis is symptomatic ICH, defined as intracranial bleeding with an associated decline in neurologic function detected on neurologic examination that cannot be ascribed to other causes. It occurs in approximately 6% of treated patients and has an associated 50% mortality. Headache, nausea, or worsening of neurologic examination findings are signs of intracranial bleeding and should prompt stopping the infusion and repeating the head CT. The main risk factors for symptomatic ICH are protocol violations, notably treatment beyond the time window and blood pressure above recommended targets. Blood pressure should be less than 185/110 mm Hg before thrombolysis, which can be achieved with intravenous labetalol or nicardipine, according to American Heart Association guidelines.

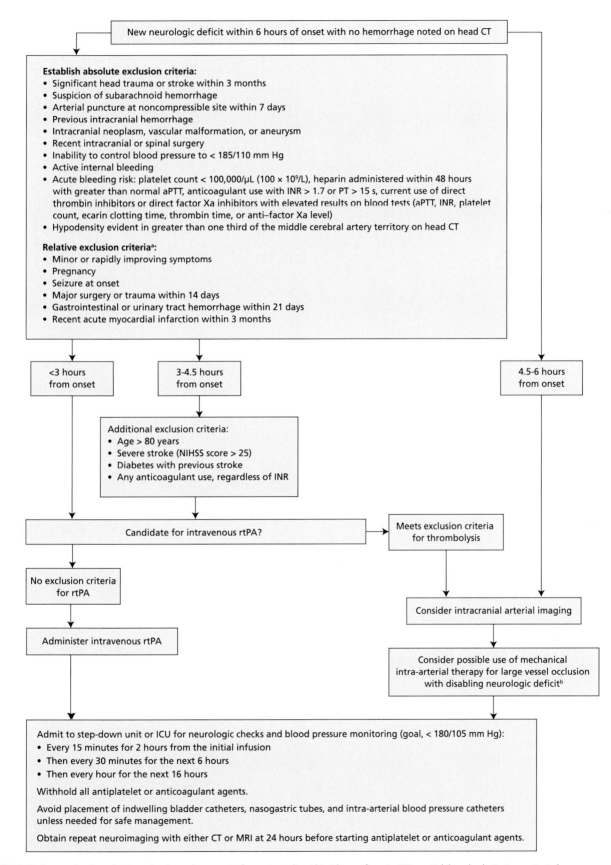

FIGURE 16. Proposed pathway for the evaluation and treatment of an acute stroke within 6 hours of onset. aPTT = partial thromboplastin time, activated; NIHSS = National Institutes of Health Stroke Scale; PT = prothrombin time; rtPA = recombinant tissue plasminogen activator.

[a]rtPA can be considered in patients with one or more relative exclusion criteria after consideration of neurologic deficits and risks versus benefits.

[b]Available evidence for the benefit of mechanical intra-arterial therapy is limited, and its appropriate use remains to be defined.

CONT.

After the initiation of intravenous thrombolysis using recombinant tissue plasminogen activator, adherence to strict monitoring protocols regarding vital signs and neurologic examination findings is required to achieve a target blood pressure less than 180/105 mm Hg and to detect signs of symptomatic ICH. Other precautions after intravenous thrombolysis include withholding all antithrombotic agents until a repeat head CT or MRI performed 24 hours after the procedure excludes ICH and monitoring for angioedema.

Antiplatelet, Anticoagulant, and Other Agents for Acute Ischemic Stroke Treatment

Most patients with ischemic stroke will arrive beyond the stated windows for intravenous thrombolysis. For most of these patients, aspirin is appropriate, but only after a dysphagia evaluation documenting the ability to safely swallow. In those unable to swallow, a rectal formulation of aspirin is available. Aspirin taken within 48 hours of ischemic stroke onset modestly reduces the risk of recurrent ischemic stroke at 2 weeks without significantly increasing the risk of intracerebral hemorrhage. No acute ischemic stroke trials have tested monotherapy with clopidogrel or the combination of aspirin and dipyridamole. However, in patients with a high-risk TIA (ABCD^2 score ≥ 4) or minor ischemic stroke (National Institute of Health Stroke Scale score ≤ 3), a 21-day course of combination aspirin and clopidogrel followed by clopidogrel monotherapy for a total of 90 days reduced the risk of subsequent stroke when administered within 24 hours of onset compared with aspirin monotherapy. No increase in the risk of ICH or differences in efficacy by subgroups was reported. Heparinoids do not reduce the risk of recurrent stroke in the acute setting for either cardioembolic or noncardioembolic stroke. Acute intravenous heparin occasionally is used in patients with rare causes of stroke, such as dissection or a hypercoagulable state, or in patients with mechanical cardiac valves if the risk of hemorrhage into the infarct is low.

Other medication classes have not been extensively studied in the acute setting. To date, no studies have been published about statins administered in the acute stroke setting. A recent trial of acute blood pressure lowering with candesartan within 36 hours showed no reduction in cardiac events or mortality but a trend toward worsening of neurologic deficits. Blood pressure lowering in patients who do not receive intravenous thrombolysis is only recommended if the blood pressure is greater than 220/120 mm Hg or if a high risk or evidence of other end-organ damage exists.

Antithrombotic Therapy After Ischemic Stroke

The management of antithrombotic agents after ischemic stroke and TIA differs from that in other ischemic atherosclerotic diseases because of the risk of hemorrhagic stroke. In patients with stroke and atrial fibrillation, anticoagulation can be started before hospital discharge if the risk of hemorrhage into the bed of the infarct is low, such as in patients with infarcts but no petechial hemorrhage, as determined by neuroimaging, or with involvement of less than one third of the middle cerebral artery distribution. For further discussion of anticoagulation in atrial fibrillation, see MKSAP 17 Cardiovascular Medicine. Warfarin is not recommended for patients with symptomatic intracranial atherosclerosis unless another high-risk condition also is identified because this drug is associated with increased mortality compared with antiplatelet agents. In all other noncardioembolic ischemic strokes, warfarin and antiplatelet agents are equivalent in terms of efficacy, although antiplatelet agents often are considered first-line agents because of ease of use.

In the nonacute setting, the combination of aspirin and clopidogrel for noncardioembolic stroke increases the risk of mortality and hemorrhagic stroke without significantly reducing the risk of ischemic stroke, compared with single-agent therapy. The combination of aspirin and dipyridamole twice daily modestly reduces the risk of recurrent ischemic stroke when compared with aspirin monotherapy, but in a large ischemic stroke secondary prevention trial, the combination of aspirin and dipyridamole was equivalent to clopidogrel monotherapy. The choice of antiplatelet agents for secondary stroke prevention is often driven by patient preference, including cost, and by risk for other medical comorbidities, given the small absolute risk differences between each agent. For noncardioembolic stroke, low-dose (81 mg/d) aspirin monotherapy is often first-line therapy for patients not previously taking antiplatelet agents. Clopidogrel or aspirin plus dipyridamole can be considered in patients who have a recurrent ischemic stroke, despite adequate control of other stroke risk factors, while taking aspirin monotherapy. The effectiveness of newer antiplatelet agents or platelet resistance assays has not been established for stroke.

KEY POINTS

- Intravenous thrombolysis is indicated within 3 hours (and can be considered within 3 to 4.5 hours) of onset of ischemic stroke in patients with a measurable deficit who meet inclusion/exclusion criteria.

- After initiation of intravenous thrombolysis, adherence to strict monitoring protocols regarding vital signs and neurologic examination findings is required to achieve a target blood pressure less than 180/105 mm Hg and to detect signs of symptomatic intracranial hemorrhage.

- For most patients with ischemic stroke who arrive at the hospital beyond the treatment window for intravenous thrombolysis, oral or rectal aspirin is usually appropriate treatment; aspirin taken within 48 hours of ischemic stroke onset modestly reduces the risk of recurrent stroke at 2 weeks without significantly increasing the risk of hemorrhage.

Hemorrhagic Stroke Treatment
Intracerebral Hemorrhage Treatment

The mainstay of therapy for acute ICH is treatment of hematoma-associated neurologic complications. Antiplatelet and antithrombotic agents should be discontinued. Given the small risk of hemorrhage with selective serotonin reuptake inhibitors, discontinuation of these agents should also be considered. In patients with hydrocephalus, external shunting of cerebrospinal fluid may be required when clinical evidence of elevated intracranial pressure is detected; osmotherapy with mannitol or hypertonic saline can be considered in patients with elevated intracranial pressure as salvage therapy. Surgical evacuation of the hematoma should be considered in patients with a cerebellar ICH with a size greater than 3 cm, particularly if evidence of neurologic worsening or brainstem compression is present. Surgical decompression for other locations can be considered on a case-by-case basis.

An additional goal of therapy in patients with ICH has been to prevent expansion of the hematoma by lowering blood pressure or using hemostatic agents. Recombinant factor VIIa therapy, however, was not associated with improved clinical outcomes in a randomized clinical trial of spontaneous ICH. In patients with a vitamin K antagonist-associated ICH, fresh-frozen plasma or prothrombin complex concentrates are recommended, as is administration of intravenous vitamin K. The appropriate treatment of ICH related to direct thrombin inhibitors or factor Xa inhibitors and the effectiveness of using platelet transfusions in antiplatelet-associated ICH have not been well established. For further details see MKSAP 17 Hematology and Oncology. In patients without elevated intracranial pressure whose systolic blood pressure is greater than 180 mm Hg or mean arterial pressure is greater than 130 mm Hg at the time of their ICH, treatment with intravenous medications can be initiated, with a target blood pressure of 160/90 mm Hg or mean arterial pressure of 110 mm Hg. Further reductions in blood pressure also may be safe. A recent trial showed that acute lowering of systolic blood pressure to less than 140 mm Hg (compared with <180 mm Hg) within 6 hours was associated with a trend to reduction of disability, without any change in adverse events or mortality. Medications that can be titrated easily, such as nicardipine or labetalol, are preferred; nitrates should be avoided because of the potential for increasing intracranial pressure.

Subarachnoid Hemorrhage Treatment

Neurologic complications in aneurysmal SAH differ according to whether they occur early (within 48 hours) or later (typically, 5-10 days) in the clinical course of the hemorrhage. In the early phase, patients often have impairments in consciousness due to hydrocephalus and require external cerebrospinal fluid shunting to alleviate and subsequently monitor intracranial pressure. A significant cause of morbidity and mortality during this phase is aneurysmal rebleeding, and thus early vascular imaging is required in all patients with SAH to diagnose any ruptured cerebral artery aneurysm. Treatment with either endovascular coiling or clipping (performed during a craniotomy) should begin early; until the aneurysm is secured, the blood pressure should be less than 140/80 mm Hg to prevent rebleeding. Other sources of early neurologic

complications include global cerebral edema and seizures; seizure prophylaxis is common in patients with SAH. Delayed cerebral ischemia due to arterial vasospasm is a significant source of later neurologic morbidity and can present with nonspecific examination findings. The patients at highest risk for developing vasospasm with subsequent delayed cerebral ischemia are those with the largest burden of blood in the basal cisterns on neuroimaging. These same patients generally have impairments in consciousness, which makes detection of subtle examination findings challenging. Although serial daily screening to identify vasospasm typically is performed with noninvasive transcranial ultrasonography during the first 2 weeks after SAH onset, CT angiography is more sensitive in detecting subtle vasospasms that may be treated with either the initiation of vasopressors to augment the blood pressure or ultimately endovascular treatment in more refractory disease. CT angiography has the additional benefit of imaging the ventricles, which will allow for detecting a change in ventricular size. Oral nimodipine improves neurologic outcomes in patients with aneurysmal SAH and is recommended in all patients with SAH for the first 21 days or until hospital discharge, whichever comes first. Cerebral vasospasm is often managed initially by inducing hypertension to prevent progression to cerebral ischemia, but only after the aneurysm has first been treated. However, clinical trial data supporting a particular target blood pressure are scant, and the American Heart Association has made no specific recommendation. In patients with clinically significant cerebral vasospasm, angiography may be necessary to confirm its severity and allow for potential therapeutic intervention.

Associated medical complications are a significant source of morbidity and mortality in SAH. Acute myocardial infarction due to contractile band necrosis in the setting of a significant sympathetic surge can occur early in the course of high-grade SAH (see Table 17) and can lead to significant reductions in systolic function, hypotension, and pulmonary edema. Respiratory failure requiring mechanical ventilation because of impaired consciousness or hypoxemia from either pneumonia or pulmonary edema is also common. Other medical complications include cerebral salt wasting syndrome, the syndrome of inappropriate antidiuretic hormone secretion, cardiac arrhythmias, and infections from pulmonary, urinary, and central venous catheters or from cerebrospinal fluid shunting sources. Given the associated level of monitoring and supportive care required for neurologic and medical complications of SAH, affected patients should be cared for in a neurologic ICU, if available.

KEY POINTS

- Surgical evacuation of the hematoma should be considered in patients with a cerebellar intracerebral hemorrhage whose size is greater than 3 cm, particularly if evidence of neurologic worsening or brainstem compression is present.

(Continued)

KEY POINTS (continued)

- Early vascular imaging is required in all patients with subarachnoid hemorrhage to evaluate for any ruptured cerebral artery aneurysm; treatment of the aneurysm with either endovascular coiling or clipping should begin early, with the blood pressure maintained at less than 140/80 mm Hg to prevent rebleeding.

Stroke Prevention

Table 18 lists the risk factors for stroke.

Primary Stroke Prevention

For a discussion of management of vascular disease risk factors and antiplatelet agents used in primary prevention of stroke, see MKSAP 17 Cardiovascular Medicine.

The approach to asymptomatic extracranial internal carotid artery stenosis has changed because of improvements in optimal medical therapy that have resulted in stroke rates close to 1% per year (compared with the previous rate of 2% per year). This lower rate seems driven by lipid-lowering therapy with statins. Aggressive risk factor control, with optimal medical therapy and comprehensive lifestyle modifications in diet, exercise habits, and tobacco use (among others), is required for all patients. Revascularization with either stenting or endarterectomy can be considered in patients with a greater than 80% stenosis and low cardiovascular risk, as long as the operative complication rate is less than 3%.

Unruptured cerebral artery aneurysms are commonly found in asymptomatic patients. A fraction of these patients have symptoms from compression of adjacent structures, such as pupillary enlargement from compression of the oculomotor nerve by a posterior communicating artery aneurysm or visual loss from compression of the optic nerve by a cavernous carotid artery aneurysm. Size, location, and a history of ruptured cerebral artery aneurysms in other locations are the principal determinants of treatment. Rupture rates from asymptomatic aneurysms without a prior history of SAH are outlined in **Table 19**. Surgical treatment with clipping or endovascular coiling can be considered in patients with aneurysms of 7 mm or greater in the posterior circulation (posterior communicating and basilar arteries) or 12 mm or greater in the anterior circulation. Regardless of aneurysmal size and location, all patients with unruptured cerebral artery aneurysms benefit from tobacco cessation and blood pressure control.

KEY POINTS

- Most patients with asymptomatic extracranial internal carotid artery stenosis should be treated with aggressive risk factor control and not stenting or elective endarterectomy, which should only be considered in patients with a greater than 80% stenosis and low cardiovascular risk (as long as the operative complication rate is less than 3%).

- In primary stroke prevention, all patients with unruptured cerebral artery aneurysms benefit from tobacco cessation and blood pressure control.

HVC

Secondary Stroke Prevention
Lifestyle and Medical Management

The treatment of modifiable vascular disease risk factors can lead to a significant decrease in the risk of recurrent

TABLE 18.	Common Risk Factors for Ischemic and Hemorrhagic Stroke		
	Ischemic Stroke/TIA	**Intracerebral Hemorrhage**	**Subarachnoid Hemorrhage**
Shared Risk Factors			
	Hypertension	Hypertension	Hypertension
	Cocaine abuse	Cocaine abuse	Cocaine abuse
	Tobacco use	Tobacco use	Tobacco use
		Arteriovenous malformation	Arteriovenous malformation
Other Risk Factors			
	Diabetes mellitus	Amyloid angiopathy	Intracranial artery dissection
	Atrial fibrillation	Decreased LDL cholesterol level	Polycystic kidney disease
	Low left ventricular ejection fraction and intracardiac thrombus	Elevated HDL cholesterol level	
	Cervicocephalic arterial dissection	Anticoagulant agent use	
	Aortic arch atheromatous disease	Antiplatelet agent use	
	Cardiac valve vegetations	Selective serotonin reuptake inhibitor use	
	Patent foramen ovale		
TIA = transient ischemic attack.			

TABLE 19. Rupture Rates Over 5 Years of Unruptured Intracranial Artery Aneurysms

Position	Size (mm)	Rupture Rate (%)
Anterior circulation aneurysm (internal carotid, anterior communicating, middle cerebral arteries)	<7	0
	7-12	2.6
	13-24	14.5
	>25	40
Posterior circulation aneurysm (posterior communicating, basilar arteries)	<7	2.5
	7-12	14.5
	13-24	18.4
	>25	50

stroke. Hypertension is a common risk factor for recurrence of all stroke subtypes, and lowering of blood pressure in patients with stroke is associated with a significant reduction in the risk for recurrence. However, the optimal goal for secondary prevention of stroke is less clear. The Eighth Joint National Committee (JNC 8) recommendations and treatment guidelines for the prevention of secondary stroke recommend antihypertensive therapy for stable patients with a sustained blood pressure of 140/90 mm Hg or greater, including those older than 60 years with preexisting cardiovascular disease. However, the benefit of initiating antihypertensive therapy in patients with stroke who have a blood pressure less than 140/90 mm Hg is uncertain. There is evidence, however, that patients with a recent lacunar infarct may benefit from a systolic blood pressure goal of less than 130 mm Hg. No specific recommendations exist regarding preferred pharmacologic agents for secondary stroke prevention. Therefore, the choice of the most appropriate antihypertensive agent is often driven by a consideration of comorbid medical conditions.

All patients with stroke require comprehensive lifestyle changes, including improving physical activity and diet and stopping tobacco use. See MKSAP 17 Nephrology for further discussion of management of hypertension, MKSAP 17 Endocrinology and Metabolism for management of type 2 diabetes mellitus, and MKSAP 17 General Internal Medicine for management of dyslipidemia. For secondary stroke prevention, statins are recommended for patients with a plasma LDL cholesterol level of 100 mg/dL (2.59 mmol/L) or higher once the ability to safely swallow has been established. Statins have been associated with an increased risk of hemorrhagic stroke and may be contraindicated in patients with a lobar ICH due to amyloid angiopathy. However, they most likely are safe in those with a deep ICH. Regardless of ICH subtype, statins are indicated for patients at high risk for ischemic events.

Surgery for Secondary Ischemic Stroke Prevention

The stroke cause with the highest risk of recurrence is symptomatic extracranial internal carotid artery stenosis, with a 26% risk of recurrent stroke at 2 years and a close to 1% per day increased risk of recurrent stroke in the first 2 weeks. Carotid revascularization, preferably within 14 days from the index event, is indicated for nondisabling strokes or TIAs in patients with symptomatic extracranial internal carotid artery stenosis in the range of 70% to 99% and can be performed with endarterectomy or angioplasty-stenting. The choice of one surgical approach is often dictated by the risk of perioperative complications or anatomic considerations. Angioplasty-stenting is often performed in patients at high risk for periprocedural cardiopulmonary complications and in those with restenosis and previous radiation therapy. In clinical trials, periprocedural stroke is reported to be higher with angioplasty-stenting than with endarterectomy, but myocardial infarction is more likely with endarterectomy. In patients with complete occlusion, none of the surgical options (carotid stenting, endarterectomy, or external carotid to internal carotid bypass) reduces the risk of recurrent stroke, and best medical therapy (including antiplatelet agents and statins) is advised. Using angioplasty-stenting also is not recommended for patients with symptomatic intracranial artery stenosis because of the high risk of periprocedural stroke and the high efficacy of optimal medical therapy.

Using surgical approaches to treat causes of cardioembolic stroke is an evolving field. For further discussion of surgical approaches to cardiac disease for stroke prevention, see MKSAP 17 Cardiovascular Medicine. **H**

KEY POINTS

- For secondary stroke prevention, statins are recommended for patients with a plasma LDL cholesterol level of 100 mg/dL (2.59 mmol/L) or higher once the ability to safely swallow has been established.

- In patients with nondisabling strokes or transient ischemic attacks who have symptomatic extracranial internal carotid artery stenosis, carotid revascularization, preferably within 14 days from the index event, is indicated for secondary stroke prevention.

Prognosis and Recovery

Neurologic Complications

Neurologic worsening can occur in patients with ischemic stroke during hospitalization as a result of stroke recurrence, hemorrhage into the area of infarction, seizures, or cerebral edema. Medical complications, particularly infections, can cause worsening of the neurologic deficit. Any patient with a change noted during neurologic examination requires repeat neuroimaging to establish any new structural lesions. Patients with a middle cerebral artery infarction involving greater than 50% of the arterial territory are at high risk for malignant cerebral infarction with associated edema and cerebral herniation. Hemicraniectomy is associated with a significant reduction in mortality and severe disability (from 76% to 25% in pooled data from three clinical trials) compared with best medical therapy

CONT.

and also should be considered early in patients with malignant cerebral infarction if they exhibit impaired alertness or have at least one pupil reactive to light.

KEY POINT

- Patients with a middle cerebral artery infarction involving greater than 50% of the arterial territory are at high risk for malignant cerebral infarction with associated edema and cerebral herniation; hemicraniectomy, which is associated with a significant reduction in mortality and severe disability compared with best medical therapy, can be considered in these patients.

Medical Complications and Stroke Units

Early mobilization and rehabilitation to a level the patient can tolerate are indicated for all survivors of stroke to improve recovery and mitigate medical complications. These patients are prone to urinary tract infections from indwelling catheters, aspiration pneumonia from dysphagia, and deep venous thrombosis (DVT). The principal cause of stroke-related mortality, these complications can be ameliorated by admission to a stroke unit, defined as (ideally) a discrete ward where a multidisciplinary team with expertise in stroke cares for these patients. Early mobilization appears to be a significant determinant of the success of stroke units, although adherence to clinical care protocols for dysphagia, DVT, and indwelling urinary catheters also are instrumental. Several bedside dysphagia screening protocols are available and should be performed before any oral intake; a formal evaluation with a speech therapist is often required. Aspiration pneumonia can be further prevented by maintaining the head of the bed at 30 degrees and instituting oral hygiene protocols. DVT prevention is required for all hospitalized stroke patients unless they are fully ambulatory. Subcutaneous unfractionated or low-molecular-weight heparin should be started in all patients with impaired mobility by hospital day 1 for ischemic stroke and by hospital day 4 (if no active bleeding is documented) in hemorrhagic stroke. For those patients at high risk for hemorrhagic complications from pharmacologic therapy, pneumatic compression stockings should be used. For further details, see MKSAP 17 Hematology and Oncology. Unless required for other reasons, indwelling urinary catheters should be removed.

KEY POINT

- Early mobilization is a significant determinant of the success of stroke units, although adherence to clinical care protocols for dysphagia, deep venous thrombosis, and indwelling urinary catheters also is instrumental.

Long-Term Prognosis and Recovery

The main predictor of stroke recovery is the severity of the neurologic deficit. Long-term follow-up evaluation shows that patients with stroke are at high risk for additional complications, including fatigue, depression, and recurrent cardiovascular disease. Survivors of stroke also are at high risk for having or developing undiagnosed obstructive sleep apnea, which can further complicate hypertension management and is a common cause of fatigue; polysomnography is helpful in diagnosis. Depression is highly prevalent in the acute and chronic setting after stroke and is one of the strongest modifiable predictors of stroke recovery.

Cognitive Impairment
Definitions, Description, and Evaluation

Cognitive impairment in older patients spans a continuum, from normal aging to dementia. Neurocognitive disorders are defined as conditions in which an acquired impairment of cognitive function occurs, with coexistent decline in function involving at least one of the following neuropsychological domains: memory/learning, complex attention, executive function, perceptual or motor abilities, language, or social cognition. Dementia is a syndrome characterized by a gradual and progressive decline in previously acquired cognitive function that results in impaired social or occupational functioning and ultimately leads to loss of independence. The diagnosis of dementia requires impairment of at least two of the previously listed neuropsychological domains. Although the incidence of dementia increases with age, this disorder is not an inevitable consequence of normal aging. Subtle cognitive decline with normal aging is common, but not universal, and should not affect independence in daily functioning. Age-associated cognitive decline is most notable for some slowing of processing speed and reaction time. Cognitive flexibility and multitasking abilities may decline with aging. Learning, or the acquisition of new information, decreases with age, but delayed recall remains relatively intact. Language comprehension and vocabulary (semantic memory) are preserved in normal aging.

Mild Cognitive Impairment

The available research suggests that a phase of cognitive impairment precedes the development of dementia. This intermediate stage between normal aging and dementia has been labeled mild cognitive impairment (MCI). In clinical practice, overlap exists between the stages, and the revised criteria for MCI further blur the line between MCI and early or mild dementia. The diagnosis of MCI is made on the basis of clinical judgment and requires the following four features: (1) subjective reports (from the patient or a reliable informant) of problems with memory, such as forgetfulness, or other cognitive difficulties; (2) objective impairment on cognitive testing in one or more cognitive domains; (3) diminished independence in daily function, with no or minimal problems with complex functional tasks, such as shopping or paying bills; and (4) no significant impairment in occupational or social functioning. The presence of significant functional deficit is what distinguishes dementia from MCI. MCI can be further subtyped as amnestic MCI or nonamnestic MCI, depending on the presence or absence of memory deficits and the number of cognitive domains that are affected (that is, a single domain versus multiple domains).

Patients with MCI have a significantly increased likelihood of conversion to dementia at a rate of 10% to 15% per year, in contrast to cognitively normal age-matched controls, who develop dementia at a rate of 1% to 2% per year. Within 6 years from the time of MCI diagnosis, approximately 80% of patients will progress to dementia. Although numerous factors have been studied, and some even have been associated with a higher risk of progression to dementia—such as baseline functional impairment, results of fluorodeoxyglucose-PET brain imaging, and the apolipoprotein E (*APOE ε4*) genotype—no reliable clinical markers exist that can predict the clinical likelihood that an individual patient with MCI will develop dementia. Similarly, no treatments or interventions have been shown to delay the onset of Alzheimer disease or other types of dementia in patients with MCI.

Neuropathologic studies have shown that most patients with amnestic MCI have pathologic findings of Alzheimer disease. The prognostic significance of nonamnestic MCI is less known. Other degenerative pathologies (such as Lewy body disease) and nondegenerative pathologies (such as vascular disease) may be the cause of MCI in a subset of patients. MCI associated with underlying Lewy body disease usually is characterized by diminished executive functioning, impairment of visuospatial abilities, or both. MCI due to vascular disease most often has a cognitive profile of impaired executive function or processing speed, with spared verbal memory. Other nondegenerative, and potentially reversible, diseases also may cause MCI, including metabolic disorders (such as hypothyroidism), vitamin B_{12} deficiency, and depression. Large-scale neuropathologic studies of MCI are not yet available to completely comprehend the full pathologic heterogeneity of the disease.

KEY POINTS

- Patients with mild cognitive impairment have a significantly increased likelihood of conversion to dementia at a rate of 10% to 15% per year.

HVC
- No reliable clinical markers or diagnostic tests can predict the likelihood that an individual patient with mild cognitive impairment will develop dementia, and no intervention has been shown to delay the onset of dementia in such a patient.

Dementia

In contrast to MCI, dementia is a progressive deterioration of cognitive function severe enough to impair occupational or social functioning. An estimated 35 million persons live with dementia worldwide, and that number is expected to triple by 2050 as life expectancy increases. Alzheimer disease is the most common type of dementia (60%-80%).

Advancing age is the major risk factor for dementia. For every 5 years after age 65 years, the prevalence of Alzheimer disease doubles. Vascular risk factors for MCI and dementia include cardiac disease, diabetes mellitus, hypertension, obesity, and tobacco use. The presence of the *APOE ε4* allele, a history of head injury, and mid- and late-life depression are additional risk factors for Alzheimer disease. Higher educational and occupational advancement are associated with a reduced risk or delayed onset of dementia.

Onset of dementia reduces one's life span. Median survival time from age of onset of dementia ranges from 3 to 12 years, with longer durations associated with earlier age of onset. Although significant interindividual variability in survival after the onset of dementia exists, disease duration tends to vary according to the underlying pathology. Persons with Alzheimer disease and dementia with Lewy bodies survive an average of 8 years after diagnosis, whereas persons with frontotemporal dementia survive an average of 6 years and persons with dementia associated with underlying vascular disease survive an average of 4 years.

Evaluation of the Patient with Suspected Cognitive Impairment

For older patients with no obvious cognitive symptoms, insufficient evidence supports routine cognitive testing. However, the following situations should prompt testing for dementia or cognitive impairment in persons age 65 years and older:

- Patients with cognitive symptoms, with or without functional impairment

- Patients who routinely miss scheduled appointments or arrive on the wrong date or at the wrong time

- Patients with inability to accurately follow instructions

- Patients with unexplained weight loss or failure to thrive

- Patients with new onset or worsening depression or anxiety, with or without cognitive symptoms

- Report from a witness, confirmed or unconfirmed by the patient, of a change in cognition, poor or decreased judgment, loss of initiative, or changes in behavior

- Patients with known risk factors for cognitive impairment (such as HIV infection or a personal history of alcohol abuse)

A careful history should focus on the evolution of symptoms, rate of progression, and functional impact on activities of daily living and work performance, if applicable. Patients with even mild restrictions in the ability to use a telephone, handle finances, use public or personal transportation, or take medications appropriately have a higher risk of progressing to dementia. Vascular risk factors, which increase the risk of cerebrovascular events, should be identified. Information on medication use and substance abuse should be elicited, and screening for depression is imperative. Multiple relationships between depression and cognitive impairment have been reported in the literature: (1) late-life depression may lead to prodromal Alzheimer disease; (2) depression may be a risk factor for future development of cognitive impairment, dementia, and Alzheimer disease (odds ratio of 1.85 for all-cause dementia); (3) cerebrovascular disease can precipitate late-life depression; and (4) cognitive impairment itself can lead to depression. More than half of patients with late-life major depression exhibit clinically significant cognitive impairment, most frequently affecting processing speed, executive function, and visuospatial ability. A history should be obtained from the patient and someone well acquainted with the patient who can provide information on current daily functioning relative to premorbid functioning. A general physical examination and a thorough neurologic examination should be performed, with motor and gait portions of the examination that evaluate for signs of parkinsonism emphasized. A detailed family history should be obtained, including any history of cognitive impairment or dementia, significant psychiatric illness in later life, motoneuron disease, or parkinsonism, because the presence of these disorders may suggest a familial neurodegenerative disease.

Although routine cognitive screening has not been recommended by the U.S. Preventive Services Task Force, the annual wellness visit covered by Medicare requires an assessment to detect cognitive impairment. Screening tests also are useful to detect cognitive impairment in patients who report cognitive difficulties. Performance on these tests can serve as a baseline and be used to monitor disease progression. Many instruments have been developed to quickly screen patients for cognitive impairment; common limitations are their low sensitivity to diagnose mild impairment, lack of validation in the primary care setting, cultural or education bias, and low reliability in distinguishing between different underlying causes. Although the Mini–Mental State Examination, on which a score less than 22 indicates dementia, has been the most extensively studied screening instrument, it is now proprietary with a cost per use. Additionally, this instrument has several weaknesses, such as a lack of sensitivity in identifying early signs of dementia and the absence of tasks that test executive function. Among the free tools that are available for clinical use, the Montreal Cognitive Assessment and "Mini-Cog" test have been validated in primary care populations; these instruments screen for impairments of executive function. Self-administered instruments, such as the Self-Administered Gerocognitive Examination and Test Your Memory examination, have been validated in memory-clinic populations to detect mild cognitive impairment and early dementia. In patients with a high intelligence quotient and normal performance on screening tests, further evaluation should be considered. Formal neuropsychological testing provides a more thorough assessment of cognitive function but is more time consuming and costly. It can provide meaningful information about the pattern and extent of cognitive impairment but should not be used in isolation to make a clinical diagnosis. Detailed neuropsychological testing is especially useful for the following patients:

1. Those with milder cognitive symptoms to determine if the cognitive difficulties are within the realm of normal age-associated cognitive decline versus MCI

2. Those with definite dementia, diagnosed on the basis of clinical impression and results of screening cognitive tests, who have clinical features overlapping two or more underlying pathologic processes

3. Those with cognitive symptoms whose clinical picture is confounded by significant depression.

Impaired performance on neuropsychological testing is determined by a patient's performance compared with healthy age- and education-matched controls. However, without premorbid results, this testing can only estimate the patient's premorbid baseline to determine cognitive areas of presumed decline; it can serve as a baseline with which to compare future test results. For patients with milder cognitive symptoms in whom the initial evaluation does not clearly indicate an early dementing process, longitudinal testing can be of value.

To identify reversible causes of cognitive decline, laboratory tests, such as a complete blood count, liver chemistry studies, thyroid function tests, and measurement of serum electrolyte, blood urea nitrogen, creatinine, and vitamin B_{12} levels, should be performed. A syphilis screening test should be performed in high-risk populations. Additional testing, such as evaluating for autoimmune disease, can be considered if relevant symptoms are present. In at-risk populations, HIV serologies should be performed. Once the presence of dementia has been confirmed, a structural neuroimaging study (MRI or CT scan) should be obtained to evaluate for nondegenerative causes that would alter management, such as cerebrovascular disease, neoplasm, subdural hematoma, or hydrocephalus. MRI and CT imaging provide similar information; however, MRI is more sensitive for detecting inflammation, infection, acute stroke, tumor, posterior fossa lesion, and characteristic imaging findings of Creutzfeldt-Jakob disease. The clinical presentation, examination findings, and differential considerations should determine the imaging study performed. Cerebrospinal fluid analysis is not part of the routine evaluation of cognitive impairment but should be considered in the following clinical situations:

- Rapidly progressive dementia
- Age of onset less than 60 years
- Malignancy or paraneoplastic disorders
- Suspicion of acute or subacute infection or of an immunosuppressed or immunodeficient state
- Positive syphilis or Lyme serology
- Systemic autoimmune disease or suspected CNS inflammatory disorder

Early-onset or rapidly progressive cognitive decline requires a more comprehensive and expedited evaluation. Brain MRI and cerebrospinal fluid (CSF) analysis should be performed promptly, and additional serologic tests and elec-troencephalography can be considered. The prion disorder Creutzfeldt-Jakob disease is the most common cause of rapidly progressive dementia, with a disease duration of less than 1 year until death. MRI can be diagnostic when diffusion-weighted or fluid-attenuated inversion recovery hyperintensi-ties involving the cortex, caudate and putamen, or thalamus are seen. CSF analysis can establish the presence of a 14-3-3 protein, and electroencephalography may reveal characteris-tics triphasic spikes. Brain biopsy is sometimes necessary to confirm the diagnosis.

KEY POINTS

HVC

- For older patients with suspected cognitive impairment who are asymptomatic, insufficient evidence supports routine cognitive testing.

- Screening for depression is imperative in the evaluation of cognitive decline.

- Once the presence of dementia has been confirmed, a structural neuroimaging study, such as an MRI or CT scan, should be obtained to evaluate for cerebro-vascular disease, neoplasm, subdural hematoma, or hydrocephalus.

Neurodegenerative Disorders

Alzheimer Disease

Alzheimer disease can be divided into three phases along a single continuum: an asymptomatic preclinical phase, a predementia phase (MCI due to Alzheimer disease), and a dementia phase.

Clinical Features

Classically, Alzheimer disease presents with the insidious development of recent memory loss. Forgetfulness of the details of recent events predominates early in the disease course. Problems with learning and retaining new informa-tion without benefit from cueing are the hallmark cognitive deficits. Aphasia is frequently seen early and is initially char-acterized by word-finding difficulties. Visuospatial dysfunc-tion also is common and often presents as episodes of becoming lost in familiar environments (geographic disori-entation) or problems in assembling objects (constructional apraxia). Executive dysfunction may manifest as impair-ment of problem-solving abilities, judgment, and multitask-ing. Atypical presentations of Alzheimer disease include early visuospatial or executive dysfunction, with relatively preserved memory.

Neurochemistry, Pathology, and Biomarkers

The pathogenesis of Alzheimer disease begins decades before the onset of clinical symptoms. Loss of choline acetyltrans-ferase, the enzyme that synthesizes acetylcholine, results in an acetylcholine deficit, which has been shown to correlate with the degree of cognitive impairment. Alzheimer disease has the following pathologic hallmarks:

1. The accumulation of neuritic plaques composed of amyloid β protein

2. The accumulation of abnormally phosphorylated tau proteins (proteins normally present in neurons that stabilize intracellular microtubules) as neurofibrillary tangles

3. Prominent neuronal loss resulting in atrophy

Biomarkers reflecting the pathophysiology of Alzheimer disease have been incorporated into recently revised diag-nostic criteria because they are assumed to be present many years before the onset of symptoms. The best validated and clinically available biomarkers are markers of neuronal degeneration or neuronal injury and markers of amyloid β deposition. However, the use of these biomarkers in the clinical setting currently has no role because of the absence of disease-modifying therapies and the cost of the advanced neuroimaging and laboratory testing.

For information on the treatment of the cognitive symp-toms of Alzheimer disease, see "Pharmacologic Therapies for Cognitive Symptoms" later in this chapter.

KEY POINTS

- Alzheimer disease can be divided into three phases along a single continuum: an asymptomatic preclinical phase, a predementia phase (mild cognitive impairment due to Alzheimer disease), and a dementia phase.

- Currently, the use of Alzheimer disease biomarkers in the clinical setting has no role because of the absence of disease-modifying therapies and the cost of advanced neuroimaging techniques and laboratory testing.

HVC

Lewy Body Disease

Lewy bodies are abnormal aggregates of proteins within neurons that occur in several neurodegenerative diseases. Lewy body disease is an umbrella term encompassing both dementia with Lewy bodies and Parkinson disease demen-tia. Dementia with Lewy bodies is the second most common cause of dementia (after Alzheimer disease) due to a neuro-degenerative disease in older patients, accounting for 20% of patients with dementia in pathologic studies. Core features are fluctuating cognition, recurrent visual hallucinations, and parkinsonism. Cognitive fluctuations include variations in both attention and level of arousal and can vary hour to hour, day to day, or week to week. The parkinsonism is typi-cally characterized by facial immobility and more axial than appendicular symptoms manifesting as postural instability and gait difficulty. Rapid eye movement sleep behavior dis-order and severe sensitivity to neuroleptic medications are significantly more common in dementia with Lewy bodies than in other dementing illnesses. Recurrent falls, depression, delusions, hallucinations, severe autonomic dysfunction, syncope, and transient unexplained loss of consciousness also commonly are present but have low specificity for dementia with Lewy bodies. Cognitive testing shows the most pronounced impairment in attention, executive function, and visuospatial function.

The distinction between dementia with Lewy bodies and Parkinson disease dementia depends on the onset of cognitive impairment relative to motor impairment. If dementia precedes, occurs concurrently with, or develops within 1 year of onset of parkinsonian motor symptoms, the diagnosis is dementia with Lewy bodies. In contrast, Parkinson disease dementia describes dementia occurring at least 1 year after a diagnosis of Parkinson disease has been well established. The parkinsonism of dementia with Lewy bodies is less responsive to levodopa than is Parkinson disease.

KEY POINTS

- Core features of dementia with Lewy bodies are fluctuating cognition, recurrent visual hallucinations, and parkinsonism with pronounced postural instability and gait difficulty.

- Dementia with Lewy bodies rather than Parkinson disease dementia is the most likely diagnosis when the dementia precedes, occurs concurrently with, or develops within 1 year of onset of parkinsonian motor symptoms.

Frontotemporal Dementia

Frontotemporal dementia (FTD) is the third most common type of neurodegenerative disorder but the second most common cause of dementia in persons younger than 65 years. The average age of onset is 50 to 60 years, but patients can develop FTD as early as their 30s; only 10% of patients with this diagnosis are age 70 years or older. FTD comprises two distinct clinical syndromes. The first, behavioral variant FTD, is associated with prominent changes in behavior, personality, or executive function. The second, primary progressive aphasia, is associated with prominent and early changes in language function and is further subclassified according to the pattern of language impairment.

The changes in social behavior and personality that occur are variable and develop insidiously, but the unifying characteristic is that there is a change. Apathy, diminished interest, loss of empathy, lack of initiative, increased emotionality, disinhibition, euphoria, impulsivity, changes in eating behaviors (such as craving more sweets and binge eating), hyperorality, and compulsiveness are the most common symptoms reported by families. Other changes include irritability, aggression, verbal abuse, hypomania, and restlessness. Similar changes in personality and behavior can be seen in the other types of dementia during the disease course, but the prominence of these symptoms early in the course of FTD helps to establish the diagnosis. Psychosis is sometimes present but is not as common.

Executive function and decision making are typically affected early in the disease. Loss of insight is typically apparent, as is poor judgment. Memory and visuospatial function are relatively spared early in the disease course, which helps to distinguish patients with FTD from those with Alzheimer disease. Atypical parkinsonism or motoneuron disease can develop in some patients with the disease.

Motoneuron disease, including amyotrophic lateral sclerosis, is seen in approximately 15% of patients preceding, simultaneous with, or after the diagnosis of FTD. Progressive supranuclear palsy (PSP) and corticobasal degeneration (CBD) are two related syndromes that may present with dementia and are pathologically related to FTD. PSP is characterized by early postural instability and falls, axial parkinsonism that is poorly responsive to levodopa, vertical gaze palsy on examination, and slurred speech. Cognitive deficits include apathy, slow processing speed, and impaired executive function. CBD is a rare disorder characterized by rigidity, akinesia, apraxia, myoclonus, dystonia, and alien-limb phenomenon (initially affecting only one limb). Cognitive deficits can be prominent and include slowed processing speed, impaired working memory, executive dysfunction, and—occasionally—aphasia. Neuroimaging in CBD may show asymmetric cortical atrophy mostly involving the parietal and posterior frontal lobes.

FTD is associated with atrophy and neuronal loss involving the frontal or temporal lobes, which are sometimes visible on neuroimaging. The underlying pathologic changes are heterogeneous and characterized by abnormal proteins that accumulate in the brain: tau, transactivating-response region DNA binding protein 43 (TDP-43), or fused-in sarcoma (FUS gene) protein. Nearly all cases of PSP and CBD are due to underling tau pathology. FTD that is associated with motoneuron disease is always due to underlying TDP-43 pathology.

The genetics of FTD also are heterogeneous. As many as 40% of patients with FTD have at least one family member with a neurodegenerative disorder. Because many associated genetic mutations have been identified, genetic testing is appropriate in patients with one or more first-degree relatives with a clinical syndrome consistent with FTD, especially those with children in whom a positive result might affect family planning. However, this testing should be performed only after genetic counseling.

KEY POINTS

- The behavioral variant of frontotemporal dementia is associated with prominent changes in behavior, personality, or executive function, and the primary progressive aphasia variant is associated with prominent and early changes in language function.

- Genetic counseling and testing are appropriate in patients with frontotemporal dementia (FTD) who have one or more first-degree relatives with a clinical syndrome consistent with FTD.

Nondegenerative Causes of Dementia

Idiopathic Normal Pressure Hydrocephalus

Idiopathic normal pressure hydrocephalus (NPH) is very rare, with an estimated incidence rate of 15 per 100,000 persons older than 50 years; an even smaller percentage of patients with NPH show sustained improvement with treatment. NPH is characterized by gait abnormalities, urinary symptoms, and cognitive decline. Accompanying neuroimaging findings include ventriculomegaly that is disproportionate to cortical atrophy in a patient without any known secondary causes of hydrocephalus, such as a history of meningitis, subarachnoid hemorrhage, or trauma. Because subcortical vascular ischemic disease can mimic the clinical symptoms and signs of NPH, MRI and a careful history that excludes hypertension, ischemic heart disease, diabetes mellitus, and dyslipidemia are essential. CSF opening pressure in patients with NPH is typically normal. Symptoms present insidiously, with peak prevalence in the seventh and eighth decades of life.

Abnormal gait is usually the first and principal symptom of NPH. This gait is characterized by a wide base, with slow, small steps and reduced foot-to-floor clearance, and can be accompanied by freezing of gait and postural instability. Urinary frequency and urgency typically precede incontinence and cognitive dysfunction. The cognitive dysfunction follows a pattern of impaired attention, psychomotor slowing, executive dysfunction, and impaired recall.

Ventriculoperitoneal shunt placement is the standard of care for NPH. Large-volume lumbar puncture or a lumbar drainage trial with cognitive and motor testing and symptom assessment before and after testing can be used to evaluate potential response to shunting. No currently available test, however, can reliably determine a positive response.

Although NPH traditionally has been considered a reversible disease if shunting is performed early in the clinical course, response to shunting is variable and infrequently sustained. Moreover, NPH is overdiagnosed, which results in a high frequency of unsuccessful procedures.

KEY POINTS

- Idiopathic normal pressure hydrocephalus is characterized by an abnormal gait that is often accompanied by urinary symptoms, cognitive decline, and ventriculomegaly on neuroimaging.

- Large-volume lumbar puncture or a lumbar drainage trial with cognitive and motor testing and symptom assessment before and after testing can be used to evaluate potential response to shunting in normal pressure hydrocephalus.

Vascular Neurocognitive Disorder

Vascular neurocognitive disorder (VND), the term now used to describe cognitive impairment of any degree (from mild cognitive impairment to vascular dementia) due to cerebrovascular disease, is the second most common cause of cognitive impairment in older persons (after Alzheimer disease). The associated clinical syndromes and underlying causes are heterogeneous. Cerebrovascular syndromes associated with cognitive decline are listed below:

- Multiple cortical infarcts, multiple subcortical infarcts, silent infarcts, or some combination of these

- Single infarcts in regions of the brain that control speech, motor functions, and senses (eloquent regions), such as lacunar infarcts involving the thalamus and basal ganglia that have vital interconnections with multiple cortical regions

- Subcortical ischemic small-vessel disease with white matter lesions that interrupt subcortical-frontal circuits or connections to distal cortical regions

- Hemorrhage, including intraparenchymal hemorrhage, subarachnoid hemorrhage, and subdural hematoma

- Hypotensive episodes that cause border-zone infarcts

- Cerebral vasculitis

Making the diagnosis of VND can be challenging because of its clinical heterogeneity. Current clinical criteria have not been validated and do not distinguish mixed causes from pure vascular causes. In contrast to the degenerative dementias, a neuropsychological profile specific to VND does not exist, and the cognitive symptoms are highly variable, depending on whether the deficits are due to microvascular or macrovascular disease. The diagnosis is made when neuroimaging or clinical history reveals evidence of a stroke or subclinical cerebrovascular disease that is responsible for impairment of at least one cognitive domain. Onset can be acute or insidious, and progression can be stepwise or gradual. Noncognitive symptoms in patients with VND are common and include focal neurologic findings, depression, pseudobulbar palsy (most commonly associated with multiple bilateral lacunar infarcts), gait abnormalities, and urinary difficulties (with the latter two symptoms explaining this disorder's confusion with NPH). Impairments of attention, executive function, and processing speed are commonly seen on neuropsychological testing, especially in patients with a subcortical vascular syndrome. Memory impairment is typically less prominent.

Treatment is aimed at identifying and treating cerebrovascular risk factors, such as smoking, diabetes mellitus, hyperlipidemia, hypertension, ischemic heart disease, atrial fibrillation, and hypercoagulable states, and at lowering stroke risk with antiplatelet or anticoagulant therapy, if indicated.

KEY POINTS

- The diagnosis of vascular neurocognitive disorder is made when neuroimaging or clinical history reveals evidence of a stroke or subclinical cerebrovascular disease that can be linked to impairment of at least one cognitive domain.

- Treatment of vascular neurocognitive disorder involves identifying and treating cerebrovascular risk factors and lowering stroke risk.

Dementia Associated with Traumatic Brain Injury

Experiencing a head injury in early or mid-life is thought to be associated with an increased risk of dementia in late life, although the association is subject to recall bias. Current evidence suggests that the severity and frequency of head injuries correlate with the risk of dementia and severity of disease.

Chronic traumatic encephalopathy, formerly known as dementia pugilistica, is a distinct progressive neurodegenerative disorder triggered by repetitive mild head injury. This disorder has most often been described in military veterans who have sustained blast or conconcussive injuries and athletes with a history of multiple concussions and subconcussions (such as boxers, football players). Chronic traumatic encephalopathy is pathologically characterized by the presence of tau-positive neurofibrillary tangles with a different distribution than is seen in Alzheimer disease. Pathologic accumulation of amyloid β protein, TDP-43, and α-synuclein protein also has been reported in a subset of patients. Symptoms develop insidiously, typically 8 to 10 years after the repeated head injuries, and are progressive. The cognitive impairment is characterized by impaired concentration, poor short-term memory, executive dysfunction, and poor judgment. Behavioral symptoms include depression, irritability, aggression, violent behaviors, emotional lability, impulsivity, and suicidality. Motor symptoms are common and include parkinsonism, unsteady gait, shuffling gait, slurred speech, and motoneuron disease.

KEY POINT

- Chronic traumatic encephalopathy is a distinct progressive neurodegenerative disorder triggered by repetitive mild head injury that typically presents with cognitive impairment and behavioral and motor symptoms.

Mixed Dementias

The combination of more than one pathology contributing to a dementia syndrome is not uncommon. Because the diagnosis of mixed dementia requires pathologic confirmation, the prevalence of this type of dementia is not entirely known. Mixed dementia is the term classically used to describe coexisting Alzheimer disease and vascular dementia. However, coexisting Alzheimer disease and dementia with Lewy bodies also is seen in 20% of patients with dementia, and Alzheimer disease is sometimes seen in patients with NPH.

Pharmacologic Therapies for Cognitive Symptoms

Although no pharmacologic disease-modifying therapy that reverses or halts neurodegeneration in any neurodegenerative dementia yet exists, two drug classes have been shown to have a positive effect in slowing the symptomatic decline: cholinesterase inhibitors and N-methyl-D-aspartate receptor antagonists. Typical benefits of these drugs in patients with dementia are mild improvements in measured cognition and performance of some activities of daily living. However, their effectiveness in improving clinically significant outcomes, such as the ability to maintain independence and reduce the need for higher levels of care, has not been established. **Table 20** lists the FDA-approved medications for treating dementia. The cholinesterase inhibitors exert their effect by inhibiting the enzymes responsible for breaking down acetylcholine, thereby increasing the levels of acetylcholine in the neuronal synapse. No clinically significant difference in effectiveness has been shown between the cholinesterase inhibitors. Relative contraindications for their use include (but are not limited to) sick sinus syndrome, left bundle branch block, uncontrolled asthma, angle-closure glaucoma, and ulcer disease. Memantine, a second-line therapeutic option, is an N-methyl-D-aspartate receptor antagonist believed to reduce glutamate-mediated neurotoxicity in the central nervous system. Memantine is often used in conjunction with a cholinesterase inhibitor and is FDA approved for moderate to severe Alzheimer disease; however, a recent trial showed that the two medications in combination were not significantly more beneficial than the cholinesterase inhibitor donepezil alone in moderate to severe Alzheimer disease.

Although no cholinesterase inhibitor is FDA approved for treating dementia with Lewy bodies and rivastigmine is the only cholinesterase inhibitor approved for Parkinson disease dementia, recent data have suggested that patients with both types of dementia benefit from treatment with cholinesterase inhibitors in terms of cognition, behaviors, and hallucinations. No drug has been shown to be beneficial for the treatment of FTD. In VND, therapy is directed at identifying and controlling vascular risk factors to minimize progression of cerebrovascular disease; evidence supporting the use of any other medication is currently insufficient. Data are similarly insufficient to support using cholinesterase inhibitors to delay progression from MCI to dementia, so their routine use for this purpose is not recommended.

KEY POINTS

- Cholinesterase inhibitors and N-methyl-D-aspartate receptor antagonists may provide mild improvements in measured cognition and performance of some activities of daily living in patients with dementia but have not demonstrated effectiveness in improving clinically significant outcomes, such as the ability to live independently.
- Cholinesterase inhibitors have not been approved to   **HVC** treat frontotemporal dementia and vascular neurocognitive disorder or to delay progression from mild cognitive impairment to dementia.

Neuropsychiatric Symptoms in Cognitive Impairment
Clinical Characteristics

Changes in behavior and mood are more common in patients with MCI and dementia than in age-matched controls. Depression, anxiety, apathy, irritability, and agitation are the

TABLE 20. FDA-Approved Medications for the Symptomatic Treatment of Dementia

Medication (route)	Mechanism of Action	Available Doses	FDA-Approved Indications		Proven Efficacy	Adverse Effects	Practical Points
			Dementia Severity	Dementia Subtype			
Donepezil (oral)	Acetylcholinesterase inhibitor	5 or 10 mg/d[a]	Mild, moderate, and severe	Alzheimer disease	Cognition, global function, ADLs, behavior	Nausea, vomiting, anorexia, diarrhea, dizziness, sleep disturbances, muscle cramps, symptomatic bradycardia	Dosages of 5 mg and 10 mg available as orally disintegrating tablet; dose in the AM to minimize risk of insomnia and vivid dreams.
Rivastigmine (oral)	Acetylcholinesterase inhibitor, butylcholinesterase inhibitor	1.5 mg, 3.0 mg, 4.5 mg, 6.0 mg BID	Mild, moderate	Alzheimer disease, Parkinson disease	Cognition, global function, ADLs, behavior	Nausea, vomiting, anorexia, diarrhea, headache	Also available in an oral solution 2 mg/mL.
Rivastigmine (transdermal)	Acetylcholinesterase inhibitor, butylcholinesterase inhibitor	4.6 mg/d, 9.6 mg/d, 13.3 mg/d	Mild, moderate	Alzheimer disease, Parkinson disease	Cognition, global function, ADLs, behavior		Typically better tolerated in terms of gastrointestinal side effects.
Galantamine (oral)	Acetylcholinesterase inhibitor, modulates nicotinic acetylcholine receptors to increase acetylcholine	Immediate release: 4 mg, 8 mg, 12 mg BID. Extended release: 8 mg/d, 16 mg/d, 24 mg/d	Mild, moderate	Alzheimer disease	Cognition, global function, behavior	Nausea, vomiting, anorexia, diarrhea, weight loss	Also available in an oral solution 4 mg/mL.
Memantine (oral)	N-methyl-D-aspartate receptor antagonist, dopamine antagonist	Immediate release: 5 mg, 10 mg BID. Extended release: 7 mg/d, 14 mg/d, 21 mg/d, 28 mg/d	Moderate, severe	Alzheimer disease	Cognition, global function, ADLs, behavior	Confusion, drowsiness, dizziness, headache, change in behavior	Also available in an oral solution 10 mg/5 mL. Interactions with trimethoprim may exist; risk of myoclonus and delirium is increased.

ADLs = activities of daily living; BID = twice daily.

[a]Although donepezil, 23 mg/d, is approved for the treatment of moderate to severe Alzheimer disease on the basis of a small improvement in scores on a neuropsychological test, no significant difference in functional outcome was observed when compared with the 10-mg dose. In addition, gastrointestinal side effects were significantly greater and the cost substantially greater. Therefore, this medication is not frequently prescribed.

most common neuropsychiatric symptoms experienced by patients with MCI. With progression of cognitive impairment, the frequency and severity of neuropsychiatric symptoms increase. Behavioral symptoms vary according to the underlying cause but are prevalent in all subtypes of dementia. Depression is common in Alzheimer disease, dementia with Lewy bodies, and vascular dementia. Apathy is most prominent in FTD and PSP but also occurs in the other dementias. A lack of motivation and indifference are often misinterpreted by family members as depression. Irritability, aggressive behaviors, and anxiety are common in Alzheimer disease and vascular dementia, whereas aberrant motor behaviors (pacing, wandering, repetitive movements, excessive fidgeting), disinhibition, and

eating disturbances are more commonly seen in FTD. Delusions are more frequent in Alzheimer disease and dementia with Lewy bodies than in FTD. Hallucinations are most common in dementia with Lewy bodies but can occur in all degenerative dementias.

Treatment of Neuropsychiatric Symptoms

Nonpharmacologic interventions can be very effective in treating the behavioral symptoms experienced by patients with dementia and should be the first-line treatment. Changes to the environment, including new caregivers, should be minimized. Structured activities should be provided and daily routines followed. Orienting tools, such as easily visualized clocks and calendars, should be used. Triggers provoking agitation or frustration should be identified and minimized. Disputing delusions or false beliefs is often ineffective, especially because patients with dementia frequently are unable to reason, rationalize, or understand logic. Therefore, validating the patient's thinking and then distracting and redirecting him or her to something more pleasant usually is more successful in dealing with behavioral problems.

When nonpharmacologic interventions alone are not effective in managing behavioral symptoms sufficiently, pharmacologic therapies may improve them. Atypical antipsychotic agents can be effective in treating agitation, aggression, delusions, and hallucinations. However, these drugs are not FDA approved for this clinical indication and have an associated black box warning due to increased cerebrovascular events and mortality rates in patients with dementia. Nevertheless, behavioral problems can jeopardize the safety of the patient or caregiver and substantially impair quality of life. The benefits versus risks of instituting medication for behaviors must be considered in each patient and discussed with the patient and his or her caregivers; the risk of death is increased by 60% in the first 10 weeks after starting antipsychotic drugs. Antiepileptic drugs, such as valproic acid, also are used off-label for the behavioral symptoms associated with dementia. Antidepressants with the fewest anticholinergic side effects can be used for depression and anxiety. Apathy is notoriously difficult to treat, but off-label medications that sometime improve this symptom include cholinesterase inhibitors and neurostimulants. Benzodiazepines are not recommended for the treatment of behavioral symptoms in patients with dementia. ◧

KEY POINTS

HVC
- Nonpharmacologic interventions are often effective in treating the behavioral symptoms experienced by patients with dementia and should be the first-line treatment.
- Atypical antipsychotic agents are effective in treating agitation, aggression, delusions, and hallucinations but have an associated black box warning due to increased cerebrovascular events and mortality rates in patients with dementia.
- Antidepressants with the fewest anticholinergic side effects can be used for depression and anxiety.

◧ Delirium

Delirium is a potentially preventable syndrome associated with other medical disorders, the adverse effects of medication, or drug withdrawal. This disorder is characterized by an acute change in cognitive functioning occurring over hours to days, with fluctuations during the course of the day. Features of delirium include inattention, disorganized thinking, executive dysfunction, altered level of consciousness (lethargy or hypervigilance), perceptual disturbances (such as hallucinations or delusions), altered psychomotor activity (hyperactivity, hypoactivity, or alternating periods of hyperactivity and hypoactivity), sleep-wake disturbances, and labile mood.

Preexisting cognitive impairment is the major predisposing factor for delirium. Additional risk factors include older age, preexisting neurologic disease (such as Parkinson disease), visual or hearing impairment, immobilization, sleep deprivation, presence of multiple medical comorbidities, alcohol abuse, and terminal illness.

Delirium complicates hospitalization for as many as 30% of patients age 65 years and older, with prevalence significantly increasing (60%-90%) for patients with Alzheimer disease. In critically ill patients, delirium is seen in as many as 80% of patients receiving mechanical ventilation. In the year following a hospitalization complicated by delirium, patients with baseline dementia experience cognitive decline at twice the rate of those without a history of delirium. The rate of incident dementia after an episode of delirium in older patients without preexisting cognitive impairment is 1.4 to 2 times that of those without a history of delirium. In addition, delirium is associated with increased length of hospital stay, increased institutionalization, and increased mortality rates both at discharge and at 1 year. The 1-year mortality rate after an episode of delirium in older patients is approximately 35%.

Delirium is underdiagnosed. Administering a delirium screening test can enhance detection of the disorder. Although many screening tools have been developed, the best validated and most reliable clinical instrument for making the diagnosis of delirium is the Confusion Assessment Method (**Table 21**) and for assessing its severity is the Delirium Rating Scale. Serial measurements can be used to monitor improvement in symptoms.

The cause of delirium in an individual patient may be one or multiple coexisting conditions (**Table 22**). Two or more underlying causes are present in as many as 50% of older patients, so a complete medical evaluation is necessary. The quest for the cause of delirium begins with a thorough medication review, a history of any illicit drug use, and testing for concurrent medical illnesses.

Treatment involves identification and correction of the underlying cause, maintaining adequate nutrition and hydration, and preventing complications. With treatment, delirium typically resolves within days; in some patients, however, more subtle cognitive dysfunction can persist for weeks to months. Environmental interventions include orienting strategies (reliance on calendars, clocks, and familiar objects in the room), promoting a normal sleep-wake cycle (having no or limited interruptions during nocturnal sleeping hours, minimizing light and noise at night, and opening curtains and encouraging activity during the daytime), identifying and correcting sensory impairments (use of dentures, glasses, and hearing aids), avoiding physical restraints, and early discontinuation of catheters and intravenous lines. No medications

TABLE 21. The Confusion Assessment Method Diagnostic Instrument[a]

Feature 1.	**Acute Onset and Fluctuating Course**
	This feature is usually obtained from a family member or nurse and is shown by a positive response to the following questions: Is there evidence of an acute change in mental status from the patient's baseline? Did the (abnormal) behavior fluctuate during the day, that is, tend to come and go, or increase and decrease in severity?
Feature 2.	**Inattention**
	This feature is shown by a positive response to the following question: Did the patient have difficulty focusing attention, for example, being easily distractible, or having difficulty keeping track of what was being said?
Feature 3.	**Disorganized Thinking**
	This feature is shown by a positive response to the following question: Was the patient's thinking disorganized or incoherent, such as rambling or irrelevant conversation, unclear or illogical flow of ideas, or unpredictable switching from subject to subject?
Feature 4.	**Altered Level of Consciousness**
	This feature is shown by any answer other than "alert" to the following question: Overall, how would you rate this patient's level of consciousness? (alert [normal], vigilant [hyperalert], lethargic [drowsy, easily aroused], stupor [difficult to arouse], or comatose [unarousable])

[a]The diagnosis of delirium by the Confusion Assessment Method requires the presence of features 1 and 2 and either 3 or 4.

Adapted with permission from Inouye SK, van Dyck CH, Alessi CA, Balkin S, Siegal AP, Horwitiz RI. Clarifying confusion: the confusion assessment method. A new method for detection of delirium. Ann Intern Med. 1990;113(12):947. [PMID: 2240918]

TABLE 22. Causes of Delirium

Drugs

  Prescription medications (such as psychotropic medications, opioids, sedative hypnotics, anticonvulsants, antiparkinsonian agents, glucocorticoids, immunosuppressants, anti-arrhythmics, antihypertensive agents, skeletal muscle relaxants, antibiotics)

  Nonprescription medications (such as NSAIDs, antihistamines)

  General anesthesia

  Alcohol or drug withdrawal

Central Nervous System Diseases

  Seizure, including nonconvulsive status epilepticus

  Acute ischemic infarction

  Intracranial hemorrhage (such as intraparenchymal hemorrhage, subdural hematoma, epidural hematoma, subarachnoid hemorrhage)

  Head injury

Metabolic Disorders

  Electrolyte disturbance

  Hyperglycemia or hypoglycemia

  Hypoxemia

  Hypercarbia

  Organ failure (such as cardiac failure, kidney impairment, liver failure)

  Endocrine (such as hypothyroidism, hyperthyroidism, hyperparathyroidism, Cushing syndrome, adrenal insufficiency)

  Nutritional (such as malnourishment, vitamin B_{12} deficiency, thiamine deficiency, niacin deficiency)

Cardiovascular Disease

  Myocardial infarction

  Hypertensive emergency

  Dysrhythmias

Infections[a]

Surgery

Trauma

Environment

  Post-acute care setting

  ICU

Other

  Acute blood loss

  Uncontrolled pain

  Fecal impaction

  Urinary retention

[a]Such as urinary tract infections, respiratory infections, cellulitis, meningitis or encephalitis, and sepsis.

CONT.

are FDA approved for the treatment of delirium. Although atypical and typical antipsychotic agents are commonly used to treat the behavioral symptoms associated with hyperactive delirium when the patient's safety is at risk, evidence of their effectiveness in this setting is limited, and these drugs have black box safety warnings when used in patients with underlying dementia. Additionally, data are insufficient to support the prophylactic use of pharmacologic agents in the prevention of delirium. Benzodiazepines can worsen delirium and are not recommended, except in the management of alcohol withdrawal.

KEY POINTS

- Treatment of delirium involves identification and correction of the underlying cause, maintaining adequate nutrition and hydration, and preventing complications.

HVC

- No pharmacologic therapy is currently FDA approved for the prevention or treatment of delirium.

Movement Disorders

Overview of Movement Disorders

Movement disorders are characterized by abnormal patterns of motor output and are broadly classified into conditions characterized by paucity and slowness of movements (hypokinetic disorders) and those marked by excessive involuntary movements (hyperkinetic disorders). Hypokinetic disorders include Parkinson disease and related disorders. Hyperkinetic movement disorders are classified according to their characteristic abnormal movements, such as tremor, tic, chorea, dystonia, and myoclonus.

Neurologic examination, particularly assessments of motor function and gait, helps distinguish the various movement disorders. Spontaneous and voluntary movements should be assessed, with attention paid to speed, amplitude consistency, and fatigability. Muscle tone should be evaluated by determining the resistance of extremities to passive movements, with special attention paid to effects of velocity and direction of movements. Hypokinetic movement disorders commonly display consistently increased tone (lead-pipe rigidity) throughout the movement of the joint, in contrast to the "give-way" hypertonia (clasp-knife phenomenon) seen with upper motoneuron lesions in which a cogwheeling component may also be present. The phenomenology of abnormal movements—especially their rhythmicity, suppressibility, randomness, directionality, and speed—can help in their classification (**Table 23**).

An examination of gait should consider the base of standing, pace of ambulation, stride length, foot clearance off the ground, postural stability, and arm swings. In Parkinson disease and other hypokinetic disorders, gait is slow, narrow based, shuffling, and associated with shortened stride length, reduced arm swings, and stooped posture. Turns may take several steps and appear stiff and unsteady. Ataxic gait is characterized by a wide base, frequent truncal swaying and veering, and impaired tandem walking on a straight line. This gait also can be accompanied by additional signs of cerebellar dysfunction, such as nystagmus, scanning and dysrhythmic speech, truncal titubation (to and fro movement), and dysmetria on finger-nose or heel-knee-shin tests.

Postural stability can best be checked by the pull test, in which the examiner throws the patient off base by pulling backward on the shoulders after a warning and the instruction to maintain balance. A positive test, characterized by toppling into examiner's arms or taking more than one corrective step, is the most reliable predictor of a risk of backward falls.

KEY POINT

HVC

- Neurologic examination, particularly assessments of motor function and gait, helps distinguish the various movement disorders.

Hypokinetic Movement Disorders

Parkinson disease is the most common type of hypokinetic movement disorder. Parkinson-plus conditions combine parkinsonism with other clinical features, such as early falling, prominent dysautonomia, or early cognitive deficits. Vascular parkinsonism results from large or small vessel ischemic or hemorrhagic lesions and is characterized by a predominant abnormality of gait disproportionate to upper extremity involvement, a history of sudden or stepwise deterioration, and absence of typical neurodegenerative progression. Medication-induced parkinsonism should be considered in patients with a history of exposure to predisposing medications, such as neuroleptic agents.

Parkinson Disease

Parkinson disease is a slowly progressive neurodegenerative disorder associated with gradual loss of dopamine-producing neurons in the substantia nigra. The pathophysiologic process in Parkinson disease involves aggregation of α-synuclein protein and formation of Lewy body inclusions in the substantia nigra and other brain regions. Several genes, including the autosomal dominant gene *LRRK2* and the autosomal recessive gene *PARK2*, have been associated with Parkinson disease in a minority of patients. In addition, exposure to certain environmental factors, including pesticides (rotenone), herbicides, well water, and excessive manganese, can increase the risk for Parkinson disease. The prevalence of this condition increases with age and is expected to significantly increase as the U.S. population ages.

Clinical Features of Parkinson Disease

The four cardinal signs of Parkinson disease are resting tremor, bradykinesia, cogwheel rigidity, and gait/postural impairment. Resting tremor is characteristically unilateral at onset and remains asymmetric. This type of tremor emerges after a few seconds of outstretched posturing of the arms and during ambulation. Bradykinesia, the core feature in Parkinson disease, consists of slowness and gradual decreasing of the amplitude of repetitive movements. A relative paucity of movement on the more affected side may be noted, including reduced facial expression, reduction in arm swing, and small handwriting (micrographia). Patients may report difficulty with both fine and gross movements. Rigidity is associated with a cogwheeling quality in the presence of tremor. In early Parkinson disease, gait and postural impairment are mild and limited to shuffling, dragging of one leg, and mild disturbance of postural reflexes at turns. A prominent impairment of gait and balance may develop at later stages, with hesitation at onset of gait and turns, freezing of gait, and severe loss of postural reflexes. Early prominent postural instability with frequent falls should raise concern for a Parkinson-plus condition. Although the initial presentation of Parkinson disease is commonly tremor predominant, a minority of affected patients may first experience an akinetic rigidity without tremor.

TABLE 23. Classification of Movement Disorders

Movement Type	Clinical Features	Causes
Hypokinetic		
Parkinsonism	Cardinal features: bradykinesia/akinesia, rigidity, resting tremor, postural instability Additional features: freezing gait, stooped posture, masked face, hypophonia	Parkinson disease, Parkinson-plus syndromes, Lewy body dementia, vascular, hydrocephalus, medications, Wilson disease, juvenile Huntington disease
Hyperkinetic		
Tremor	Rhythmic oscillations of a body part, can occur at rest or with action (postural or kinetic), intention tremor amplitude increased near target	At rest: parkinsonism (see above) Postural and kinetic: enhanced physiologic tremor, essential tremor Intention tremor: cerebellar For more information, see Table 29

Dystonia	Sustained, stereotyped, and directional twisting and posturing movements of various body parts; can be focal, segmental, or generalized; transient improvement possible with a sensory trick ("geste antagoniste")	Idiopathic or primary dystonia
		
		  Generalized: positive for *DYT1*
		
		  Segmental: Meige syndrome (facial and oromandibular dystonia)
		
		  Focal: torticollis, blepharospasm, writer's cramp
		
		Dopa-responsive
		
		  Damage to the basal ganglia: anoxic injury, postencephalitic, dystonic cerebral palsy
		
		Medication-induced
		
		  Acute dystonic reaction, tardive dystonia

Chorea	Random, nonrepetitive, quick, unsustained, purposeless movements with a flowing dance-like pattern	Huntington disease, postinfectious (Sydenham chorea), chorea gravidarum, autoimmune (systemic lupus erythematosus, antiphospholipid syndrome), hyperglycemia, vascular, drug-induced, neuroacanthocytosis
Hemiballismus	Unilateral high-amplitude proximal flailing, choreiform movements of limbs	Lesions of contralateral subthalamic or other parts of basal ganglia (usually stroke)
Athetosis	Slow convoluted writhing movements of fingers and toes Pseudoathetosis similar but elicited by eye closure	Early life damage to basal ganglia (hypoxic, kernicterus, vascular) Pseudoathetosis caused by proprioceptive pathway lesions
Tic	Stereotyped, brief, purposeless, rapid movements that break the flow of normal movements; common premonitory urges; can be simple or complex, motor or vocal	Tourette syndrome, autism, developmental delay syndromes, Huntington disease
Myoclonus	Rapid, shock-like, jerky movements of isolated body parts	Metabolic (uremia, hepatic failure, electrolyte imbalance), serotonin syndrome, postanoxic, Creutzfeldt-Jakob disease, corticobasal degeneration Sleep-related (hypnic jerks, nocturnal myoclonus), myoclonic epilepsies
Akathisia	Inner restlessness associated with repetitive movements	Drug-induced, restless legs syndrome
Psychogenic	Highly variable, inconsistent, distractible, acute onset, episodic, tremor frequency suggestive of different frequencies, most fixed dystonias	Conversion disorder, malingering, factitious illness, somatoform disorder

In addition to symptoms affecting motor systems, Parkinson disease also is associated with a wide variety of nonmotor symptoms, ranging from autonomic dysfunction to problems with sleep, mood, and cognition (**Table 24**). Some nonmotor symptoms, including hyposmia (diminished sense of smell), constipation, and rapid eye movement (REM) sleep behavior disorder (acting out of dreams secondary to loss of normal muscle paralysis during the dream phase of sleep), may precede onset of motor symptoms by years.

TABLE 24. Nonmotor Symptoms of Parkinson Disease

Type of Complication	Symptoms
Cognitive	Bradyphrenia (slow processing), mild subcortical cognitive impairment, and dementia possible at advanced stages
Affective and behavioral	Depression, anxiety, apathy, psychosis, drug-related impulse control disorder, dopamine dysregulation syndrome (craving for dopaminergic medications)
Sleep related	Sleep fragmentation, rapid eye movement sleep behavior disorder, restless legs syndrome, excessive daytime sleepiness, sleep-wake reversal, drug-related sleep attacks
Autonomic	Constipation, postural hypotension, bladder and sexual dysfunction, sialorrhea, seborrhea, excessive sweating, hyposmia
Musculoskeletal	Truncal and cervical flexion posturing, camptocormia (truncal flexion during standing and walking), frozen shoulder, striatal hand deformities (dystonic joint deformities, including flexion of metacarpophalangeal joints and extension of proximal interphalangeal joints), fall-related injuries
Pain related	Painful dystonia, painful rigidity, mechanical pain, central and visceral pain

Cognitive impairments in Parkinson disease are subcortical, which implies that they primarily involve slow processing speed, impaired short-term memory, and attention deficits with relative sparing of cortical functions, such as language and declarative memory. These impairments are typically mild in the early stages of the disease but can progress to dementia in the later stages. Early dementia within the first year of the appearance of motor parkinsonism is a hallmark of dementia with Lewy bodies (see Lewy Body Disease in Cognitive Impairment).

Diagnosis of Parkinson Disease

The diagnosis of Parkinson disease is made on the basis of history and clinical examination. Diagnostic criteria require the presence of bradykinesia with at least one other cardinal feature (resting tremor, rigidity, or postural instability) and the absence of red flags for atypical forms of parkinsonism (**Table 25**). An MRI of the brain is recommended to rule out vascular lesions and hydrocephalus. Single photon emission CT (SPECT) of the brain using ioflupane-123, a ligand for a dopamine transporter, may reveal reduced ligand uptake in the basal ganglia as a result of degeneration of dopamine terminals. However, the sensitivity of this test is not superior to that of an expert clinical assessment, and it should be reserved only for patients in whom the differentiation between Parkinson disease and essential tremor or drug-induced parkinsonism is not feasible on clinical grounds. The test cannot distinguish between Parkinson disease and Parkinson-plus conditions.

TABLE 25. Red Flags for Atypical Forms of Parkinsonism

Red Flags	Features
Dysautonomia	Prominent orthostatic hypotension, urinary incontinence, impotence, sweating dysfunction (mild autonomic deficits potentially seen in early Parkinson disease)
Abnormal eye movements	Supranuclear vertical gaze palsy (which can be overcome by the oculocephalic maneuver), slowness of vertical saccades
Prominent early cognitive impairment	Dementia within first year of onset (mild cognitive impairment common in Parkinson disease and dementia, may develop in a notable subgroup of patients in advanced stages)
Visual hallucinations	Early and not provoked by medications (levodopa-induced hallucinations seen in Parkinson disease, especially in later stages)
Early prominent postural instability and falls	Within first year of onset
Prominent gait ataxia	With or without additional cerebellar deficits (dysmetria, nystagmus)
Symmetric or markedly asymmetric involvement	Parkinson disease characteristically asymmetric at onset and throughout its course
	Lack of asymmetry indicative of atypical parkinsonism
	Very severe asymmetric involvement; possibly suggestive of corticobasal degeneration and usually associated with severe fixed dystonic posturing, myoclonus, apraxia, and sensory cortical deficits
Rapid onset and stepwise deterioration	More suggestive of vascular parkinsonism (Parkinson disease associated with slow onset and gradual course)
Lack of response to levodopa[a]	Most important red flag of atypical parkinsonism

[a]Must not be secondary to adverse effects or insufficient dosing of medication.

Treatment of Parkinson Disease

Currently, no medication with proven efficacy is available to slow the progression of Parkinson disease. Recent studies have shown the beneficial role of rigorous daily exercise in improving motor fitness and gait, and thus physical activity or physical therapy should be encouraged in all patients with the disease. Research is under way to determine whether specific exercise regimens, such as resistance or aerobic exercises, provide a neuroprotective effect.

Pharmacologic therapy should be tailored to optimize each patient's motor, social, and intellectual functioning and to minimize any adverse effects (**Table 26**). Early symptoms may not need treatment, but a bothersome tremor, decreased dexterity, increased rigidity, and slowness are reasons to consider treatment. In patients with mild symptoms, monotherapy with monoamine oxidase type B inhibitors can be considered as

TABLE 26. Medications for Parkinson Disease	
Medication Class	**Clinical Indication**
Dopamine substrate (levodopa)	Most effective treatment for motor deficits
	Initial therapy in older patients (>70 years) and in those with severe motor symptoms, gait freezing, or falls
	Second-line treatment in younger patients who have not benefitted from dopamine agonists

Decarboxylase inhibitors
  Carbidopa
  Benserazide[a]
	Suppression of peripheral adverse effects of levodopa

Dopamine agonists
  Pramipexole
  Ropinirole
  Rotigotine (patch)
  Bromocriptine
  Pergolide
  Apomorphine (injection)
  Cabergoline[a]
  Lisuride[a]
  Piribedil[a]
	First-line treatment in younger patients; adjuvant therapy to limit total dose of levodopa

Catechol-*o*-methyltransferase inhibitors
  Entacapone
  Tolcapone
	Counteracting of wearing-off phenomenon, prolongation of levodopa effect

Monoamine oxidase type B inhibitors
  Selegiline
  Rasagiline
	Initial therapy in mild cases, potentiation of levodopa effect, tremor

Glutamate antagonist Amantadine	Dyskinesia, tremor, fatigue

Anticholinergic agents
  Trihexyphenidyl
  Benztropine
  Biperiden
	Tremor, mild benefit against parkinsonism but avoid use in old age and dementia

[a]Available in Europe.

initial therapy, but the benefit of these agents is usually modest. Dopaminergic medications, including levodopa (the precursor molecule converted to dopamine) and dopamine agonists (agents that activate dopamine D_2 receptors in the absence of dopamine), are the most effective drugs to control the key motor deficits in Parkinson disease. Levodopa generally is used in combination with the decarboxylase inhibitor carbidopa to block levodopa's peripheral adverse effects outside the central nervous system. Eventually, all patients with Parkinson disease will require the benefit of levodopa. The initial use of dopamine agonists instead of levodopa in younger patients (age <65-70 years) is encouraged by many experts in an effort to delay levodopa-related complications, such as motor fluctuations (caused by the wearing off of the beneficial effects of the medication before the next dose is administered) and medication-induced dyskinesia (involuntary choreic movements). These complications emerge in as many as 50% of patients treated for more than 5 years with levodopa and may reflect disease progression rather than duration of exposure to levodopa.

Dopamine agonists are associated with higher risk of specific adverse effects, including impulse control disorder, punding, sleep attacks, ankle edema, hallucinations, and confusion, that may limit their use, especially in older patients. Impulse control disorder is the increased tendency for compulsive behaviors, such as excessive gambling, shopping, or hypersexuality, and all patients taking dopamine agonists should be monitored for this complication. Punding is a complex prolonged, purposeless, and stereotyped behavior (such as collecting, sorting, cataloguing, or assembling and disassembling common objects) that can become disruptive. Sleep attacks involve falling asleep without warning and can cause motor vehicle collisions. Dopamine agonists all have similar efficacy and can be used interchangeably, but no rationale supports their use in combination.

Levodopa should be started as initial therapy in older patients and as replacement or additional therapy in younger patients who did not benefit or had adverse effects from dopamine agonists. Also, gait impairment and freezing that can increase the risk of falls mandate initiation of levodopa therapy. The immediate-release formulations of levodopa provide a higher peak dose effect than similar doses of sustained-release formulations. Therefore, immediate-release formulations commonly are used during the wake cycle and sustained-release formulations, if needed, at nighttime. However, sustained-release levodopa or dopamine agonists can be added to immediate-release levodopa to provide more sustained levels of dopamine receptor activation, thereby delaying the development of levodopa-related motor complications. A typical initial dose of levodopa is 300 mg/d divided into three doses, with most patients benefitting from a slow titration to minimize adverse effects; further dose adjustment should be made on an individual basis.

As Parkinson disease progresses, the medication regimen should be adjusted to address progressive motor deficits and minimize evolving medication-related complications. For patients in whom the motor benefits of medication wear off quickly, strategies include either using a greater frequency of immediate-release levodopa dosing or using sustained-release levodopa. Other options include adding a dopamine agonist, a catechol-O-methyltransferase inhibitor, or a monoamine oxidase type B inhibitor. In patients with dyskinesia, adding amantadine may help a subset of patients. In patients with prominent tremor, anticholinergic medications may provide some additional benefit, but their high adverse effect profiles limit their use, especially in patients with cognitive impairment and in older patients.

Medication-induced psychosis, especially visual hallucinations, is another adverse effect of dopaminergic medications. Treatment strategies include monitoring for infection and metabolic derangement and discontinuing anticholinergic drugs, amantadine, or dopamine agonists. Discontinuing catechol-*O*-methyltransferase and monoamine oxidase type B inhibitors also can be considered but may worsen the wearing-off phenomenon. A reduction in levodopa dosing may be required. When necessary, the preferred antipsychotic agents are clozapine and quetiapine.

Deep brain stimulation (DBS) surgery is a treatment based on the delivery of electrical stimulation to targeted brain regions. The stimulation delivered can modulate abnormal activity within target regions. For example, subthalamic nucleus DBS can disrupt abnormal rhythmic activity within that region and should be considered in patients with Parkinson disease who have sustained motor benefit from levodopa but are limited by disabling medication-related adverse effects that are refractory to medical management. In this select group, DBS can be highly effective in reducing motor complications, such as wearing off and dyskinesia, while providing motor benefits comparable to those of levodopa. Patients with atypical parkinsonism, major cognitive deficits, and unstable mood disorder should not receive DBS. Patients who meet the criteria for DBS should be referred to a movement disorder neurologist for an "on/off" medication evaluation (**Figure 17**). Also, patients

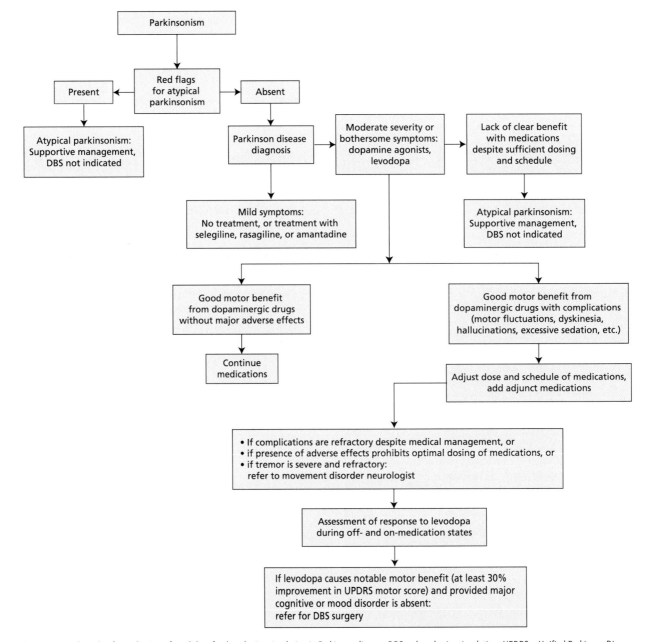

FIGURE 17. Algorithm for evaluation of candidacy for deep brain stimulation in Parkinson disease. DBS = deep brain stimulation; UPDRS = Unified Parkinson Disease Rating Scale.

should be advised that levodopa-refractory symptoms, including speech deficits and postural instability, typically do not improve with DBS, with the potential exception of a refractory tremor. DBS targets in Parkinson disease include the subthalamic nucleus and globus pallidus interna, with the former being more amendable to a reduction in medication dose.

KEY POINTS

- Parkinson disease, the most common type of hypokinetic movement disorder, is characterized by four cardinal signs: resting tremor, bradykinesia, cogwheel rigidity, and gait or postural impairment.

HVC
- The diagnosis of Parkinson disease is made on the basis of history and clinical examination and requires the presence of bradykinesia with at least one other cardinal feature (resting tremor, rigidity, or postural instability) and the absence of red flags.

HVC
- Single photon emission CT of the brain should be reserved for differentiating Parkinson disease from drug-induced parkinsonism in patients with an atypical clinical picture.

HVC
- Recent studies have shown the beneficial role of rigorous daily exercise in improving motor fitness and gait in patients with Parkinson disease, and thus physical activity or physical therapy should be encouraged in all patients with the disease.

- Dopaminergic medications, including levodopa and dopamine agonists, are the most effective drugs to control the key motor deficits in Parkinson disease.

- Deep brain stimulation surgery is highly effective for patients who have had a sustained motor benefit from levodopa but are limited by adverse effects of the medication.

Parkinson-Plus Syndromes

Parkinson-plus syndromes account for nearly 10% of patients with clinical parkinsonism. The diagnosis usually is suggested by the presence of defining features, a faster progression, and the absence of levodopa responsiveness. The primary syndromes involved are progressive supranuclear palsy (PSP), multiple system atrophy (MSA), and corticobasal degeneration (CBD). PSP is defined by parkinsonism with oculomotor abnormalities, including impairment of vertical saccades and supranuclear vertical gaze palsy, the latter of which can be overcome by passive head movements (such as the oculocephalic maneuver). Patients with PSP also exhibit facial dystonia (with a characteristic surprised appearance), axial rigidity, and prominent postural instability with early falls. MSA comprises three subtypes that are characterized by a combination of parkinsonism and prominent dysautonomia (Shy-Drager syndrome), cerebellar ataxia (MSA-C), or dystonia (MSA with predominant parkinsonism [formerly known as striatonigral degeneration], or MSA-P). CBD may present with markedly asymmetric parkinsonism and often is associated with dystonia,

myoclonus, cortical sensory deficits, and cognitive deficits, including impairment in motor planning (apraxia), calculation, and left-right distinction. A brain MRI in a patient with CBD may reveal asymmetric cortical, particularly parietal, atrophy, although this finding may be absent at earlier stages.

KEY POINT

- Parkinson-plus syndromes include progressive supranuclear palsy, multiple system atrophy, and corticobasal degeneration.

Drug-Induced Parkinsonism

A number of drugs, especially dopamine receptor-blocking antipsychotic agents, can cause parkinsonism (**Table 27**). This complication is usually reversible but may not resolve for as long as 6 months after drug cessation. Drug-induced parkinsonism may be distinguishable from idiopathic Parkinson disease on the basis of the symmetry of symptoms and the absence of typical nonmotor features. For drug-induced extrapyramidal complications of dopamine blockers (**Table 28**), see later discussion of Other Drug-Induced Movement Disorders in Hyperkinetic Movement Disorders.

KEY POINT

- Drug-induced parkinsonism may be distinguished from idiopathic Parkinson disease on the basis of the symmetry of symptoms and the absence of typical nonmotor features.

Hyperkinetic Movement Disorders

Major hyperkinetic movement disorders are discussed in the following paragraphs. For additional hyperkinetic disorders, see Table 23.

Essential Tremor

Tremor is characterized by rhythmic and oscillatory movement and classified on the basis of its association with rest or

TABLE 27. Medications Causing Drug-Induced Parkinsonism	
Medication Class	**Examples**
Common	
Antipsychotic agents	Typical: haloperidol, chlorpromazine
	Atypical: risperidone, olanzapine, ziprasidone, aripiprazole
Antiemetic agents	Metoclopramide, prochlorperazine
Dopamine depleters	Tetrabenazine, reserpine
Uncommon	
Mood stabilizers, antiepileptic drugs	Lithium, valproic acid
Other	Amiodarone, flunarazine, SSRIs including fluoxetine
SSRIs = selective serotonin reuptake inhibitors.	

TABLE 28. Extrapyramidal Complications of Dopamine D$_2$ Receptor Blockers

Type of Movement Disorder	Symptoms
Acute Reactions (Reversible)	
Acute dystonia	Immediate dystonic spasms; often involves the neck, face, larynx, and eyes (oculogyric crisis); rapid reversal with intravenous diphenhydramine
Acute akathisia	Immediate sensation of restlessness with urge to constantly move and pace
Subacute or Chronic Syndrome (Reversible)	
Parkinsonism	Similar to Parkinson disease, dose dependent, resolves within months after removal of the causative agent, symmetry and absence of nonmotor features, which favors a drug-induced over idiopathic cause
Tardive Syndromes (Late Onset, May Be Irreversible)	
Tardive dyskinesia	Repetitive stereotyped choreiform movements, oral-facial-lingual predominance, also can affect the extremities and trunk
Tardive dystonia	Sustained dystonic posturing commonly affecting the face, neck, trunk, and arms; extensor axial dystonia common
Tardive akathisia	Chronic sensation of restlessness with urge to constantly move and pace
Other Disorders	
Withdrawal emergent syndrome (reversible)	Dyskinesia starting after withdrawal from neuroleptic agents, stops within a few months, differential diagnosis of tardive dyskinesia masked by antipsychotic agents and only appearing after their removal (dyskinesia may become persistent)
Neuroleptic malignant syndrome (treatable emergency)	Idiosyncratic, rapid onset and progression, rigidity, dystonia, hyperthermia, rhabdomyolysis, and altered mental status

action (**Table 29**). Essential tremor is a common movement disorder that typically presents with a bilateral upper extremity postural and action tremor. Common features include a reduction of tremor amplitude with alcohol, an age of onset in late adolescence or middle age, a slow progression, and the possible development of neck and vocal tremors. Family history is positive for tremor in 50% of affected patients. Although the tremor remains stable or exhibits minor progression over time in most affected patients, a subset may experience progressive worsening of the tremor that can markedly disrupt feeding, handwriting, and fine manual tasks. A fraction (4%) of patients with a long-standing history of essential tremor may develop parkinsonism over time; some, but not all, of these patients may have Lewy body

pathology on autopsy (which also is characteristic of patients with Parkinson disease).

Essential (or action) tremor should be distinguished from enhanced physiologic tremor (see Table 29). This latter type of tremor is present but unnoticeable in most persons; when enhanced by triggers, such as medications, caffeine, toxins, thyroid disease, exertion, or anxiety, it can appear similar to essential tremor. Evaluation of patients with action tremor should include identification and removal of any potential causative medications (**Table 30**) and assessment of thyroid function. Patients younger than 40 years should undergo testing for Wilson disease with serum ceruloplasmin and 24-hour urine copper measurements and with slit lamp examination for Kayser-Fleischer rings (**Figure 18**). Atypical causes of action tremor include dystonic tremor, rubral tremor, and fragile X tremor ataxia syndrome (see Table 29).

The treatment of essential tremor is symptomatic. Mild low-amplitude tremor may not require treatment unless it causes unacceptable social embarrassment. For more disabling tremors, the two most effective medications are propranolol and primidone. If these first-line therapies are not effective, adding other agents, including clonazepam, topiramate, gabapentin, and nimodipine, may provide additional tremor control in some patients. Injection with botulinum toxin can benefit some patients with refractory tremor, especially those with prominent neck or voice tremor. Use of this drug for limb tremor is limited by its adverse effect of weakness. DBS of the thalamus (specifically, the ventral intermediate nucleus) should be considered in patients with refractory disease and can provide significant benefit.

KEY POINTS

- Essential tremor is common and presents with bilateral upper extremity action tremor in late adolescence or middle age, progresses slowly, and typically has reduced amplitude with alcohol ingestion.

- Mild essential tremors may not need treatment; more disabling tremors may be treated symptomatically with propranolol and primidone.

Dystonia

Dystonia involves sustained, stereotyped, and directional twisting and posturing movements of various body parts. Generalized dystonias involve multiple body parts, including the lower extremities, whereas focal and segmental dystonias have a restricted distribution and usually spare the lower extremities. The onset of generalized dystonias commonly occurs at a young age (<25 years) and may have various causes, including metabolic and genetic disorders and ischemic and infectious damage to the basal ganglia. All patients with primary generalized dystonia should be challenged by a short trial with low-dose levodopa to screen for dopa-responsive dystonia, a rare but treatable cause of generalized dystonia. Young adults with progressive dystonia should be screened for Wilson disease, especially in the presence of

TABLE 29. Classification of Tremors

Tremor Type	Disease Association	Features
Resting Tremor[a]		
Parkinsonian resting tremor	Parkinson disease	Re-emergence of tremor after a short delay with outstretched posturing and during ambulation, associated with other parkinsonian signs (rigidity, bradykinesia, gait impairment)
	Atypical, drug-induced, and vascular parkinsonism	Similar to Parkinson disease; tremor sometimes symmetric; red flags for atypical parkinsonism sometimes present
Dystonic tremor	Dystonia	Associated with dystonic posturing; seen both at rest and with action; position dependent with a null point at which tremor stops
Action Tremor		
Postural and kinetic tremors[b]	Essential tremor	Present in the outstretched arm position and with various actions; commonly (but not universally) associated with a positive family history and an improvement in symptoms with alcohol
	Enhanced physiologic tremor	Normal low-amplitude, high-frequency tremor seen in association with triggers, such as stress, drugs, and thyroid disease; similar to essential tremor but resolves with resolution of underlying physiologic stressor
Intention tremor[c]	Cerebellar disease	Tremor during movements that increases in amplitude as hand approaches target (also known as terminal tremor); possible association with other cerebellar symptoms, including dysmetria
	Severe essential tremor	
	Fragile X tremor ataxia syndrome	Neurodegenerative disease seen in older men with a family history of mental retardation in young males and premature ovarian failure in females; symptoms of (intention) tremor, ataxia, parkinsonism, neuropathy, and dementia
Rubral tremor	Cerebellar outflow disorders (multiple sclerosis, stroke, traumatic brain injury)	Coarse proximal tremor present at rest, worse with posturing (especially large-amplitude and proximal tremors in the "wing-beating" position with elbows flexed), and most severe during movements.
Task-specific tremor	Primary writing tremor	Only present with specific task
Orthostatic tremor	Orthostatic tremor	High-frequency tremor emerging in the legs only during standing (orthostatic position); resolving with sitting or action

[a]Tremor present with the affected extremity resting unsupported.

[b]Postural tremor is present with the arm in an outstretched position, and kinetic tremor is present during reaching, writing, and other movements.

[c]Intention tremor is a specific subtype of kinetic tremor that becomes very prominent near target, exhibiting a crescendo of increased severity at the terminal section of the movement path.

TABLE 30. Medications Causing Drug-Induced Action Tremor

Medication Class	Examples
β-Adrenergic agonists	Albuterol, terbutaline, theophylline
Stimulants	Amphetamines, methylphenidate, nicotine, caffeine
Mood stabilizers/ antiepileptic drugs	Lithium, valproic acid, carbamazepine
Neuroleptic agents	Haloperidol, olanzapine (postural and at rest)
Tricyclic antidepressants	Amitriptyline
Selective serotonin reuptake inhibitors	Fluoxetine
Immunosuppressant agents	Cyclosporine, tacrolimus
Other agents	Amiodarone, procainamide, mexiletine, levothyroxine, verapamil, atorvastatin, glucocorticoids

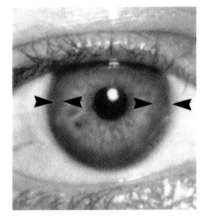

FIGURE 18. Kayser-Fleischer ring (bracketed by arrowheads) in the cornea of a patient with Wilson disease indicating copper deposition in the Descemet membrane of the iris.

other associated findings, such as tremor, parkinsonism, and elevated levels of liver enzymes. The most common type of generalized dystonia is associated with mutation in the dystonia 1 gene (*DYT1*).

The most common focal dystonias include cervical dystonia (spasmodic torticollis), eyelid dystonia (blepharospasm), vocal cord spasmodic dysphonia, and task-specific hand dystonia (writer's cramp and musician's dystonia). Transient improvement of dystonic movement by a sensory trick ("geste antagoniste"), such as specific sensory stimuli (gently touching the involved area with the hand), provides further diagnostic clues.

Medications used for treatment of dystonia include anticholinergic agents, benzodiazepines, and baclofen. The benefit of pharmacotherapy in dystonia, however, is limited. In focal dystonias, including torticollis, injection with botulinum toxin is an effective treatment and is potentially superior to other medications. In primary generalized dystonia, DBS of the globus pallidus interna can markedly improve dystonia. Among patients with generalized dystonias, those with a positive *DYT1* mutation show the best response to DBS.

KEY POINTS

- Dystonia involves sustained, stereotyped, and directional twisting and posturing movements of various body parts.

- In focal dystonias, including torticollis, injection with botulinum toxin is an effective treatment and is potentially superior to use of other medications.

Choreiform Disorders and Huntington Disease

Chorea consists of random, nonrepetitive, flowing dance-like movements and can be caused by medications (such as antipsychotic agents and estrogen-containing drugs), endocrine derangement (as in thyrotoxicosis and acute hyperglycemia), pregnancy (chorea gravidarum), streptococcal infection (Sydenham chorea), autoimmune disease (systemic lupus erythematosus and antiphospholipid syndrome), and neurodegenerative disorders involving the basal ganglia. Huntington disease is the most common neurodegenerative cause of generalized chorea and is associated with progressive parkinsonism, gait impairment, impulsiveness, psychiatric disorders, and dementia. This condition, which is confirmed by genetic testing, is transmitted in an autosomal dominant manner, and its expression derives from the length of a repeat section (trinucleotide repeat) on chromosome 4 known as the *huntingtin* gene. The disease is caused when the repeat length exceeds a certain threshold; generational transmission often is associated with the phenomenon of "anticipation," in which the disease starts at an earlier age in a child because of increased repeat length compared with that of the parent. Because no disease-modifying treatment is available, Huntington disease is treated symptomatically.

KEY POINT

- Chorea consists of random, nonrepetitive, flowing dance-like movements and can be caused by medications, endocrine derangement, pregnancy, streptococcal infection, autoimmune disease, and neurodegenerative disorders involving the basal ganglia

Tic Disorders and Tourette Syndrome

Tics are stereotyped, brief, rapid movements that break the flow of normal movements. Partially suppressible, tics may be generated to achieve transient relief from preceding uncomfortable focal sensations (premonitory urges). Tics usually start during childhood and range from simple to complex motor movements. Most patients achieve full remission or significant reduction of tics by adulthood.

Tourette syndrome is characterized by childhood onset, persistence of multiple complex motor tics for at least 1 year, and presence of vocal tics. Echolalia (repetition of others' words) and coprolalia (utterance of obscenities) are rare but classic forms of complex vocal tics. The specific cause of the syndrome remains unclear but may involve genetic influences causing disruption of the basal ganglia–frontal cortex network. Common comorbidities include attention-deficit hyperactivity disorder, obsessive compulsive disorder, and mood disorders. Treatment options include reassurance (often appropriate in mild disease), cognitive behavioral therapy, and treatment of psychiatric comorbidities. Anti-tic medications are indicated when tics cause educational, occupational, or social dysfunction.

Although only the antipsychotic agents pimozide and haloperidol have been approved by the FDA to treat severe Tourette syndrome, other commonly used agents for this condition include the α_2-adrenergic agonists clonidine and guanfacine; benzodiazepines; the dopamine-depleting agent tetrabenazine; topiramate; and—in patients with refractory disease—the antipsychotic agents aripiprazole, ziprasidone, and risperidone. The risk of tardive dyskinesia is a concern when antipsychotic agents are used in adulthood. Botulinum toxin may provide an additional option for certain simple (blinking) or potentially dangerous (cervical whiplashing) tics.

KEY POINTS

- Tourette syndrome is characterized by childhood onset, persistence of multiple complex motor tics for at least 1 year, and presence of vocal tics.

- Treatment of Tourette syndrome includes reassurance (often appropriate in mild disease), cognitive behavioral therapy, and treatment of psychiatric comorbidities

Restless Legs Syndrome and Sleep-Related Movement Disorders

Restless legs syndrome (RLS) is a common movement disorder characterized by discomforting sensations in the legs at rest or when falling asleep, an urge to move the legs, and immediate relief after moving the legs or walking. Patients with RLS should be screened for iron deficiency and receive iron supplements in the presence of deficiency or even low-normal serum ferritin levels (<45 ng/mL [45 µg/L]). Certain drugs, such as selective serotonin reuptake inhibitors and dopamine-blocking agents, can worsen RLS. Stimulants should be avoided late in the day. The most effective treatments are dopamine agonists, specifically pramipexole, ropinirole, and the rotigotine patch. Adverse effects of these medications, such as impulse control disorder, may limit their use. Other dopamine agonist complications include the development of augmentation (that is, symptoms begin to appear earlier in the day) and rebound (that is, symptoms return with greater intensity as the dose wears off). Use of long-acting formulations can lessen both of these complications. Other pharmacologic options include levodopa, gabapentin, opioids, benzodiazepines, and carbamazepine.

Periodic limb movements of sleep are brief triple flexion movements of the lower legs that repeat several times in 20-second cycles during early sleep. This disorder is very common and can occur independently or be associated with RLS, sleep-disordered breathing, or narcolepsy. The diagnosis is made by polysomnography. Treatment is not required unless severe sleep fragmentation occurs.

In REM sleep behavior disorder, patients do not experience normal muscle paralysis during the REM phase of sleep and, as a result, tend to physically act out their dreams; this tendency leads to shouting, kicking, punching, and similar behaviors during sleep. The diagnosis is based on the report of a bed partner or results of polysomnography. The main disorder in the differential diagnosis is nocturnal epilepsy. Highly effective treatment options include clonazepam and melatonin. In recent years, REM sleep behavior disorder has been identified as a strong predictor of future development of Parkinson disease and other α-synuclein–related disorders, such as multiple system atrophy and dementia with Lewy bodies.

KEY POINTS

- Patients with restless legs syndrome should be screened for iron deficiency and receive iron supplements in the presence of deficiency or even low-normal serum ferritin levels.

- The most effective treatments of restless legs syndrome are dopamine agonists, specifically pramipexole, ropinirole, and the rotigotine patch

Other Drug-Induced Movement Disorders
Tardive Dyskinesia

Medications that block dopamine D_2 receptors can cause various extrapyramidal adverse effects, ranging from acute dystonic reaction to parkinsonism and tardive dyskinesia (see Table 28). Tardive dyskinesia is associated with characteristic choreiform and dystonic craniofacial movements, but involvement of other body parts, including the neck and trunk, also

is possible. Removal of the causative medication is key to treatment, but symptoms of tardive dyskinesia can take months to resolve or may become permanent. A longer duration and higher dose of the causative medication, older age, and female sex carry a higher risk of permanent dyskinesia. Although typical antipsychotic agents (such as haloperidol) pose the highest risk of developing tardive dyskinesia, this disorder also can occur with the chronic use of many atypical antipsychotic drugs, the antiemetic agent metoclopramide, and the tricyclic antidepressant amoxapine. All patients taking any of these agents must first be warned of this potential complication. Pharmacologic treatment of tardive dyskinesia is often unsatisfactory, but options include clonazepam, tetrabenazine, anticholinergic agents, and clozapine.

Neuroleptic Malignant Syndrome

Neuroleptic malignant syndrome (NMS) is a life-threatening disorder caused by an idiosyncratic exposure to therapeutic doses of dopamine-blocking agents. NMS pathophysiology involves a sudden decrease in dopamine D_2 receptor activity, but the mechanism underlying this decrease is unclear. This condition has rapid onset and progression and is characterized by hyperthermia, rhabdomyolysis, altered mental status, and extrapyramidal symptoms, including rigidity and dystonia. Treatment of NMS involves the removal of the causative agent and supportive management; medical options include the muscle relaxant dantrolene (to relieve muscle breakdown) and dopamine agonists, such as bromocriptine

A similar syndrome can occur in the setting of rapid withdrawal from chronic dopaminergic treatment, as in hospitalized patients with Parkinson disease. **H**

KEY POINTS

- Medications that block dopamine D_2 receptors can cause various extrapyramidal adverse effects, ranging from acute dystonic reaction to parkinsonism and tardive dyskinesia.

- Removal of the causative medication is key to treating tardive dyskinesia, but symptoms can take months to resolve or may become permanent.

- Neuroleptic malignant syndrome is a life threatening disorder caused by an idiosyncratic reaction to dopamine-blocking agents that presents with hyperthermia, rhabdomyolysis, altered mental status, and extrapyramidal symptoms, including rigidity and dystonia.

Multiple Sclerosis
Spectrum, Pathophysiology, and Epidemiology

Multiple sclerosis (MS) is an autoimmune condition that results in immune-mediated damage to structures in the central nervous system (CNS). Autopsy studies have shown the widespread effects of MS on the brain, spinal cord, and optic nerve. The pathologic hallmarks of MS are focal areas of inflammation and demyelination in white matter tracts, sometimes associated with damage to glial structures and axonal transection. The neurologic symptoms and disability experienced by patients with MS are consequences of these pathologic processes.

MS generally has a younger age of onset than most chronic neurologic conditions, with most patients experiencing their first symptoms between the ages of 20 and 40 years. However, pediatric and older age–onset MS can occur. Patients with MS are mostly female, with a female to male ratio of approximately 3:1, according to most epidemiologic studies.

Multiple genetic and environmental factors contribute to the risk of MS. Genome-wide assays have identified risk alleles in genes for the major histocompatibility complex, interleukin-2 receptor, and interleukin-7 receptor, among many others. Despite the large number of genes involved, however, no specific genetic markers are diagnostic of MS. Twin studies show a concordance of 25% in monozygotic twins and 2.4% in dizygotic twins. Geographic location before adolescence is a clearly established environmental factor, with the highest risk of MS found in northern latitudes.

KEY POINT

- Multiple sclerosis is an autoimmune condition resulting in immune-mediated damage to structures in the central nervous system that is characterized by young age of onset (20-40 years) and a 3:1 female predominance.

Presenting Signs and Symptoms

The symptoms of MS are thought to occur as a result of the functional interruption by inflammatory lesions of critical axonal tracts. In most patients, focal lesions occur intermittently and acutely and lead to the rapid onset of clinical symptoms, often termed a relapse or "flare." Relapses tend to evolve over the course of a few days and often last for weeks to months before improving. Improvement in symptoms may represent remyelination of demyelinated areas and increased recruitment of other brain regions to substitute for areas of more extensive injury.

Because MS can affect nearly any part of the CNS, myriad symptoms can occur. The most common clinical manifestations of an MS relapse are optic neuritis, myelitis, and brainstem/cerebellar symptoms. Optic neuritis, or inflammation of the optic nerve, often presents as a subacute visual deficit in one eye along with pain with eye movement. An ophthalmologic examination will reveal a reduction in visual acuity, a scotoma or visual field deficit, and color desaturation (resulting in a decreased ability to discriminate colors). Pupillary examination will reveal an afferent pupillary defect, which results in paradoxical dilation of the pupil when light is rapidly shifted from the unaffected to the affected eye. If the anterior portion of the optic nerve is involved, funduscopic examination may also reveal papillitis (inflammatory changes in the retina causing a flared appearance of the optic disc).

Myelitis, or focal inflammation within the spinal cord, usually manifests as sensory or motor symptoms below the affected spinal level. Some patients also may experience a tight, band-like sensation around the chest or abdomen during the acute inflammatory process; Lhermitte sign, a shock-like sensation radiating down the spine or limbs induced by neck movements; and urinary frequency, urgency, or retention. Unlike other spinal cord processes, MS generally causes a partial myelitis, and thus symptoms of a full-cord transection are exceedingly rare. Physical examination often reveals focal weakness and possibly reduced sensation below a specific spinal level (sensory level). Muscle tone can be flaccid in the acute setting, but often spasticity is noted subsequently on muscular examination.

Disruption of vestibular or cerebellar pathways can lead to ataxia and vertigo; appendicular or truncal ataxia also can be seen, with dysmetria on finger-to-nose testing and difficulties with tandem gait. Brainstem involvement also can result in eye movement abnormalities and cause symptoms of diplopia or oscillopsia (a sensation of jerking of the visual field). Dysconjugate eye movements, nystagmus, and internuclear ophthalmoplegia (inability to adduct one eye and nystagmus in the abducting eye) sometimes are seen on oculomotor examination.

In addition to the development of acute and subacute focal symptoms, MS can also result in subtle chronic symptoms because of widespread cortical demyelination and atrophy, commonly manifested as cognitive dysfunction and mental and physical fatigue. In contrast to cerebrovascular disease, MS generally is not associated with cortical syndromes, such as aphasia and neglect.

Many patients with MS also experience the Uhthoff phenomenon, which is transient worsening of baseline neurologic symptoms with elevations of body temperature. Similar to electrical conductance, neuronal conductance is reduced at elevated temperatures, which allows a magnification of symptoms from previously demyelinated lesions. Uhthoff phenomenon events should be differentiated from relapses because they do not represent new inflammatory events and do not require direct treatment. Any patient with suspected relapse should be screened for intercurrent infection.

KEY POINT

- The most common clinical manifestations of a multiple sclerosis relapse are optic neuritis, myelitis, and brainstem/cerebellar symptoms; subtle chronic symptoms also can develop because of widespread cortical demyelination and atrophy, often manifested as cognitive dysfunction and mental and physical fatigue.

Diagnosis of Multiple Sclerosis
Diagnostic Criteria and Testing

No MS-specific diagnostic biomarkers are available; therefore, confirming the diagnosis of MS requires a full assessment of clinical symptoms, ancillary testing, and exclusion of other conditions in the differential diagnosis. The official diagnostic criteria for MS, known as the McDonald criteria, provide guidelines about the proper integration of clinical and diagnostic evidence. The McDonald criteria require evidence of CNS demyelination disseminated in both space and time. These criteria can be satisfied by a combination of documented clinical relapses, signs on physical examination, and the distribution of lesions on an MRI. Because MRI is the main diagnostic tool in MS, the McDonald criteria also provide guidance about which abnormalities are specific to MS, which is critical because many other disorders also cause brain lesions on MRI. **Figure 19** shows examples of each of the five lesion types that meet these criteria: periventricular, juxtacortical, infratentorial (brainstem and cerebellum), spinal cord, and contrast enhancing. Knowledge of the location and type of lesions that are specific to MS is critical because other common conditions, such as migraine, microvascular ischemic disease, and head trauma, can also cause white matter lesions on MRI. However, these conditions do not cause lesions that meet the McDonald criteria requirements in terms of location and conformation. Proper application of the diagnostic criteria as they apply to MRI findings can prevent unnecessary neurologic testing, referrals, and misdiagnoses.

In addition to MRI, ancillary testing can be used to show objective evidence of demyelinating lesions. Reduced evoked potential conduction velocity on electrophysiologic testing—such as visual evoked potentials, brainstem auditory evoked potentials, and somatosensory evoked potentials—can be used as surrogate markers for demyelinating lesions in CNS white matter pathways. Optic coherence tomography is being increasingly used to confirm optic nerve damage; this testing uses near-infrared light to quantify the thickness of the retinal nerve fiber layer in the optic disc and the thickness of the macula. Reduced thickness in these regions is seen in patients with MS, most severely in patients with previous optic neuritis, but also in those who have not had this syndrome.

Cerebrospinal fluid (CSF) testing can be helpful when the diagnosis of MS is not clear but is not required for diagnosis if the full McDonald criteria have been met and other causes have been excluded. The CSF of approximately 85% to 90% of persons with MS contains oligoclonal bands not present in their serum and also an elevated IgG index and synthesis rate. Additionally, mild elevations in the CSF leukocyte count or protein level are sometimes present.

KEY POINTS

- The diagnosis of multiple sclerosis (MS) requires evidence of central nervous system demyelination disseminated in both space and time; MRI is the main diagnostic tool in MS.

- Cerebrospinal fluid testing can be helpful when the diagnosis of MS is not clear but is not required for diagnosis if the full McDonald criteria have been met and other causes have been excluded.

HVC

Differential Diagnosis of Multiple Sclerosis

Whenever the diagnosis of MS is being considered, conditions that mimic the disorder should be part of the differential diagnosis (**Table 31**). Various rheumatologic, inflammatory, infectious, and metabolic disorders can cause neurologic symptoms and MRI changes that sometimes are incorrectly diagnosed as MS. Knowledge of the other potential diagnoses in the differential and their distinguishing features can help reduce misdiagnoses and inappropriate referrals.

Clinical Course of Multiple Sclerosis

The potential clinical phenotypes of MS are shown in **Figure 20**. Most patients with MS (approximately 85%) initially experience a relapsing-remitting course. Those who do not meet the full diagnostic criteria for MS after a first event are said to have had a clinically isolated syndrome (CIS). Because disease-modifying therapies for MS have been shown to be useful in CIS for reducing the risk of

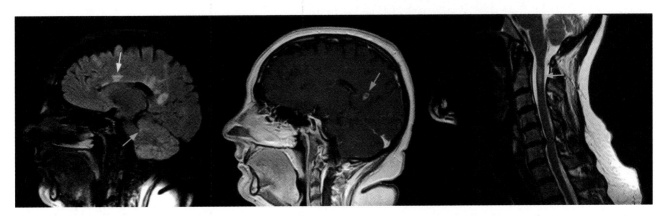

FIGURE 19. Characteristic lesions seen on MRI in multiple sclerosis. *Left*, sagittal fluid attenuated inversion recovery (FLAIR) brain sequence revealing periventricular (*yellow arrow*), juxtacortical (*red arrow*), and infratentorial (*green arrow*) lesions. *Center*, sagittal T1 brain image after administration of intravenous contrast; MS lesions are typically either silent or dark on T1 imaging, but those lesions that enhance with contrast (*orange arrow*) do so because of active inflammation within that lesion. *Right*, sagittal T2 scan of the cervical spine showing a lesion at approximately the C2 level (*blue arrow*).

TABLE 31.	Differential Diagnosis of Multiple Sclerosis
Disorder	**Notes**
Other demyelinating diseases	
ADEM	Monophasic, often postinfectious syndrome causing large, diffuse areas of inflammatory CNS demyelination
	Characterized by fevers and encephalopathy, typically with focal neurologic symptoms, that help differentiate this entity from MS
	More common in children (rare in adults)
Neuromyelitis optica (Devic disease)	Antibody-mediated inflammation directed at aquaporin-4 antibody channels in the CNS that results in inflammatory demyelination in the optic nerve and spinal cord
	Can be differentiated from MS by NMO IgG antibody testing and by its lack of significant brain involvement, large and longitudinally extensive spinal cord lesions, and profound CSF leukocytosis
Idiopathic transverse myelitis[a]	Monophasic, often postinfectious syndrome causing spinal cord inflammation
	Differentiated from MS by the presence of symptoms and findings unique to the underlying systemic disorder in addition to any neurologic symptoms
Systemic inflammatory diseases	
SLE	Can cause encephalopathy and white matter changes on MRI, often follows a relapsing-remitting course
Sjögren syndrome	Can cause an NMO-like disorder (with optic neuritis and myelitis), multiple cranial neuropathies, and a small-fiber neuropathy
Sarcoidosis	Causes granulomatous inflammation in the parenchyma and meninges of the brain and spinal cord
	Occasionally associated with myelopathy
Metabolic Disorders	
Adult-onset leukodystrophies	Rare
	Include adrenoleukodystrophy and metachromatic leukodystrophy
	May cause white matter changes and progressive neurologic symptoms
	Family history typically present
Vitamin B_{12} deficiency	Can cause optic neuropathy, cognitive changes, and subacute combined degeneration of the spinal cord (spasticity, weakness, and vibratory and proprioceptive sensory loss)
Copper deficiency	Can cause a myelopathy identical to that of vitamin B_{12} deficiency
Infections	
HIV infection, Lyme disease, and syphilis	Can cause encephalopathy and myelopathy
	Can be diagnosed with appropriate serologic and CSF analysis
HTLV	Causes a slowly progressive myelopathy with thoracic spinal cord atrophy
	Sometimes termed tropical spastic paraparesis because more common in patients in equatorial latitudes
Vascular disorders	
Sporadic and genetic stroke syndromes (hypercoagulability disorders)	Microvascular ischemic diseases potentially causing nonspecific white matter changes on MRI that are often confused with MS
	Distinguished from MS by age, other vascular risk factors, and findings on neurologic examination
CNS vasculitis	Primary type diagnosed by catheter angiography or tissue biopsy
	Can present with both stroke-like changes and meningeal contrast enhancement on MRI
Susac syndrome	Causes a small-vessel arteriopathy that causes dysfunction of the retina and cochlea and corpus callosum lesions seen on MRI
	Subacute clinical progression, without remission or relapse
Migraine	Subcortical white matter lesions sometimes present and often confused with MS lesions
	CADASIL a possible diagnosis in patients with a familial syndrome of migraine, subcortical strokes, mood disorders, and early dementia

(Continued on the next page)

TABLE 31. Differential Diagnosis of Multiple Sclerosis *(Continued)*

Disorder	Notes
Neoplasia (primary CNS neoplasm [gliomas or lymphomas] or metastatic disease)	Neoplasms with progressively worsening symptoms and neuroimaging findings
	Brain biopsy indicated when imaging cannot differentiate neoplasms from demyelinating disease
Paraneoplastic syndromes	May cause progressive cerebellar ataxia or myeloneuropathy (neuropathy affecting the spinal cord and peripheral nerves)
	Personality and mental status changes in addition to seizures and movement disorders possible with paraneoplastic limbic encephalitis
	Diagnosis often made on the basis of antibody testing and evaluation for metastases
Somatoform disorders	Psychiatric disorders presenting with neurologic-like symptoms that are due to somatization, conversion, and similar conditions
	Neurologic evaluation findings normal

ADEM = acute disseminated encephalomyelitis; CADASIL = cerebral autosomal dominant arteriopathy with subcortical infarcts and leukoencephalopathy; CNS = central nervous system; CSF = cerebrospinal fluid; HTLV = human T-lymphotropic virus; MS = multiple sclerosis; NMO = neuromyelitis optica; SLE = systemic lupus erythematosus.

ªFor more information on idiopathic transverse myelitis, see Spinal Cord Disorders.

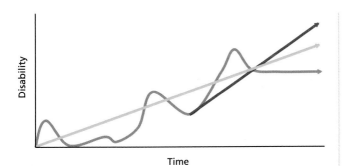

FIGURE 20. Visual representation of the three clinical phenotypes of multiple sclerosis. Most patients with MS will experience a relapsing-remitting course (*blue line*) at disease onset. Relapses initially do not result in significant permanent disability; however, as time goes on, residual disability accrues. Some patients with a relapsing-remitting course will continue in this manner and eventually plateau at a consistent level of disability. However, some will transition to a secondary progressive course (*red line*), in which disability accrues over time without clear relapsing or remitting events. Patients with primary progressive MS (*green line*) never experience any relapsing-remitting events, instead undergoing progressive disability accumulation from the start.

conversion to clinically definite MS by approximately 50%, stratification of the risk of conversion is helpful in making treatment decisions. Patients with brain lesions on MRI at the time of their CIS have a 10-year risk of conversion to clinically definite MS of approximately 90%, whereas the risk of those without brain lesions is only 10% to 20%.

Symptoms of an MS relapse tend to peak after a few days to weeks and are followed by a period of recovery that may take weeks to months. In the first few years of MS, significant or complete recovery is common. Eventually, however, recovery diminishes and permanent disability can accumulate. In approximately 50% to 60% of patients with an initial relapsing-remitting course, relapses become infrequent or cease completely after a median of 10 to 15 years, but neurologic disability continues to accrue in a slowly progressive manner. This latter disease stage is termed secondary progressive MS.

Approximately 15% of patients with MS never experience a relapse but instead have progressive disability accumulation from the time of disease onset. This clinical phenotype is termed primary progressive MS. Although this subtype often presents later in life (fifth or sixth decade), rapid disability accumulation can occur. Although early studies of the natural history of the disease type had implicated sex and age at onset as predictors of rapid progression, recent studies have only supported early disability accrual as a predictor of long-term progression rates.

In addition to the classic MS subtypes, the recent increased availability of MRI has led to the identification of radiologically isolated syndrome; this term describes the disease in patients without demyelinating symptoms but with incidental MRI changes that satisfy the radiologic requirements of the McDonald diagnostic criteria for MS. Although the official diagnosis of MS cannot be made in the absence of demyelinating symptoms, patients with these incidental MRI changes are thought to be at high risk for later conversion to clinically definite MS. The diagnosis, prognosis, and treatment of radiologically isolated syndrome are controversial and the subjects of ongoing research.

KEY POINT

- Patients who do not meet the full diagnostic criteria for multiple sclerosis (MS) after a first event (clinically isolated syndrome) but have brain lesions on MRI have a 10-year risk of conversion to clinically definite MS of approximately 90%.

Treatment of Multiple Sclerosis
Lifestyle Modifications and General Health Care
Although some patients with MS avoid physical activity because of disability and fatigue, strengthening, stretching, and aerobic exercise is recommended. Maintenance of an

active healthy lifestyle and muscular fitness can mitigate disability to some extent and preserve appropriate muscle tone. Physical therapy and home exercise programs are useful in this regard, especially after a clinical relapse. Although symptoms can appear worse with exertion-related body temperature increases (Uhthoff phenomenon), patients with MS should be assured that neurologic injury will not result. In patients with significant Uhthoff phenomenon, minimization of discomforting symptoms can be achieved with strategies aimed at avoiding heat exposure or cooling the body.

Exercise also can help preserve bone health, which is vital given the increased risk of osteoporosis in patients with MS. The threefold to sixfold increased rate of reduction of bone mineral density seen in patients with MS is likely due to various factors, such as reduced physical activity, increased rates of vitamin D deficiency, and the effects of repeated glucocorticoid use. Vitamin D and calcium supplementation can help minimize this effect.

The use of vitamin D has additional benefits for patients with MS. The links between vitamin D deficiency and MS pathophysiology have been clearly established, with reduced serum vitamin D levels predicting future accumulation of new lesions on MRI. A recent randomized trial of the addition of vitamin D supplements to interferon-beta treatment showed that this supplementation reduced the accumulation of MRI lesions compared with placebo. Because of these data, vitamin D supplementation is now suggested for all patients with MS, although the ideal dosing regimen and serum 25-hydroxyvitamin D level are still unknown.

Because the risk of an MS relapse is increased at the time of systemic infections and because of the immunosuppressive nature of some of the newer MS medications, steps to prevent infection also are recommended. Current MS treatment guidelines suggest vaccination against influenza and maintenance of standard immunizations. Patients with MS with bladder dysfunction should be provided strategies to reduce the risk of urinary tract infection, such as intermittent catheterization or prophylactic antibiotics.

Smoking cessation is strongly advised for all patients with MS because of the threefold increased risk of conversion to secondary progression associated with cigarette smoking.

Because of the age and female sex of many patients with MS, issues related to pregnancy and lactation often must be addressed. Fortunately, the estrogenic state of pregnancy actually has an immunomodulatory effect that tends to reduce autoimmunity and result in the reduced MS relapse rates seen during pregnancy. However, the risk of relapse in the first three months after delivery is significantly increased. Despite this fact, repeated studies have shown that not only does pregnancy not cause additional permanent disability, but multiparous women seem to have better long-term MS outcomes than nulliparous or uniparous women. The impact of breastfeeding on MS relapse risk remains controversial, with various studies providing conflicting evidence.

KEY POINTS

- Maintenance of an active healthy lifestyle and strengthening, stretching, and aerobic exercise are recommended for all patients with multiple sclerosis to mitigate disability and preserve appropriate muscle tone. **HVC**

- Vitamin D supplementation, annual influenza vaccination, and maintaining a routine immunization schedule are recommended for all patients with multiple sclerosis. **HVC**

- Smoking cessation is strongly advised for all patients with multiple sclerosis because of the threefold increased risk of conversion to secondary progression associated with cigarette smoking. **HVC**

Treatment of Acute Exacerbations

A true MS relapse is likely when patients with the disease experience new or worsening neurologic symptoms lasting greater than 24 hours. Transient symptoms lasting minutes to hours, however, should not be considered a true relapse. Before initiation of treatment for an MS relapse, the possibility of a pseudorelapse (transient worsening of underlying neurologic symptoms in the setting of infection or systemic illness) should be considered. If a pseudorelapse is suspected, tests should be performed to discover and treat any occult infections or metabolic disturbances, which often results in resolution of neurologic symptoms.

Confirmed relapses typically are treated with high-dose glucocorticoids. Treatment is traditionally administered intravenously with methylprednisolone, 1 g/d for 3 to 5 days. However, recent studies have shown equivalency between this dose of intravenous glucocorticoids and oral prednisone, 1250 mg/d, and thus this alternative strategy is gaining wider use, especially given its reduced cost and ease of administration. The typical adverse effects of short-term, high-dose glucocorticoids are insomnia, hyperglycemia, a metallic taste, gastritis, fluid retention, irritability, and, on rare occasions, psychosis. Frequent glucocorticoid treatment should be avoided because it places patients at risk for the long-term adverse effects of these drugs, such as osteopenia and early cataracts. Relapses that are refractory to glucocorticoid treatment may respond to rescue therapy with plasmapheresis. **H**

KEY POINT

- Confirmed relapses of multiple sclerosis typically are treated with high-dose glucocorticoids.

Disease-Modifying Therapies

Definitive treatment of MS relies less on addressing relapses as they occur than on preventing relapse occurrence (and the associated accrual of disability) in the first place. This prevention is achieved with MS disease-modifying therapies, a series of immunomodulatory or immunosuppressive medications that have been shown to reduce the risk of relapse, disability progression, and new MRI lesion formation. Twelve disease-modifying therapies have been approved by the FDA for use in relapsing-remitting MS (**Table 32**), each differing in their route of administration, mechanism of action, and potential adverse effects. Additionally, the interferon beta preparations and glatiramer acetate have been shown to delay conversion to clinically definite MS in those with CIS. Unfortunately, the options are far more limited for those with progressive forms of MS; mitoxantrone is the only FDA-approved therapy for those with secondary progressive MS, and no therapies have proven benefit in primary progressive MS.

Choosing an appropriate therapy from these options depends on patient tolerability, risk stratification, and disease activity. Treatment decisions in MS often are made in discussion between an experienced specialist (a general neurologist or MS specialist) and the patient. No clear consensus exists about how to select the appropriate therapy, what defines treatment failure, or how to decide the order in which medications should be introduced. Generally, most physicians recommend self-injection medications (one of the interferon beta preparations or glatiramer acetate) as first-line agents, given their favorable risk profiles. Patients who are unable to tolerate these medications or in whom the medications are ineffective are often then switched to agents with better efficacy profiles (such as the oral or intravenous options outlined in Table 32), although this greater efficacy comes with greater potential risks.

The interferon beta preparations (beta-1a and beta-1b) use an immunomodulatory cytokine that shifts immune responses away from autoimmunity and increases the integrity of the blood-brain barrier. Interferon beta-1a is typically administered either once weekly by intramuscular injection or

TABLE 32.	Disease-Modifying Therapies for Multiple Sclerosis			
Medication	**Route of Administration**	**Potential Adverse Effects**	**Recommended Monitoring**	**Pregnancy Category**[a]
Interferon beta-1a (three formulations) and interferon beta-1b (two formulations)	Intramuscular or subcutaneous injection	Flu-like symptoms, fatigue, depression, increased spasticity, transaminitis, rare autoimmune hepatitis, and injection site reactions	CBC and liver chemistry testing every 3-6 months	C
Glatiramer acetate	Subcutaneous injection	Injection site reactions, lipoatrophy of skin at injection sites, and rare systemic panic attack-like syndrome	None	B
Natalizumab	Intravenous	Black-box warning of increased risk of PML, common adverse effects of headache and chest discomfort, and rare hepatotoxicity, infusion reactions and anaphylactic reactions	Rigorous, regimented, industry-sponsored monitoring (TOUCH™ program) and JC virus antibody testing	C
Alemtuzumab	Intravenous	Infusion reactions, including headache and rash; upper respiratory, urinary tract, and herpes virus infections; autoimmune thrombocytopenic purpura and autoimmune thyroid disease.	Pretreatment screening for varicella vaccination, thyroid function monitoring every 3 months, and monthly urinalysis and CBC and serum creatinine measurement	C
Fingolimod	Oral	Transaminitis, lymphopenia, increased risk of serious herpesvirus infection, hypertension, bradycardia (usually only with the first dose), and macular edema	Cardiac monitoring after administration of first dose, ophthalmologic screening, liver chemistry testing, and CBC	C
Dimethyl fumarate	Oral	Diarrhea, nausea, abdominal cramping, flushing, and lymphopenia	Frequent monitoring of CBC in first 6 months after administration and every 6 months thereafter	C
Teriflunomide	Oral	Alopecia, respiratory infections (including TB), pancreatitis, transaminitis, lymphopenia, hypertension, and peripheral neuropathy	Frequent CBC monitoring, hepatic panel, serum amylase and lipase measurements, and blood pressure determination in the first 6 months, every 6 months thereafter.	X
Mitoxantrone	Intravenous	Black-box warnings for cardiotoxicity and acute myeloid leukemia; other adverse effects of infection, nausea, oral sores, alopecia, menstrual irregularities, and blue discoloration of urine	Required monitoring of cardiac function by echocardiography or multigated radionucleotide angiography before each infusion and regular CBC	D

CBC = complete blood count; PML = progressive multifocal leukoencephalopathy; TB = tuberculosis.

[a]Pregnancy categories: B, animal studies suggest fetal risk; C, animal studies suggest adverse fetal effects; D, evidence of human fetal risk; X = documented fetal abnormalities.

three times weekly by subcutaneous injection, whereas interferon beta-1b is administered every other day by subcutaneous injection. A pegylated formulation of interferon beta-1a (peginterferon beta-1a) administered by twice-monthly subcutaneous injection also has recently been approved by the FDA. The interferons have been shown to reduce the relapse rate by approximately one third over 2 years compared with placebo and to have positive effects on disability progression and MRI findings. Head-to-head studies have shown general equivalence for most of the interferons, although more frequent administration resulted in slightly increased efficacy of one or the other in some studies.

Glatiramer acetate, a copolymer of four amino acids, is administered daily by subcutaneous injection. This medication likely has multiple mechanisms of action that result in immunomodulation. Glatiramer acetate and high-dose interferon betas exhibit similar reductions in relapse rates compared with placebo and are equivalent in head-to-head studies. Combining glatiramer acetate with an interferon-beta provides no added benefit to what either drug achieves alone.

Natalizumab is a monoclonal antibody that is administered by once-monthly intravenous infusion. Natalizumab binds to a cellular adhesion molecule on activated T-cells that is required for transmigration into the CNS. Natalizumab is a highly effective medication, reducing relapse rates by approximately two thirds compared with placebo over 2 years and slowing 2-year disability progression by approximately 40%. Despite its efficacy, natalizumab is typically limited to use as a second-line agent because of the risk of development of progressive multifocal leukoencephalopathy, a CNS demyelinating infection caused by reactivation of the JC virus. The overall risk is approximately 1:1000 but is significantly higher in patients who have previous exposure to immunosuppressant agents or chemotherapy and those who have elevated serum titers of antibodies against the JC virus. Stratification of risk by treatment history and JC virus antibody testing is thus an important step before initiating natalizumab.

Alemtuzumab is an anti-CD52 monoclonal antibody that causes complement-mediated lysis of circulating lymphocytes. It is administered as an infrequent intravenous infusion (once per day for 5 consecutive days and then again for 3 consecutive days 1 year later). Alemtuzumab reduces relapse rates and the risk of disability progression by approximately half and also significantly reduces the accumulation of new lesions and brain atrophy on MRI, compared with the interferon beta preparations. Because of significant safety concerns (see Table 32), alemtuzumab administration requires intensive safety monitoring and risk modification. Its increased risk of herpetic viral infections can be reduced with use of prophylactic antiviral agents.

Fingolimod is a once daily pill that results in sequestration of activated lymphocytes in lymph nodes. Fingolimod reduces relapse rates by approximately half over 2 years compared with placebo and also reduces the risk of disability progression and accumulation of new MRI lesions. Fingolimod

requires first-dose monitoring because of the first-dose bradycardia that occurs in most patients and should not be used in patients with heart block.

Teriflunomide is a once daily pill that exerts an immunosuppressive effect by inhibiting a mitochondrial enzyme involved in pyrimidine synthesis in rapidly dividing cells. Compared with placebo, teriflunomide reduces relapse rates by one third and also reduces the risk of disability progression and the accumulation of new MRI lesions over 2 years.

Oral dimethyl fumarate exerts its immunomodulatory effects by modulating the nuclear factor–like 2 transcriptional pathway. Twice daily dosing is approved for use in relapsing-remitting MS and has been shown to reduce relapse rates by slightly less than one half and to reduce the risk of disability progression and new MRI lesion development over 2 years.

Mitoxantrone is an anthracenedione chemotherapeutic agent that exerts an immunosuppressive effect by reducing lymphocyte proliferation. Although this medication has been shown to reduce relapse rates and is the only drug ever to have had any success in reducing the rate of disability accumulation in those with secondary progressive MS, the risks of cardiac toxicity and secondary leukemia have significantly limited its use.

KEY POINTS

- Interferon beta preparations and glatiramer acetate are immunomodulatory, disease-modifying medications used to treat multiple sclerosis that reduce the risk of relapse, disability progression, and new MRI lesion formation.

- Natalizumab is a highly effective medication that reduces relapse rates in multiple sclerosis by approximately two thirds compared with placebo and slows disability progression by approximately 40% but is used only as a second-line agent because it can cause progressive multifocal leukoencephalopathy.

Symptomatic Management

Adequate management of MS requires the treatment of symptoms that remain chronic after previous relapses or progression. Symptomatic pharmacologic and nonpharmacologic interventions (**Table 33**) can increase the quality of life of patients with MS.

Spasticity is a frequent consequence of damage to the corticospinal tract in MS. This symptom manifests clinically as increased muscle tone, painful muscle cramps, spasms, and contractures. Spasticity can be reduced by using muscle relaxants, such as baclofen, tizanidine, or cyclobenzaprine. Gabapentin also has been used successfully to reduce spasms in MS. For severe spasticity, botulinum toxin or implantable intrathecal baclofen pumps also can be used.

Treatment of neuropathic pain frequently involves the use of many of the same medications used to treat painful diabetic neuropathy. Although newer medications, such as pregabalin and duloxetine, have been used successfully for this type of

TABLE 33.	Symptomatic Management in Multiple Sclerosis	
Symptom	**Nonpharmacologic Management**	**Pharmacologic Management**
Spasticity	Physical therapy, stretching, massage therapy	Baclofen (oral or intrathecal pump), tizanidine, cyclobenzaprine, gabapentin, benzodiazepines, carisoprodol, botulinum toxin
Neuropathic pain	N/A	Gabapentin, pregabalin, duloxetine, tricyclic antidepressants, tramadol, carbamazepine, topiramate, capsaicin patch
Fatigue	Proper sleep hygiene, regular exercise	Modafinil, armodafinil, amantadine, amphetamine stimulants
Depression	Individual or group counseling	Antidepressants (such as SSRIs, SNRIs, tricyclic antidepressants, antipsychotic agents)
Cognitive dysfunction	Cognitive rehabilitation and accommodation strategies	No proven therapy
Impaired mobility	Physical and occupational therapy; use of braces, canes, rolling walkers, or electrostimulatory walk-assist devices	Dalfampridine
Urinary urgency/ frequency	Timed voids, avoidance of caffeine	Oxybutynin, tolterodine
Urinary retention	Manual pelvic pressure, intermittent catheterization	None
Pseudobulbar affect	None	Dextromethorphan-quinidine
Limb tremor	Occupational therapy	Botulinum toxin

N/A = not applicable; SNRIs = serotonin–norepinephrine reuptake inhibitors; SSRIs = selective serotonin reuptake inhibitors.

pain, less expensive generic alternatives, such as tricyclic antidepressants and gabapentin, are equally effective and well tolerated. Treatment of trigeminal neuralgia, a common neuropathic pain syndrome in MS, is discussed in more detail in Headache and Facial Pain.

Chronic fatigue is a very common symptom in MS. The fatigue associated with MS can have various causes, such as depression, insomnia, or other comorbid conditions. However, patients with MS without these conditions also can experience significant fatigue, which is often described as a sensation of mental exhaustion, frequently occurring in the midafternoon. Lifestyle adjustments, such as improving sleep hygiene, getting regular exercise, and treating depression, can sometimes resolve this symptom. For those with refractory fatigue, stimulant medications can be used. The most common medications of this type used in MS are modafinil, armodafinil, and amantadine. For fatigue that is refractory to these medications, amphetamine stimulants, such as methylphenidate, also can be considered.

Depression also is a common symptom in patients with MS, and the suicide rate is elevated in those with MS compared with those with depression for other reasons. The depression that occurs in MS is likely multifactorial, involving the emotional response to dealing with a chronic disease, the consequences of demyelinating lesions and inflammatory cytokines, and the adverse effects of treatments (such as the interferon betas). Clinicians should be vigilant for signs of depression and have a low threshold for initiating antidepressants and offering referrals to psychiatry and individual or group therapy programs.

Cognitive dysfunction occurs in at least 50% of patients with MS. The most common deficits involve short-term memory, processing speed, and executive function. Cognitive disability has a significant effect on the employability of patients with MS and can reduce their overall quality of life. Unfortunately, no trials of pharmacologic therapy to reduce or prevent cognitive dysfunction in MS have yet been successful, including trials of memantine and donepezil. Formal neuropsychological testing and cognitive rehabilitation and accommodative strategies (such as creating checklists to overcome memory deficits) sometimes can be of benefit.

Maintenance of mobility in patients with MS is essential in maintaining overall quality of life, and maintenance of an active, healthy lifestyle can help stave off future disability. Physical and occupational therapy is useful to ensure gait safety and improve walking ability and endurance. Assistive aids, such as braces, canes, walkers, and electrostimulatory walk-assist devices, can be useful for many patients. Pharmacologic therapy with dalfampridine, a voltage-gated potassium channel antagonist, has been shown to improve walking speed, leg strength, and gait in approximately 40% of patients with baseline gait impairment. This medication likely functions by accentuating and amplifying action potentials, which allows for signal transmission through demyelinating lesions in the corticospinal tract. As a consequence of this method of action, however, dalfampridine has the rare adverse effect of seizures and should not be used in patients with kidney impairment, given the reduced clearance of the drug and resultant potentially higher rate of seizures.

CONT.

Bladder dysfunction occurs in many patients with MS. Urinary frequency and urgency are more readily managed than other patterns of bladder dysfunction and are often amenable to abstinence from caffeine, timed voids, and anticholinergic medications, such as oxybutynin or tolterodine. Patients with urinary hesitancy or retention can be more difficult to treat, however, because anticholinergic agents can worsen retention and lead to predisposition to urinary tract infections. Those with mixed bladder symptoms should be evaluated by a urologist, and intermittent catheterization should be considered.

Pseudobulbar affect, a less common symptomatic manifestation of MS, can act as a significant impediment to social interaction in patients with MS. This symptom manifests as uncontrolled fits of laughter or crying that occur without distinct or appropriate triggers. A successful trial of the combination agent dextromethorphan-quinidine has led to FDA approval of the use of this pharmacotherapy for pseudobulbar affect in MS. **H**

KEY POINTS

- Spasticity can be reduced in multiple sclerosis by using muscle relaxants, such as baclofen, tizanidine, or cyclobenzaprine; severe spasticity may respond to botulinum toxin or implantable intrathecal baclofen pumps.

HVC
- Although newer medications, such as pregabalin and duloxetine, have been used successfully to treat neuropathic pain in multiple sclerosis, less expensive generic alternatives, such as tricyclic antidepressants and gabapentin, are as effective and well tolerated.

- Depression is a common symptom of multiple sclerosis (MS), and the suicide rate is elevated in patients with depression from MS compared with depression from other causes.

Disorders of the Spinal Cord

Presenting Symptoms and Signs of Myelopathies

The vital anatomy of the spinal cord and its susceptibility to injury because of its small diameter make recognizing and resolving spinal injury in a timely manner crucial. Spinal cord disorders, or myelopathy, can occur as a result of extrinsic (external compression) or intrinsic (intramedullary) pathology.

The presenting signs and symptoms of spinal cord injury often occur at or below the site of the lesion. When injury to the corticospinal tracts occurs, spastic paresis or paralysis is possible, manifesting as weakness, hyperreflexia, muscle spasms, and extensor plantar responses. Involvement of the distal spinal cord and lower roots (cauda equina syndrome)

can involve weakness of the lower motoneuron type, with decreased muscle tone and areflexia. A detailed sensory examination in suspected spinal cord injury is critical, including ascending pinprick testing throughout the entire torso and neck, because myelopathies often result in a distinct sensory level below which sensation can be altered or lost. This typically correlates anatomically with the level of injury and thus helps with localization and directed spinal imaging. Loss of perianal sensation in particular is a key finding that suggests cauda equina syndrome. Gait is abnormal in most patients with myelopathy and sometimes can be an isolated presenting sign in mild progressive myelopathy. Findings can range from a subtle spastic gait or sensory ataxia to complete paralysis.

Many patients with myelopathy will report pain at the level of the compressive disease, and focal tenderness to percussion over the spinal column may be elicited. Some also describe squeezing or banding sensations around the chest or abdomen near the level of compression that sometimes lead to unnecessary cardiac, pulmonary, or gastrointestinal evaluations and delay in appropriate diagnosis. Patients also can experience disruptions in bowel and bladder function and loss of sphincter tone.

KEY POINTS

- When injury to the corticospinal tracts occurs, spastic paresis or paralysis is possible, manifesting as weakness, hyperreflexia, muscle spasms, and extensor plantar responses.

- Involvement of the distal spinal cord and lower roots (cauda equina syndrome) can involve weakness of the lower motoneuron type, with decreased muscle tone and areflexia.

- Myelopathies often result in a distinct sensory level below which sensation can be altered or lost, and this finding typically correlates anatomically with the level of injury and helps with localization and directed spinal imaging.

Compressive Myelopathies

Clinical Presentation

H

Spinal cord compression can result from acute or chronic causes. Prompt evaluation and confirmation of suspected acute spinal cord compression with appropriate neuroimaging studies should occur in an urgent manner. Immediate treatment may be necessary to prevent severe and irreversible neurologic injury.

The most common clinical presentation is neck or back pain, followed by weakness, sensory changes, and bowel and bladder dysfunction. Examination often reveals upper motoneuron signs (weakness, spasticity, hyperreflexia, and extensor plantar responses), but lower motoneuron signs (atrophy, hyporeflexia) also can occur at or below the level of compression. Specific signs and symptoms can provide clues about the cause of the compression. Patients with fevers and focal tenderness, especially those who have had recent instrumentation surgery to the back, may have an epidural abscess. Patients with a history of neoplasm and focal back pain should arouse concern for metastatic disease (**Figure 21**) or pathologic vertebral fracture. Patients receiving anticoagulation may have myelopathic symptoms from an epidural hematoma.

Patients with chronic spinal stenosis due to osteoarthritic degenerative spinal disease frequently have chronic myelopathic symptoms, most often involving the cervical and lumbar spines; thoracic spine symptoms are quite uncommon. Most patients with chronic compressive myelopathy will report progressive leg weakness, spasticity, distal numbness, and bladder impairment at presentation. Some with lumbar stenosis may describe symptoms resembling vascular claudication (pseudoclaudication) with exertional groin, thigh, or buttock pain and possibly weakness or numbness. Compressive myelopathy thus should be considered in older patients with gait dysfunction or weakness. **H**

KEY POINT

- Prompt evaluation and confirmation of suspected acute spinal cord compression with appropriate neuroimaging studies should occur in an urgent manner because immediate treatment may be necessary to prevent severe and irreversible neurologic injury.

Diagnosis

MRI of the spinal cord in the suspected location of injury is the preferred means of diagnosing compressive myelopathy and can sometime reveal its cause. CT myelography is useful when MRI is not feasible (as in patients with implantable devices) but is difficult to obtain on an emergent basis, cannot be used in patients with contrast dye allergies or impaired kidney function, and may not directly establish the cause of the compression.

KEY POINT

- MRI of the spinal cord is the preferred method to diagnose compressive myelopathy.

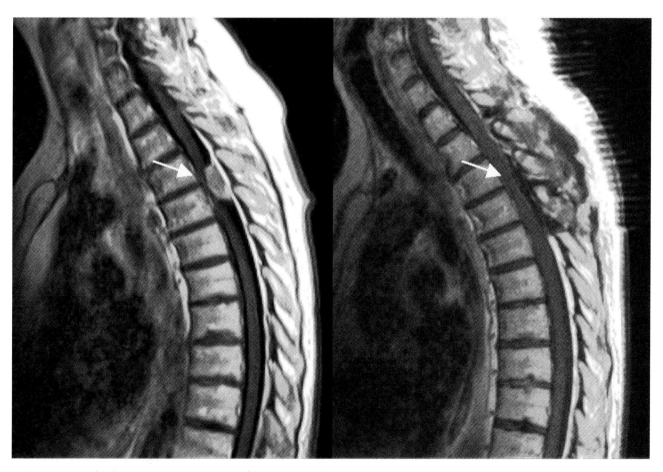

FIGURE 21. Spinal cord compression due to a tumor. MRI of the thoracic spine of a 60-year-old woman with progressive lower extremity weakness. A postcontrast T1 image (*left*) shows spinal cord compression by a mass lesion (*arrow*). *Right,* compression was relieved (*arrow*) after surgical resection. Pathologic analysis of the lesion suggested meningioma.

Treatment

Surgical decompression is typically required to treat spinal cord compression. Medical therapies can complement surgical treatment, depending on the underlying cause. For example, epidural hematoma or abscess may require management of the bleeding diathesis or antibiotics. These complementary treatments, however, should not replace necessary neurosurgical intervention. Glucocorticoids have no role in treating spinal cord compression caused by infection or hematoma. However, several trials have shown the benefits of high-dose intravenous glucocorticoids administered within the first 8 hours of traumatic spinal cord injury.

Spinal cord compression from metastatic disease requires emergent use of high-dose glucocorticoids and subsequent treatment with surgical decompression followed by radiation for most tumor types. Clinical trials have shown the superiority of surgical decompression in optimizing ambulation. However, certain radiosensitive tumor types, such as leukemia, lymphoma, myeloma, and germ cell tumors, may not require initial surgical decompression and may be treated urgently with radiation therapy. Surgical intervention is also sometimes deferred in patients with a poor prognosis for long-term survival or with a low functional status and in those without a distinct neurologic deficit.

For chronic cervical or lumbar stenosis or acute disk herniations, physical therapy and symptomatic management of spasticity and pain (with oral or injected medications) can control symptoms in most patients. However, surgical decompression may also be required for those refractory to medical management. See MKSAP 17 General Internal Medicine for more information.

KEY POINTS

- High-dose intravenous administration of glucocorticoids within the first 8 hours of traumatic spinal cord injury improves outcomes.
- Urgent surgical decompression followed by glucocorticoids and radiation therapy is typically required to treat spinal cord compression due to metastatic disease.
- Radiosensitive tumor types, such as leukemia, lymphoma, myeloma, and germ cell tumors, often may be treated urgently with radiation therapy alone.

Noncompressive Myelopathies

Noncompressive myelopathy can be caused by many inflammatory, infectious, metabolic, vascular, and genetic disorders. The most common cause is multiple sclerosis (see Multiple Sclerosis) and associated inflammatory and demyelinating disorders (such as neuromyelitis optica and sarcoidosis).

Idiopathic Transverse Myelitis

Idiopathic transverse myelitis (TM) (**Figure 22**) is a monophasic inflammatory and demyelinating myelopathy affecting a portion of the spinal cord. Idiopathic TM usually is considered a para- or postinfectious inflammatory response.

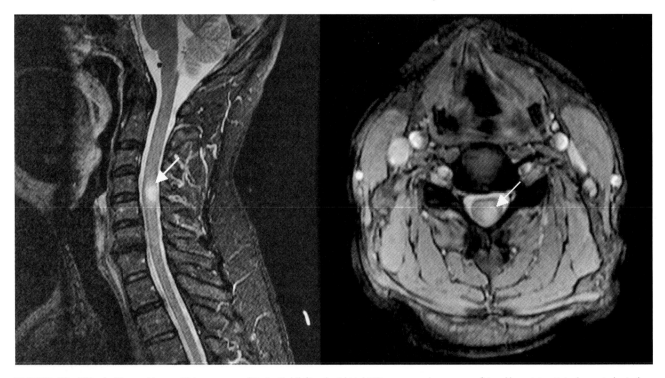

FIGURE 22. MRIs of a 53-year-old man with transverse myelitis. Sagittal (*left*) and axial (*right*) T2 sequences show an area of signal hyperintensity in the cervical spinal cord (*arrows*), mostly posterior with lateral extension to the left hemicord. This pattern could be consistent with disorders that have a predilection for the posterior columns, such as vitamin B$_{12}$ and copper deficiencies and neurosyphilis, although inflammatory transverse myelitis and multiple sclerosis can also affect this region.

CONT.

Affected patients frequently experience a subacute onset of weakness, sensory changes, and bowel or bladder dysfunction, which is sometimes preceded by back pain or a thoracic banding sensation.

Diagnostic criteria for idiopathic TM require the presence of clinical features of the syndrome, evidence of inflammation (either leukocytosis in the cerebrospinal fluid or contrast enhancement on MRI), and exclusion of other potential causes. A recent consensus statement outlined the characteristics distinguishing true idiopathic TM from TM due to other causes (such as multiple sclerosis or neuromyelitis optica). The predictive signs of idiopathic TM were listed as complete myelitis (symptoms related to complete rather than partial transection of the cord), a lack of either oligoclonal bands or elevated IgG index in the cerebrospinal fluid, and the absence of lesions on brain MRI. Distinguishing idiopathic TM from TM due to multiple sclerosis or neuromyelitis optica is imperative because idiopathic TM does not relapse after approximately 30 days from symptom onset and does not require long-term immunomodulatory therapy. The standard of care for acute interventions for idiopathic TM is derived from experience in other demyelinating and inflammatory disorders and multiple small, open-label trials. The consensus-based treatment of idiopathic TM is acute infusion of intravenous methylprednisolone, 1 g/d for 3 to 7 days. This therapy is intended to result in cessation of the inflammatory damage to the spinal cord and allow for recovery of neurologic function. Patients whose disease is refractory to glucocorticoids may benefit from plasmapheresis or cyclophosphamide.

Potential infectious causes of nonidiopathic TM are herpes simplex virus, varicella zoster, West Nile virus, human T-lymphotropic virus, Lyme disease, and neurosyphilis. HIV infection also can cause a TM-like syndrome at the time of seroconversion or a chronic degenerative vacuolar myelopathy in patients with chronic low CD4 counts. Additionally, mycobacterium tuberculosis can infect the meninges and spinal cord and cause myelopathic symptoms. These infectious causes should be considered when evaluating patients with TM and excluded, as appropriate. Treatment should be directed against the particular infection present. The addition of glucocorticoids to treat these disorders is controversial but may be indicated when infections are associated with significant concomitant spinal cord edema (as is sometimes true in tuberculosis). **H**

KEY POINT

- The consensus-based treatment of idiopathic transverse myelitis is acute infusion of intravenous methylprednisolone, 1 g/d for 3 to 7 days; patients whose disease is refractory to glucocorticoids may benefit from plasmapheresis or cyclophosphamide.

Subacute Combined Degeneration

Severe vitamin B_{12} deficiency (see MKSAP 17 Hematology and Oncology) can cause subacute combined degeneration, which is dysfunction of the corticospinal tracts and dorsal columns of the spinal cord. This entity manifests as a spastic paresis with reduced vibration and position sense and ataxia. MRIs may show increased signal in the affected white matter pathways, which usually is restricted to specific white matter tracts without signs of inflammatory change. Besides a low serum vitamin B_{12} level, laboratory study results usually show an elevated serum methylmalonic acid level, an elevated serum homocysteine level, and (potentially) a macrocytic anemia. Because clinical symptoms of vitamin B_{12} deficiency sometimes occur with low-normal serum levels of vitamin B_{12}, these other supportive laboratory values also should be obtained when a high index of suspicion for subacute combined degeneration exists. Abnormal findings should provoke an evaluation for their cause. Replacement of vitamin B_{12} usually halts progression of the disease but generally does not reverse existing symptoms. Copper deficiency, whether due to nutritional deficiency, malabsorption, or zinc toxicity, also can cause subacute combined degeneration and, thus, should be considered in patients with suggestive symptoms. **H**

KEY POINT

- In patients with subacute combined degeneration, results of laboratory studies usually show a low serum vitamin B_{12} level, an elevated serum methylmalonic acid level, an elevated serum homocysteine level, and macrocytic anemia.

Vascular Disorders

Vascular disorders also can lead to noncompressive myelopathy. Infarcts in the territory of the anterior spinal artery may occur as a result of atherosclerosis or embolism and typically present as sudden-onset flaccid paralysis, with preservation of vibration and position sense (because the posterior columns are not supplied by this artery). Prolonged hypotension during cardiovascular or aortic surgery also sometimes cause watershed infarcts in the area where the anterior spinal artery meets with the most prominent radicular artery (artery of Adamkiewicz), which is part of the vascular supply of the thoracic spinal cord.

Dural arteriovenous fistulas of the spinal vascular supply can either result in a chronic myelopathy due to venous congestion or cause spinal infarcts due to altered vascular dynamics or thrombosis. These fistulas are most common in men older than 50 years, especially those with previous spinal surgery. Catheter-based angiography is still considered the gold-standard diagnostic tool for dural arteriovenous fistulas. Abnormal vascular flow voids also are sometimes noted on spinal MRI. These malformations can be treated with endovascular procedures or surgical ligation. **H**

KEY POINT

- Dural arteriovenous fistulas causing noncompressive myelopathy of the spinal cord can be treated with endovascular procedures or surgical ligation.

Genetic Testing

Genetic testing should be considered in those with a family history of myelopathy. Hereditary spastic paraplegia comprises a group of rare hereditary disorders that cause chronic, progressive, ascending weakness and spasticity, often beginning in childhood or adolescence. Genetic screening is available, but no treatment currently exists. Female carriers of X-linked adrenoleukodystrophy can develop adrenomyeloneuropathy, a degenerative condition of the spinal cord and peripheral nerves. In clinical situations in which one of these disorders is being considered, involvement of a genetic counselor is indicated.

Neuromuscular Disorders
Peripheral Neuropathies
Overview

Peripheral nervous system disorders can be distinguished from central nervous system disorders on the basis of clinical features and confirmed with specific diagnostic studies (**Table 34**). Neuromuscular disorders include peripheral neuropathy, myopathy, neuromuscular junction disease, plexopathy, radiculopathy, and motoneuron disease. See **Table 35** for further information.

Classification, Findings, and Diagnosis

Peripheral neuropathies are disorders of sensory, motor, and autonomic nerves. At presentation, patients may have negative (loss of sensation) or positive (paresthesia, dysesthesia, and pain) sensory symptoms, weakness, or dysautonomia (orthostatic symptoms, altered sweating, urinary symptoms, impotence, and gastroparesis). Physical examination may reveal deficits in various sensory modalities, flaccid weakness, hyporeflexia, and ataxia.

Peripheral neuropathies can be classified on the basis of distribution of sensorimotor deficits (symmetric versus asymmetric, distal versus proximal, focal versus generalized), pathology (demyelinating versus axonal), size of nerve fibers involved (large versus small fibers), family history, and autonomic involvement (**Figure 23**). Small-fiber neuropathies involve small, unmyelinated nerve fibers and affect pain and temperature sensation and autonomic function; large-fiber neuropathies are associated with the loss of joint position and vibration sense and sensory ataxia.

TABLE 34.	Features Distinguishing Peripheral from Central Nervous System Disorders	
Features	**PNS Disorder**	**CNS Disorder**
Onset	Subacute or insidious	Sudden (stroke) or gradual (mass lesions)
Pattern of weakness	Focal or multifocal (in the territory of the affected nerve, plexus, or root) or generalized	Entire limb, unilateral, or with a pyramidal pattern of weakness[a]
Atrophy	Yes (at times prominent)	No (or mild, if related to disuse)
Fasciculations	Yes	No
Tone	Decreased or normal	Increased (spastic) or normal
Pattern of sensory symptoms	Focal or multifocal (in the territory of the affected nerve, plexus, or root) or stocking-glove in distribution	Entire limb or unilateral
Type of sensory symptoms	Positive symptoms (paresthesia, dysesthesia, or allodynia[b]) more frequent, but negative symptoms (numbness) possible	Negative symptoms more frequent, but positive symptoms possible
Dissociated sensory loss	Pain/temperature and vibration/proprioception deficits travel together	Dissociation of pain/temperature and vibration/proprioception deficits possible with spinal and brainstem lesions
Deep tendon reflexes	Diminished or normal	Increased
Pathologic reflexes	Absent	Present, including extensor plantar response, Hoffmann sign,[c] knee cross adduction, jaw jerk, snout, and clonus
Additional localizing symptoms	Cramps	Headache, seizures, and visual and language-related symptoms
EMG	Abnormal	Normal

CNS = central nervous system; EMG = electromyography; PNS = peripheral nervous system.

[a]Pyramidal weakness is caused by upper motoneuron lesions and affects extensors more than flexors in the upper limbs and flexors more than extensors in the lower limbs.

[b]Paresthesia is an abnormal spontaneous sensation, such as tingling, burning, or electrical sensation. Dysesthesia is an unpleasant sensation provoked by neutral stimuli, such as light touch or contact of clothes. Allodynia is pain provoked by nonnoxious stimuli.

[c]Hoffmann sign is positive if thumb is flexed in response to flicking or snapping of the distal phalanx of the middle finger.

TABLE 35. Common Symptoms and Signs of Neuromuscular Disorders

Symptoms and Signs	Differential Diagnosis
Weakness	
Distal extremities	Dying-back polyneuropathy (as in diabetes mellitus)
Proximal extremities	Myopathy, polyradiculopathy
Multifocal with pain (mononeuropathy multiplex)	Vasculitis, rheumatoid arthritis, diabetes
Focal asymmetric	ALS, inclusion body myositis, radiculopathy, multifocal motor neuropathy
Fluctuating	Myasthenia gravis
Ocular	Myasthenia gravis, mitochondrial myopathy
Bulbar (tongue, palate, lips)	ALS, myasthenia gravis, inclusion body myositis
Cranial nerves (especially III and VII)	Diabetes, Lyme disease, sarcoidosis, HIV infection
Neck extensors	ALS, myasthenia gravis (including with anti-MuSK antibody)
Fasciculations	ALS, GBS, radiculopathy
Sensory	
Stocking-glove gradient	Generalized polyneuropathies
Dermatomal pattern	Radiculopathy, peripheral nerve lesion
Distal pain without hyporeflexia or weakness	Small fiber neuropathy
Marked proprioceptive loss in single limb	Dorsal root ganglionopathy (cancer, Sjögren syndrome, HIV infection)
Autonomic	
Decreased sweating, early satiety, constipation, impotence, erectile dysfunction, orthostatic hypotension, resting tachycardia	Diabetes, amyloidosis, autoimmune dysautonomia (antiganglionic acetylcholine receptor antibody), paraneoplastic

ALS = amyotrophic lateral sclerosis; GBS = Guillain-Barré syndrome; MuSK = muscle-specific kinase.

Laboratory tests in all patients with a suspected peripheral neuropathy should include a complete blood count, erythrocyte sedimentation rate determination, serum protein electrophoresis with immune fixation, thyroid function tests, and measurement of hemoglobin A_{1C}, fasting plasma glucose, and serum vitamin B_{12} levels. Analysis of cerebrospinal fluid (CSF) is helpful if Guillain-Barré syndrome, demyelinating neuropathy, or mononeuropathy multiplex is suspected. Genetic testing can identify hereditary neuropathies in patients with a positive family history. Special laboratory testing can be considered in specific settings (**Table 36**).

Electromyography (EMG), which for the purpose of this discussion includes both nerve conduction studies (assessing electrical conduction through the nerves) and needle electrode examination (assessing the electrical activity pattern within muscles), can confirm the presence of neuropathy and distinguish between axonal and demyelinating forms. EMG also can differentiate neuropathy from myopathy and radiculopathy from plexopathy (see later discussions). Nerve biopsy is indicated only in a small subset of neuropathies when concern for vasculitic, infectious, or infiltrative neuropathy exists. Small-fiber neuropathies, which typically have normal EMG and nerve biopsy findings, can be diagnosed with autonomic testing, including a quantitative sudomotor axon reflex test and skin biopsy, to assess intraepidermal nerve fiber density. The cause of peripheral neuropathy remains unknown in nearly one third of patients (cryptogenic neuropathy).

KEY POINTS

- Electromyography, including both nerve conduction studies and needle electrode examination, can confirm the presence of neuropathy, differentiate between axonal and demyelinating forms, and distinguish neuropathy from myopathy and radiculopathy from plexopathy.
- Nerve biopsy is indicated only in a small subset of neuropathies when concern for vasculitic, infectious, or infiltrative neuropathy exists

HVC

Mononeuropathies

Mononeuropathies generally involve a single nerve. A common type is meralgia paresthetica, a compressive neuropathy of the lateral femoral cutaneous nerve that causes isolated anterolateral thigh numbness without weakness. Diagnosis is clinical and treatment is conservative. Mononeuropathy multiplex involves multiple nerves at different sites and can indicate vasculitis, especially when pain is prominent. Plexopathies involve multiple sensory and motor nerves simultaneously at the brachial or lumbosacral plexus. Diagnosis is based on clinical pattern, EMG findings, and additional laboratory testing (see Table 36). Treatment is based on the specific cause.

Carpal Tunnel Syndrome

Carpal tunnel syndrome is caused by focal compression of the median nerve at the wrist. Initial presentation typically includes sensory symptoms in the thumb and second and third digits, with possible radiation to the whole hand. With progression, weakness of thumb abduction and opposition and thenar atrophy may be noted. Symptoms are exacerbated by prolonged wrist flexion or extension. The physical examination finding with the greatest likelihood ratio is the presence of hypalgesia in the distribution of the median nerve (LR, 3.1). The likelihood ratios for Tinel and Phalen signs are only 1.4 and 1.3, respectively. Treatment is supportive and usually involves wrist bracing, occupational therapy, anti-inflammatory medications, and—in patients with severe pain—glucocorticoid injections.

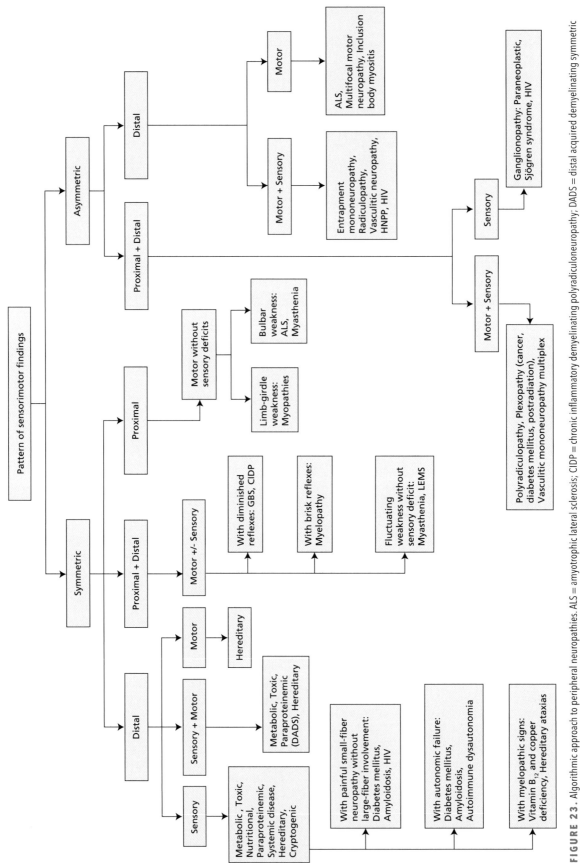

FIGURE 23. Algorithmic approach to peripheral neuropathies. ALS = amyotrophic lateral sclerosis; CIDP = chronic inflammatory demyelinating polyradiculoneuropathy; DADS = distal acquired demyelinating symmetric neuropathy; GBS = Guillain-Barré syndrome; HNPP = hereditary neuropathy with predisposition to pressure palsy; LEMS = Lambert-Eaton myasthenic syndrome.

TABLE 36. Additional Laboratory Testing in Peripheral Neuropathy

Cause	Clinical Presentation	Laboratory Testing
Diabetes mellitus, impaired glucose tolerance	Distal symmetric polyneuropathy, mononeuropathy, lumbosacral radiculoneuropathy	Glucose tolerance test; hemoglobin A_{1c} measurement
Uremia, thyroid disease, anemia	Distal symmetric polyneuropathy	Hematocrit; serum creatinine, TSH, and free thyroxine (T_4) measurements
Collagen vascular disease, polyarteritis nodosa, vasculitis, Sjögren syndrome	Vasculitic mononeuropathy multiplex, ganglionopathy (in Sjögren syndrome)	ESR; rheumatoid factor; serum antinuclear antibody, ANCA, anti-Ro/SSA, and anti-La/SSB antibody measurements
Syphilis	Posterior column disease resembling large-fiber neuropathy	RPR; CSF VDRL
Paraproteinemia associated with MGUS, amyloidosis, lymphoproliferative disease	Symmetric sensory demyelinating neuropathy; other variants also possible, including symmetric axonal sensory neuropathy, multifocal motor neuropathy, cranial neuropathy	SPEP; UPEP; IFE; serum free light chain measurement
Vitamin B_{12} or copper deficiency	Myeloneuropathy with brisk reflexes	Serum copper, vitamin B_{12}, and methylmalonic acid measurements
CIDP, GBS	Progressive polyradiculoneuropathies	Serum antiganglioside antibody and CSF cell and protein measurements
Miller Fisher variant of GBS	Ophthalmoplegia, ataxia, areflexia	Serum anti-GQ1b antibody measurement
Multifocal motor neuropathy	Asymmetric, pure motor weakness	Serum anti-GM1 antibody measurement
Distal acquired demyelinating symmetric neuropathy	Distal sensory loss, tremor, sensory ataxia	SPEP; IFE; serum anti-MAG antibody measurement
Amyloidosis	Autonomic and small-fiber neuropathy	Abdominal fat pad biopsy; transthyretin gene testing (in familial disease)
Infectious neuropathy	Variable, cranial nerve palsy, myelopathy, flaccid paralysis (in West Nile virus)	Serum HIV antibody and Lyme antibody and CSF West Nile virus antibody measurements
Toxic neuropathy	Symmetric sensory or sensorimotor neuropathy, acute motor neuropathy (in lead poisoning)	Serum lead, arsenic, mercury, and thallium measurements; 24-hour urine excretion of heavy metals
Celiac disease	Sensory neuropathy and ataxia	Anti–tissue transglutaminase antibody and anti-endomysial antibody measurements
Porphyria	Acute painful polyradiculopathy	Urine porphobilinogen and δ-aminolevulinic acid measurements
Fabry disease	Painful small-fiber neuropathy	α-Galactosidase measurement
Paraneoplastic disease	Subacute progressive sensory neuropathy, ganglionopathy	Serum anti-Hu and anti-CRMP5 measurement; testing for CSF oligoclonal bands

ANCA = anti–neutrophil cytoplasmic antibody; CIDP = chronic inflammatory demyelinating polyradiculoneuropathy; CRMP5 = collapsin response mediator protein 5; CSF = cerebrospinal fluid; ESR = erythrocyte sedimentation rate; GBS = Guillain-Barré syndrome; IFE = immune fixation electrophoresis; MAG = myelin-associated glycoprotein; MGUS = monoclonal gammopathy of unknown significance; RPR = rapid plasma reagin; SPEP = serum protein electrophoresis; TSH = thyroid-stimulating hormone; UPEP = urine protein electrophoresis.

If the diagnosis is uncertain or symptoms are persistent, EMG can differentiate the cause from radiculopathy, confirm median nerve compression, and quantify the severity of nerve injury. In the presence of refractory pain, weakness, or EMG evidence of active denervation, decompression surgery is recommended.

Bell Palsy

Bell palsy is idiopathic paralysis of the facial nerve that leads to complete unilateral facial paralysis. This disorder is distinct from a central weakness, such as stroke, in which forehead and periorbital muscles are spared because of bilateral innervation of the upper face. Hyperacusis and impaired taste may occur in Bell palsy. When the presentation is classic and without any additional neurologic deficits, brain imaging and routine laboratory testing are not necessary. However, Bell palsy can have a secondary cause, such as diabetes mellitus, vasculitis, Lyme disease, sarcoidosis, HIV infection, and compressive or infiltrative malignancies. In the presence of suggestive clinical features, therefore, determination of the hemoglobin A_{1c} value, erythrocyte sedimentation rate, and—in endemic areas—Lyme antibody titer should be considered. If symptoms worsen or do not improve by 2 months after symptom onset or if any new deficit develops, further assessment with brain MRI and additional testing for secondary causes is required.

Treatment with oral prednisone within the first 72 hours expedites both the speed and the rate of full recovery. In contrast, treatment with antiviral therapy alone has no benefit. Artificial tears should be used and a nighttime eye patch applied for corneal protection. A treatment course of several weeks is common, with complete recovery in 70% to 90% of affected patients. Older age and diabetes mellitus have a negative effect on prognosis. A few patients develop synkinesis (concomitant movement of perioral and periorbital muscles) as a result of aberrant reinnervation.

Brachial and Lumbosacral Plexopathies

Common causes of brachial and lumbosacral plexopathies include diabetes, cancer, radiation, and trauma. Imaging is mandatory to rule out structural lesions and malignancy. Idiopathic brachial plexitis is subacute severe pain and weakness that peak within 2 weeks. This type of plexopathy is associated with marked atrophy; a triggering event, such as infection or surgery, usually precedes its presentation. Spontaneous recovery over an extended period of time (as long as 2 years) is common.

KEY POINTS

HVC • Meralgia paresthetica, a compressive neuropathy of the lateral femoral cutaneous nerve that causes isolated anterolateral thigh numbness without weakness, can be clinically diagnosed and treated conservatively.

HVC • Carpal tunnel syndrome can be diagnosed clinically by the presence of hypalgesia in the distribution of the median nerve; initial treatment involves wrist bracing, occupational therapy, and anti-inflammatory medications.

HVC • Bell palsy is idiopathic paralysis of the facial nerve that leads to complete unilateral facial paralysis; patients with a classic presentation and no other neurologic deficits can be diagnosed without brain imaging and laboratory testing.

HVC • Early treatment of Bell Palsy with oral prednisone (within 72 hours of symptom onset) improves outcomes; antiviral therapy does not affect prognosis.

Polyneuropathies

Polyneuropathies preferentially affect distal parts of the longest nerves, a result of increased metabolic vulnerability of distal axons that gives rise to the dying-back phenomenon (axonal degeneration at the most distal point of the axon). Symptom onset typically is in the feet, and a stocking-glove gradient of sensory deficits is usually present. Polyneuropathies affecting large nerve fibers can be associated with loss of proprioception, weakness, and diminished reflexes. In contrast, polyneuropathies affecting small nerve fibers are associated

with pain, dysesthesia, and autonomic deficits but no weakness or proprioceptive deficit.

Neuropathies of Diabetes Mellitus and Impaired Glucose Tolerance

Diabetes can cause various types of neuropathy (Table 37). The most common pattern is symmetric distal sensory or sensorimotor. Either small or large fibers can be affected. Autonomic neuropathy can be prominent in diabetes and lead to profound orthostatic hypotension, impotence, gastroparesis, and potentially dangerous unawareness of hypoglycemic symptoms. Diabetic mononeuropathy can involve cranial nerves or predispose patients to entrapment neuropathies, such as carpal tunnel syndrome. Diabetic amyotrophy, also known as proximal lumbosacral radiculoneuropathy, is associated with subacute painful involvement of the lumbosacral plexus. Prominent proximal lower extremity weakness and muscle wasting with weight loss are typical. Unlike polyneuropathy, diabetic amyotrophy is not related to glycemic control or diabetes duration. Recovery is slow, usually taking between 3 and 36 months.

Diagnosis of diabetic peripheral neuropathy is clinical. EMG can reveal a distal and symmetric axonal sensorimotor polyneuropathy. Dysautonomia can be confirmed by autonomic testing. Other forms of diabetic neuropathy can be diagnosed on the basis of clinical findings, EMG results, and exclusion of alternative causes. Although the prevalence and severity of neuropathy correlate with the duration of diabetes,

TABLE 37. Peripheral Nerve Dysfunction in Diabetes Mellitus	
Classification	**Signs and Symptoms**
Autonomic neuropathy	Orthostatic hypotension, early satiety, nausea and vomiting (gastroparesis), constipation (colonic dysmotility), erectile dysfunction, hyperhidrosis, or hypohidrosis
Proximal lumbosacral radiculoneuropathy (diabetic amyotrophy)	Severe pain followed by weakness and muscle wasting in proximal lower extremities, weight loss, possible occurrence with or without proximal sensory loss
Mononeuropathy	Sensory loss, paresthesia or pain in the distribution of a single nerve followed by weakness (median or peroneal nerve), cranial nerve palsy (especially cranial nerves III, VI, or VII)
Radiculopathy	Sensory loss, pain and weakness in the distribution of nerve roots, thoracic radiculopathy causing patchy truncal numbness is common
Sensorimotor peripheral neuropathy	Asymptomatic (sometimes), distal length-dependent sensory loss and weakness, often painful, possible loss of ankle reflex
Small-fiber neuropathy	Burning distal extremity pain without weakness, may be non-length dependent, spares ankle reflex

the association between glucose intolerance and neuropathy (especially involving the small fibers) has become increasingly recognized. A sizeable number of patients with glucose intolerance (11%-25%) show evidence of small-fiber neuropathy on specialized testing, but most of these patients are clinically asymptomatic; some (5%-10%) are symptomatic, experiencing symmetric distal pain and paresthesia. Therefore, screening for glucose intolerance should be performed in patients without diabetes who have distal sensory neuropathy on presentation.

Tight glycemic control and minimizing cardiovascular risk factors can slow the progression and improve the symptoms of diabetic neuropathy. Treatment of painful neuropathies resulting from diabetes or other causes is symptomatic. Tricyclic antidepressants (amitriptyline, nortriptyline), serotonin–norepinephrine reuptake inhibitors (venlafaxine, duloxetine), antiepileptic drugs (pregabalin, gabapentin, valproic acid), opioids (tapentadol), and topical capsaicin are commonly used. Only pregabalin, duloxetine, and tapentadol (extended release) have FDA approval for painful diabetic neuropathy, but these agents are all costly, and other less expensive options, such as tricyclic antidepressants, should be tried first. Although opioids can be used for severe acute pain, their long-term use should be limited to truly refractory pain.

Hereditary Neuropathies

Hereditary neuropathies commonly present as slowly progressive distal weakness, numbness without pain or paresthesia, areflexia, and ataxia. Foot deformities, such as hammertoes, high arches, and distal leg atrophy ("stork legs") are common (**Figure 24**). The most common inherited neuropathy, Charcot-Marie-Tooth disease type 1, is demyelinating and associated with palpable peripheral nerves and uniform slowing of motor nerve conduction velocities on EMG; type 2 is axonal. Both types can be confirmed with genetic testing. Hereditary neuropathy with predisposition to pressure palsy is a form of hereditary neuropathy that presents with recurrent acute and reversible mononeuropathies caused by nerve compression at susceptible pressure sites (such as the elbows, wrists, and knees). Affected patients should be instructed to avoid compressive positions.

Inflammatory Polyradiculoneuropathies
Guillain-Barré Syndrome

Guillain-Barré syndrome (GBS) is an autoimmune, primarily demyelinating polyradiculoneuropathy that presents with acute generalized weakness and rapid progression over several days or weeks. GBS is thought to be caused by an infection-induced (most commonly, *Campylobacter jejuni*) aberrant autoimmune response targeting peripheral nerves and spinal

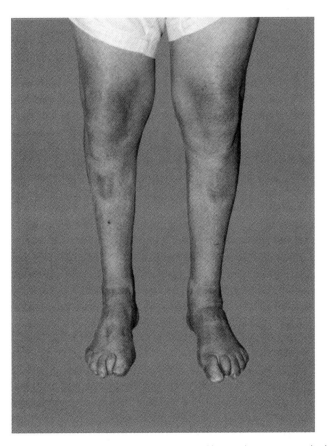
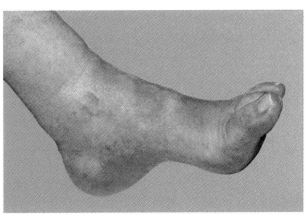

FIGURE 24. High arches, hammertoes, and distal leg atrophy in a patient with inherited neuropathy.

H
CONT.

roots. Half of patients with GBS have serum antibodies against gangliosides, which are components of peripheral nerves. Weakness is ascending, starting in the lower extremities and spreading to the upper limbs and bulbar and respiratory muscles. Diffuse areflexia is a key diagnostic clue. Paresthesia is common, but true sensory deficits are rare. Low back pain, a result of nerve root inflammation, can be prominent initially. Dysautonomia is common and may cause life-threatening labile blood pressure and arrhythmias. Because of the risk of dysautonomia and the possibility of respiratory failure, all patients with GBS should be hospitalized for respiratory and cardiovascular monitoring. Variants of GBS include a paraplegic variant, with weakness limited to the legs; a pharyngeal-cervical-brachial variant, with relative sparing of the legs; and the Miller Fisher variant, with multiple cranial neuropathies and ataxia.

The differential diagnosis of GBS includes myasthenic crisis, acute myelopathies, Lyme disease, West Nile virus, carcinomatous and sarcoid meningitis, acute lead neuropathy, botulism, and tick paralysis. The diagnosis is made on the basis of clinical features and results of CSF analysis, which reveal a classic pattern of a highly elevated protein level with a normal or mildly elevated leukocyte count (albuminocytologic dissociation) in 90% of patients. Although EMG confirms the diagnosis when it shows a predominantly demyelinating pattern, results may initially be normal. MRI of the lumbar spine is not mandatory but may reveal evidence of spinal root enhancement.

Therapy includes supportive management and, in most patients who experience severe progressive symptoms, treatment with either plasmapheresis or intravenous immune globulin (IVIG). Both therapies are equally effective and shorten the time to recovery by as much as 50%. Compared with IVIG, plasmapheresis has a faster mode of action but is less convenient and potentially requires longer hospitalization. Retreatment with IVIG is indicated if symptoms deteriorate after initial improvement or stabilization. Glucocorticoids are not beneficial in GBS and may even slow the recovery. Prognosis is favorable in 80% of patients, but relapse occurs in 6% and requires repeated treatment.

Chronic Inflammatory Demyelinating Polyradiculoneuropathy

Chronic inflammatory demyelinating polyradiculoneuropathy (CIDP) is a chronic and treatable autoimmune neuropathy. The classic presentation involves generalized areflexia and progressive or relapsing symmetric sensory and motor neuropathy. CIDP initially can present similarly to GBS, but symptoms do not stabilize after 4 weeks and continue to evolve over more than 2 months. Sensory symptoms and proximal weakness are more common in CIDP than in GBS. CIDP may be isolated or occur in the setting of a number of systemic conditions, including diabetes, lymphoma, and HIV infection. CSF and EMG findings are comparable to those in GBS. In the setting of diagnostic uncertainty, nerve biopsy can differentiate CIDP

from vasculitis or amyloidosis. Treatment options include prednisone, immunosuppressive therapies, and periodic IVIG or plasmapheresis.

Critical Illness Neuropathy

Critical illness neuropathy is common in patients with prolonged stays in the ICU because of sepsis or multiorgan failure. Besides a lengthy stay in the ICU, risk factors include prolonged mechanical ventilation and prolonged use of neuromuscular blocking agents; sepsis is not a risk factor. Typical features of critical illness neuropathy include failure to wean from the ventilator and generalized or distal lower extremity weakness.

This condition is differentiated from critical illness myopathy by the absence of myopathic changes on EMG and a normal serum creatine kinase (CK) level. However, the two conditions can occur simultaneously. A normal CSF protein level also distinguishes this disorder from GBS.

Treatment is supportive. Tight glycemic control and early physical therapy can be protective and reduce morbidity. Most patients fully recover, but a sizable percentage (30%) experience significant residual weakness. **H**

Systemic Neuropathy

Certain metabolic, nutritional, toxic, infectious, and paraneoplastic disorders can provoke neuropathy (**Table 38**). Copper and vitamin B_{12} (cobalamin) deficiencies, most often caused by bariatric surgery, intrinsic factor antibodies, and a restrictive (usually vegetarian) diet, can damage peripheral nerve and spinal cord structures (see Disorders of the Spinal Cord). Vitamin B_1 deficiency can lead to an axonal sensorimotor neuropathy and should be treated with aggressive thiamine supplementation. Alcohol abuse can cause a distal axonal neuropathy that is often painful and sometimes complicated by superimposed nutritional deficiencies.

Paraproteinemic Neuropathy

Paraproteinemic neuropathy often presents as a symmetric distal sensory neuropathy and occurs in the setting of monoclonal gammopathy of undetermined significance (MGUS), multiple myeloma, amyloidosis, cryoglobulinemia, and other hematologic malignancies (see MKSAP 17 Hematology and Oncology). Paraproteinemic neuropathy is identified by the presence of monoclonal immunoglobulins (M-band paraproteins) and is treated by managing the underlying condition. Paraproteinemia also can be associated with other forms of neuropathy, including sensorimotor, cranial, or multifocal motor neuropathy. Therefore, patients with various forms of peripheral neuropathy should be screened for paraproteinemia.

Amyloid Neuropathy

Amyloidosis is characterized by extracellular deposition of amyloid protein in various tissues, including the peripheral nerves. This disorder is characterized by marked autonomic

TABLE 38.	Neuropathies Related to Systemic Disease
Metabolic	
Uremia	
Liver disease	
Hypothyroidism	
Acromegaly	
Critical illness (multifactorial)	
Nutritional	
Vitamin B$_{12}$ deficiency	
Vitamin B$_1$ deficiency	
Vitamin B$_3$ deficiency	
Vitamin B$_6$ excess	
Vitamin E deficiency	
Copper deficiency	
Infectious	
HIV	
Lyme disease	
Leprosy	
Sarcoidosis (granulomatous)	
Rheumatologic and Vasculitic	
Systemic lupus erythematosus	
Rheumatoid arthritis	
Polyarteritis nodosa	
Sjögren syndrome	
Mixed connective tissue disease	
Paraproteinemic and Paraneoplastic	
Monoclonal gammopathy of undetermined significance (MGUS)	
Polyneuropathy, organomegaly, endocrinopathy, monoclonal protein, and skin lesions (POEMS)	
Amyloidosis	
Multiple myeloma	
Lymphoma	
Paraneoplastic neuropathy and ganglionopathy	

dysfunction and small-fiber neuropathy. Common symptoms include distal pain and paresthesia, orthostatic symptoms, gastroparesis, urinary incontinence, and impotence.

Primary amyloidosis is associated with monoclonal proteins, whereas familial amyloidosis is secondary to a genetic mutation.

Monoclonal Gammopathy of Undetermined Significance

Both isolated MGUS and MGUS related to hematologic malignancies (10%) are associated with neuropathy. MGUS with IgM gammopathy is linked to an immune-mediated neuropathy

characterized by distal sensory loss, ataxia, and tremor (distal acquired demyelinating symmetric [DADS] neuropathy). Half of patients with DADS neuropathy have antibodies against myelin–associated glycoprotein, and these patients respond poorly to therapy. The other half respond favorably to glucocorticoids, IVIG, plasmapheresis, or rituximab. Additionally, paraproteinemic neuropathy with IgG or IgA has a favorable response to plasmapheresis.

KEY POINTS

- Diagnosis of diabetic peripheral neuropathy is clinical. **HVC**
- Low doses of tricyclic antidepressants, such as amitriptyline and nortriptyline, are a cost-effective, first-line treatment option for patients with painful peripheral neuropathy. **HVC**
- In 90% of patients with Guillain-Barré syndrome, cerebrospinal fluid analysis reveals a classic pattern of a highly elevated protein level with a normal or a mildly elevated leukocyte count (albuminocytologic dissociation); therapy includes supportive management plus intravenous immune globulin or plasmapheresis.

Amyotrophic Lateral Sclerosis

Amyotrophic lateral sclerosis (ALS) is a fatal disease involving motoneurons and is associated with progressive weakness and muscle wasting. ALS often presents with focal weakness, muscle twitches or cramping, or difficulties with speech or swallowing. The disease progresses relentlessly, eventually culminating in death from respiratory failure within several years. ALS is characterized by upper motoneuron signs (such as hyperreflexia, spasticity, and an extensor plantar response) coexistent with lower motoneuron findings (such as atrophy and fasciculation). Sensory deficits are characteristically absent. Frontotemporal dementia sometimes is present.

Diagnosis is based on clinical findings, EMG results, and exclusion of alternative causes. MRI of the brain and spinal cord can help exclude stroke and cervical cord compression and will occasionally reveal a T2 bright signal in bilateral corticospinal pathways suggestive of ALS. The differential diagnosis includes Lyme disease, hyperparathyroidism, thyrotoxicosis, and multifocal motor neuropathy. Benign fasciculation syndrome, which is associated with widespread fasciculations and (sometimes) cramping but not with weakness or upper motoneuron signs, should not be confused with ALS.

Treatment is supportive. Riluzole, a glutamate release inhibitor, may slow the progression of ALS by a modest 3 months. Monitoring of liver function is recommended during riluzole therapy. Percutaneous endoscopic gastrostomy can improve quality of nutrition and prolong survival and should be considered before patients reach the advanced stage of the disease. Respiratory support includes noninvasive methods, such as biphasic positive airway pressure, and should be started in the presence of respiratory symptoms or hypercarbia. It also is essential to discuss prognosis and establish goals of care with patients and families, thereby avoiding unnecessary diagnostic and therapeutic measures.

HVC

KEY POINTS

- Amyotrophic lateral sclerosis (ALS) is a fatal disease involving the motoneurons that is associated with progressive weakness and muscle wasting for which treatment is supportive; it is essential to discuss prognosis and establish goals of care with patients and families, thereby avoiding unnecessary diagnostic and therapeutic measures.

- Riluzole, a glutamate release inhibitor, may slow the progression of amyotrophic lateral sclerosis by a modest 3 months.

Neuromuscular Junction Disorders

Myasthenia Gravis

Myasthenia gravis (MG) is an autoimmune disease directed against the postsynaptic neuromuscular junction. Onset is most common in the third decade of life in women and after age 50 years in men. Fluctuating, painless, and fatigable weakness involving the cranial, cervical, respiratory, and limb muscles is typical. Ocular involvement is sometimes the initial presentation of MG, but half of patients with only ocular symptoms at first will develop generalized weakness within 2 years; the other half will have limited disease. Bulbar weakness is common, either as the initial presentation or with progression of the disease. Physical examination can reveal ptosis, diplopia on sustained gaze, bilateral facial paresis, flaccid dysarthria, cervical weakness, and fatigable extremity weakness. The presence of respiratory symptoms should prompt close monitoring of respiratory parameters (vital capacity and negative inspiratory force) because of the risk of rapid respiratory failure (myasthenic crisis). Myasthenic crisis can occur as part of the natural history of extraocular MG or be triggered by external factors, including infection, surgery, and medications (aminoglycosides, fluoroquinolones, magnesium, β-blockers, or calcium channel blockers).

Diagnosis of MG is based on clinical findings, detection of disease-specific antibodies (acetylcholine receptor antibodies in 90% of patients with MG and anti–muscle-specific kinase [MuSK] antibodies in another 5% [with 5% of patients remaining antibody negative]), and EMG findings (such as a characteristic decremental response to repetitive stimulation). CT of the chest should be obtained in patients with MG to screen for thymoma, a tumor associated with the disease.

First-line treatment options in stable patients include the cholinesterase inhibitor pyridostigmine, glucocorticoids, and immunosuppressant agents. Pyridostigmine monotherapy may be sufficient in patients with mild disease but should be avoided in those with acute respiratory failure because the drug increases respiratory secretions. Glucocorticoids can transiently worsen any weakness and

should be started at a lower dosage with slow upward titration in the presence of moderate weakness. In patients with severe weakness, initiation of acute treatment with IVIG or plasmapheresis must precede any glucocorticoid treatment. Glucocorticoid-sparing disease-modifying medications, such as azathioprine, mycophenolate mofetil, and cyclosporine, are mainstays of long-term maintenance therapy in patients with advanced disease. Myasthenic crisis and refractory disease should be treated with plasmapheresis or IVIG. MG associated with anti–MuSK-positive antibodies is typically refractory to pyridostigmine and requires more aggressive immunosuppressive therapy; patients with anti–MuSK-positive antibodies also respond well to plasmapheresis or IVIG.

Thymectomy should be performed in all patients with thymoma. Benefits of thymectomy in other patients are not firmly established, but some experts recommend it for patients with generalized MG who are younger than 65 years and within 3 years of diagnosis.

KEY POINTS

- Myasthenic crisis and refractory myasthenia gravis should be treated with plasmapheresis or intravenous immune globulin.

- Thymectomy should be performed in all patients with myasthenia gravis who have a thymoma.

Lambert-Eaton Myasthenic Syndrome

Lambert-Eaton myasthenic syndrome is an autoimmune disorder caused by autoantibodies against voltage-gated calcium channels located at the presynaptic neuromuscular junction. This condition has a presentation similar to MG except that weakness improves with exercise, and hyporeflexia and dysautonomia are present. Diagnosis is confirmed by detection of serum anti–voltage-gated calcium channel antibodies and the EMG finding of facilitation of motor response to rapid repetitive stimulation. Malignancy, especially small cell lung cancer, is found in as many as 60% of patients with Lambert-Eaton myasthenic syndrome. Therapy consists of treating any underlying malignancy or, in nonparaneoplastic disease, immunosuppression.

KEY POINT

- Malignancy, especially small cell lung cancer, is found in as many as 60% of patients with Lambert-Eaton myasthenic syndrome.

Myopathies

Overview

Myopathies are disorders of the skeletal muscles. Diagnosis requires a systematic approach involving clinical history, measurement of muscle-related serum marker (CK and aldolase) levels, EMG, muscle biopsy, and, in certain patients, genetic and imaging tests.

Most myopathies involve symmetric weakness of the proximal limb muscles. An atypical distribution of weakness in ocular, bulbar, and distal limb muscles may point to a specific cause. Normal sensory and reflex examination can differentiate myopathy from neuropathy. Many myopathies are painless; the presence of pain should prompt investigation of metabolic, toxic, and infectious causes. Rapid progression is suggestive of inflammatory, toxic, or endocrine myopathies, whereas most hereditary myopathies have a stable or slowly progressive course. Mitochondrial myopathies may present with fluctuating weakness and ocular and bulbar involvement.

The serum CK level is elevated in many forms of myopathy and can be followed to monitor disease activity and response to treatment. Mild elevation of the serum CK level (<5 times normal) is not specific to myopathies and can be seen in ALS, CIDP, muscle trauma (falls, post-EMG), and persistent elevation of the serum CK level ("benign hyperCKemia"). Aldolase is a less specific marker of myopathy and can also indicate hematologic or hepatic disease. EMG can help confirm the presence of myopathic changes (such as low amplitude, short duration, and polyphasic motor unit potentials) and determine distribution of involved muscles. Muscle biopsy is the most helpful test to confirm the diagnosis, but in some hereditary myopathies, genetic testing can provide the confirmation without the need for biopsy. The serum CK level should be checked before EMG to prevent procedure-related false-positive results.

KEY POINTS

- Painful myopathies should prompt investigation of metabolic, toxic, and infectious causes.

- The serum creatine kinase level is elevated in many forms of myopathy and can be followed to monitor disease activity and response to treatment.

Inflammatory Myopathy

Idiopathic inflammatory myopathies include polymyositis, dermatomyositis, and inclusion body myositis. Polymyositis and dermatomyositis present with acute or subacute proximal muscle weakness. Involvement of cervical extensor and respiratory muscles can occur in later stages. Muscle pain and tenderness may be present in half of affected patients. Diagnosis is based on a highly elevated serum CK level, myopathic changes on EMG, and inflammatory findings on a muscle biopsy. Biopsy reveals endomysial inflammation in polymyositis and perimysial and perivascular inflammation in dermatomyositis. Dermatomyositis can further be distinguished by its distinct cutaneous manifestations, such as periorbital heliotrope rash and Gottron papules on the hands. Autoantibodies are found in 90% of patients with polymyositis and dermatomyositis.

Inclusion body myositis has a slowly progressive course and has a predilection to affect distal upper extremity flexor, quadriceps, and bulbar muscles. Presentation can be asymmetric and mimic ALS, but upper motoneuron signs are absent. Muscle biopsy reveals inflammation and characteristic inclusion bodies. This condition has a poor response to treatment.

For more information on inflammatory myopathy, see MKSAP 17 Rheumatology.

Endocrine-Related Myopathy

Hypothyroid myopathy can cause diffuse myalgia, proximal muscle weakness, and elevation of the serum CK level. Myoedema, the transient development of an edematous lump in a muscle in response to external percussion, may be seen on examination, as can depressed and delayed reflexes. In contrast, hyperthyroidism can lead to myopathy associated with brisk reflexes, fasciculations, and ophthalmoplegia. Hyperparathyroidism, Addison disease, Cushing disease, and acromegaly also can cause myopathy. Vitamin D deficiency can cause reversible proximal muscle weakness, myalgia, fatigue, and osteomalacia-related bone pain.

Glucocorticoid-Induced Myopathy

Glucocorticoid-induced myopathy usually is seen in patients receiving chronic high-dose treatment. Proximal weakness and myalgia are present. Testing reveals normal serum CK levels and normal EMG findings. In patients treated with glucocorticoids for inflammatory myopathies, persistence of weakness after normalization of the serum CK level may indicate glucocorticoid-induced myopathy. Glucocorticoid-free drug holidays may help decrease the risk of myopathy.

Critical illness myopathy is most often associated with use of intravenous glucocorticoids during prolonged stays in the ICU. However, this condition also may be triggered by prolonged inactivity and exposure to neuromuscular blockade. Patients have profound painless generalized weakness that may impede being weaned off a ventilator. The serum CK level is elevated, which helps to distinguish critical illness myopathy from its less common counterpart critical illness neuropathy. Treatment is supportive and should include weaning off glucocorticoids. H

KEY POINT

- Treatment of critical illness myopathy is supportive and should include weaning off any glucocorticoids.

Toxic Myopathy

Toxic myopathy often presents with painful proximal weakness that progresses rapidly. Statins can cause subacute toxic myopathy associated with rhabdomyolysis. The lipophilic statins, including simvastatin, atorvastatin, and lovastatin, have a higher propensity to cause this problem than the hydrophilic agents pravastatin, rosuvastatin, and fluvastatin. The risk of myopathy increases with higher dosage, the addition of fenofibrate or gemfibrozil, and the addition of cytochrome P3A4 inhibitors (including macrolides, cyclosporine, and itraconazole). Serum CK levels can be mildly or highly elevated. Coenzyme Q_{10} supplementation has been used to protect against statin myopathy, but its benefit remains uncertain. Ethanol, interferon, antiretroviral agents, and antimalarial drugs also cause toxic myopathy.

Inherited Myopathies

Inherited myopathies include muscular dystrophies, channelopathies, and metabolic, congenital, and mitochondrial myopathies. Many of these conditions start early in life, but some present in adulthood. Milder forms of muscular dystrophy, such as Becker and Emery-Dreifuss muscular dystrophy, survive into adulthood and should be closely monitored for cardiac complications. Myotonic dystrophies are associated with myotonia, an impairment of muscle relaxation causing stiffness and a delayed hand-grip release. Myotonic dystrophy type 1 causes distal weakness and is associated with cataracts, frontal balding, and cognitive impairment. Myotonic dystrophy type 2 is milder and causes proximal weakness. Mitochondrial myopathy can present with significant variability and may cause fatigue, myalgia, ophthalmoplegia, and various extramuscular manifestations. The estimated prevalence of mitochondrial myopathies is between 6 and 16 per 100,000 persons, and their presence should be suspected in the presence of multiorgan involvement and maternal transmission. Isolated mild myopathy is less common. Other adult-onset metabolic myopathies can present with isolated exercise-induced weakness, cramps, and myoglobinuria; they include many deficiencies of key metabolic pathways, such as glycogen storage and fatty acid oxidation.

Neuro-oncology

Intracranial Tumors

Intracranial tumors commonly present with new-onset seizures or headache. Rapidly progressing tumors also can present with focal neurologic deficits, including hemiparesis, hemineglect, or a visual field cut. Some tumors, particularly those affecting the frontal lobes and primary central nervous system (CNS) lymphomas (which affect the brain diffusely), can present with sometimes subtle changes in personality, behavior, or cognition. Symptoms of headache, lethargy, nausea, vomiting, and visual changes should prompt concern for a mass lesion causing increased intracranial pressure.

The neurologic examination of a patient with a suspected brain tumor should include an assessment of attention, language, and neglect and also visual field testing. A funduscopic examination should be performed to detect papilledema resulting from increased intracranial pressure. On cranial nerve examination, partial oculomotor nerve palsy (suggested by a dilated, nonreactive pupil) may indicate pressure on the brainstem or early herniation. Unilateral or bilateral abducens nerve palsy can be a sign of increased intracranial pressure. Other cranial nerve findings suggest the direct involvement of the brainstem. Multiple cranial nerve palsies can occur in leptomeningeal disease. Strength, sensation, and coordination should be carefully assessed; deficits may or may not be present, depending on the location of the lesion. Tone and deep tendon reflexes will be decreased acutely with a rapidly progressive lesion affecting the contralateral corticospinal tracts and will be increased with chronic lesions. The plantar response may be extensor contralateral to the lesion. Normal findings on neurologic examination do not exclude the presence of a brain tumor in patients with a concerning history, but focal findings and, particularly, findings of increased intracranial pressure necessitate a more urgent evaluation.

The differential diagnosis of an intracranial tumor includes any space-occupying lesion (such as an abscess, toxoplasmosis, or tuberculoma), sarcoidosis, a demyelinating disease, a vascular malformation, and radiation necrosis. The most useful diagnostic test in a patient with a suspected brain tumor is a contrast-enhanced MRI of the brain. In many instances, specific signal characteristics on the MRI suggest the diagnosis of a primary CNS tumor and even the specific pathology (**Table 39**). CT scans, which more effectively image blood and calcium, are indicated when intracranial bleeding or tumor-related calcification or bone erosion are suspected. PET and MRI spectroscopy can help predict tumor grade or distinguish a tumor from another mass lesion, but these tests are not definitive, are expensive, and are rarely necessary.

Lumbar puncture usually is not necessary in patients in whom the clinical history and MRI findings suggest a primary brain tumor. A lumbar puncture is indicated if the differential diagnosis includes a CNS mass lesion thought to be the result of infection, inflammatory or demyelinating disease, or primary CNS lymphoma. Lumbar puncture is contraindicated if clinical or imaging signs of herniation are present.

Ultimately, a tissue sample often is needed to make a definitive tissue diagnosis of a primary brain tumor. The decision to biopsy a lesion is based on the entire clinical picture. In suspected low-grade or benign tumors, serial MRI scanning is sometimes favored over a biopsy or resection. When an infectious source (such as an abscess or a tuberculoma) is strongly suspected, antibiotic treatment may be attempted before biopsy. In patients with a systemic malignancy and multiple brain lesions suggestive of brain metastases, biopsy usually is not needed for diagnosis.

Glucocorticoids are often used for symptomatic treatment of cerebral edema related to CNS mass lesions. This treatment can be life-saving in patients with impending herniation. However, glucocorticoids also can impede the diagnostic evaluation. For example, they can alter contrast enhancement on an MRI and significantly decrease the sensitivity of brain biopsy results in primary CNS lymphoma. Whenever possible, glucocorticoids should be deferred until after biopsy in patients with suspected CNS lymphoma.

TABLE 39.	Clinical and Radiographic Features of Intracranial Tumors			
Tumor Type	**Typical Age at Onset**	**Imaging Findings**	**Treatment**	**Median Survival**
Metastatic tumor	60+ y	Multifocal lesions at gray-white matter junction; ring enhancement with contrast	Radiation, with or without surgery	10-16 mo
Glioma				
Astrocytoma		Infiltrating white matter lesion	Surgery	
Low-grade (fibrillary)	30-50 y	No enhancement	Surgery, with or without radiation	7-8 y
Anaplastic	35-55 y	Contrast enhancement	Surgery and radiation, with or without temozolomide	3-4 y
Glioblastoma multiforme	45-65 y	Possible hemorrhage, possible multifocal or "butterfly" lesions (bihemispheric)	Surgery and radiation and temozolomide (in older patients, sometimes only one modality is used)	12-15 mo
Oligodendroglioma	30-50 y	Infiltrating white matter lesion; vague contrast enhancement with a "honeycomb" pattern and calcifications that are best seen on CT scan	Surgery and chemotherapy (carmustine or temozolomide), with or without radiation	
Low grade				6-10 y
Anaplastic				3-4 y
Meningioma	50-65 y	Extra-axial (that is, not in the brain parenchyma); calcified, with diffusely enhancing "lightbulb" sign	Possible surgery, possible artery embolization, possible radiation (rare)	
Benign				Rarely limits life expectancy
Atypical				13 y
Anaplastic				3-4 y
Schwannoma	40-50 y	Cerebropontine angle; contrast enhancement	Possible surgery	Rarely limits life expectancy
Dysembryoplastic neuroepithelial tumor	<20 y	Temporal lobe; intracortical location often with small cysts. Contrast enhancement is rare. May be confused with low-grade glioma.	Surgery if intractable seizures, mass effect, or changes on serial MRIs are present	Rarely limits life expectancy
Ganglioglioma	<30y	Temporal lobe; homogeneous or nodular contrast enhancement	Surgery	Rarely limits life expectancy if complete resection possible
Ependymoma	30-40 y[a]	Posterior fossa or spinal cord lesion; contrast enhancement and calcifications, with or without hydrocephalus	Possible surgery, possible radiation	15-20 y
Medulloblastoma	20-30 y[a]	Posterior fossa (cerebellum); contrast enhancement and hydrocephalus	Surgery and radiation, with or without chemotherapy	17-18 y
Primary central nervous system lymphoma		Homogeneous white matter lesion; diffusely enhancing, periventricular, and often multifocal	Chemotherapy (methotrexate), with or without radiation	
Immunocompetent	45-70 y			1-4 y
AIDS-related	30-40 y		Antiretroviral therapy	1-2 y

[a]Age range given is for adult presentation; tumor is most common in children.

KEY POINTS

- The most useful diagnostic test in a patient with a suspected brain tumor is a contrast-enhanced MRI of the brain.

- Glucocorticoids can be life-saving in patients with a mass lesion and impending herniation but can also alter contrast enhancement on an MRI and significantly decrease the sensitivity of brain biopsy results in primary CNS lymphoma.

Metastatic Brain Tumors

Brain metastases are the most common type of intracranial tumor in adults. The tumors most likely to metastasize to the brain are lung cancer, breast cancer, and melanoma. Metastatic brain tumors are often multiple but can be solitary. Typically located at the gray-white matter junction, these tumors exhibit ring enhancement with contrast. The suspicion of a metastatic brain lesion should prompt evaluation for a primary tumor and appropriate cancer staging.

Primary Central Nervous System Tumors

Primary Central Nervous System Gliomas

After metastatic tumors, the second most common intracranial tumors are glial tumors that arise from the supporting tissues that surround neurons. These tumors include astrocytomas, oligodendrogliomas, and ependymomas. Glioblastoma multiforme (World Health Organization grade IV astrocytoma) is the most common and the most aggressive primary CNS tumor.

KEY POINT

- Glioblastoma multiforme is the most common and most aggressive primary CNS tumor.

Primary Central Nervous System Lymphoma

Primary CNS lymphoma (PCNSL) is a non-Hodgkin lymphoma that can affect any part of the CNS but commonly presents as a focal supratentorial lesion. Visual symptoms are common because of frequent tumor involvement of the optic radiations. PCNSL most commonly affects immunocompromised patients but can occur in patients with intact immune systems. An association with the Epstein-Barr virus has been noted. Pathologic analysis, usually of a brain biopsy specimen, is required to make a diagnosis of PCNSL. Diffuse large B cell lymphoma is typical. Cerebrospinal fluid (CSF) cytology can be diagnostic in 10% of patients, although repeated samples often are necessary. Ocular involvement in the vitreous or retina may be seen in 10% to 20% of patients and can be detected with a slit lamp examination and confirmed by vitreal biopsy.

KEY POINT

- Pathologic analysis, usually of a brain biopsy specimen, is required for diagnosis of primary central nervous system lymphoma.

Meningioma

Meningiomas are benign tumors that arise from the meningeal coverings of the brain. They are the most common extra-axial (that is, not in the brain parenchyma) intracranial lesion in adults; other extraparenchymal tumors include schwannomas. Meningiomas are typically slow-growing tumors that often are discovered incidentally; clinical signs generally are subtle. These tumors have characteristic imaging features, including intense homogeneous contrast enhancement ("lightbulb" sign), areas of calcification, and a dural tail, which is thickening of the dura adjacent to the mass (**Figure 25**).

KEY POINT

- Meningiomas are extraparenchymal tumors that can be identified by characteristic radiographic features such as homogeneous enhancement with contrast ("lightbulb" sign).

Management of Intracranial Tumors

Management of Metastatic Brain Tumors

Patients with multiple brain metastases typically are treated with whole-brain radiation, which is associated with a modest increase in survival and control of local tumor growth and symptoms. Stereotactic radiosurgery (radiation administered to a focal area of brain) also is being used with or without whole-brain radiation to minimize neurotoxicity. Surgical resection has become a major initial management option for patients with a solitary, accessible brain metastasis and controlled extracranial disease. Surgery is the best way to rapidly control mass effect from a tumor and tumor-related edema.

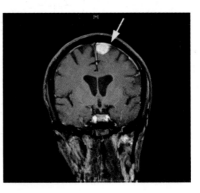

FIGURE 25. Coronal postcontrast T1-weighted MRI showing a left parafalcine meningioma. The tumor enhances homogeneously with contrast, which makes it look like a "lightbulb." Note the "dural tail" (*arrow*).

CONT.

This treatment typically is followed by whole-brain radiation and/or stereotactic radiosurgery.

KEY POINT

- Patients with multiple brain metastases typically are treated with whole-brain radiation, whereas those with a single brain metastasis are usually candidates for surgical resection.

Management of Primary Central Nervous System Gliomas

Whenever possible, the first intervention for primary CNS gliomas is total or near-total resection. The extent of resection is correlated with long-term outcomes. Surgical resection also provides relief of any mass effect and pathologic specimens for diagnosis and prognosis. Patients with glioblastoma multiforme (World Health Organization grade IV astrocytoma) typically receive adjuvant radiation and chemotherapy. Photon radiation is administered to a focal field around the tumor (including a small margin) rather than whole-brain radiation to limit toxicity. Oral temozolomide, an alkylating agent, given in combination with focal radiation has been shown to improve 2- and 5-year survival rates in patients with glioblastoma multiforme compared with radiation alone. Currently, no established standard of care for treatment of grade III gliomas exists. After surgery, chemotherapy and/or radiation often are used and may prolong survival and time to tumor progression. In patients with grade II gliomas, the risks of adjuvant therapies have to be weighed against the potential benefits, particularly in younger patients who typically have longer survivals and greater potential for secondary complications of treatment (such as neurotoxicity or secondary malignancies from radiation or chemotherapy).

Molecular testing of the tumor has had an increasing role in the treatment and prognosis of primary CNS gliomas.

KEY POINT

- Whenever possible, the first intervention for primary central nervous system gliomas is total or near-total resection.

Management of Primary Central Nervous System Lymphoma

The management of primary central nervous system lymphoma (PCNSL) is distinct from the management of CNS gliomas. Resection is not indicated and has been shown to worsen patient outcomes in PCNSL. In patients with PCNSL and HIV infection, the first intervention should be to start antiretroviral therapy; for those who have undergone organ transplantation, immunosuppressive therapy should be stopped, if possible. PCNSL is sensitive to both radiation and chemotherapy. Because PCNSL distribution is universally diffuse throughout the brain, whole-brain (and not focal) radiation is necessary. Most clinicians use systemic methotrexate-based chemotherapy followed

by radiation, although in older patients, radiation sometimes is not used because of the risk of neurotoxicity. Although PCNSL is very sensitive to glucocorticoids, these drugs should be avoided early in the disease because they can limit the usefulness of biopsy and subsequent tissue diagnosis.

KEY POINT

- Resection of primary central nervous system lymphoma is not indicated and can worsen patient outcomes.

Management of Meningiomas

Patients with small, asymptomatic meningiomas without evidence of invasion of other intracranial structures and without surrounding edema are usually followed clinically and radiographically, with a first follow-up MRI performed 3 to 6 months after the tumor is identified to ensure that it is not an atypical meningioma exhibiting rapid growth. Patients with large or symptomatic tumors, tumors that invade surrounding parenchyma, or tumors that grow over time may be considered for surgery and/or radiation therapy. If intervention is indicated, surgical resection is usually the first-line therapy, followed by radiation for higher-grade tumors or tumors that could not be resected completely. Rarely, arterial embolization is used to shrink large tumors before resection.

KEY POINT

- Small asymptomatic meningiomas can be followed conservatively with an initial repeat MRI at 3 to 6 months. **HVC**

Medical Management of Complications of Primary Central Nervous System Tumors

Glucocorticoids often are used to decrease the mass effect associated with edema caused by CNS tumors or by the radiation used to treat them. Drug courses should be kept short to minimize the potentially severe adverse effects of long-term use. All patients taking glucocorticoids should receive calcium and vitamin D supplementation, and bisphosphonates are indicated for those at highest risk of osteoporosis. All patients receiving chronic glucocorticoids or prolonged daily temozolomide should receive prophylaxis for *Pneumocystis jirovecii* pneumonia.

Venous thromboembolism is a common and potentially lethal complication of CNS tumors. Low-molecular-weight heparin is recommended for secondary prevention in patients with these tumors and venous thromboembolism. Inferior vena cava filters should be reserved only for patients with an absolute contraindication to anticoagulation.

Prophylactic use of antiepileptic drugs (AEDs) is not recommended in most patients with brain tumors. AEDs can be used in those with brain tumors and one or more seizures. In these patients, nonenzyme-inducing AEDs, such as lacosamide, lamotrigine, levetiracetam, and valproic acid, are preferred because of their limited interaction with commonly used chemotherapeutic agents.

HVC

KEY POINTS

- For patients with central nervous system tumors who are receiving chronic glucocorticoid or prolonged daily temozolomide therapy, prophylaxis against *Pneumocystis jirovecii* pneumonia is appropriate.

- Prophylactic use of antiepileptic drugs is not recommended in most patients with brain tumors.

Paraneoplastic Neurologic Syndromes

Paraneoplastic neurologic syndromes (PNSs) are a heterogeneous group of conditions affecting multiple targets in the neuraxis of patients with cancer. Symptomatic progression is typically subacute (over a period of weeks). An immune reaction to the primary tumor is thought to be responsible for the generation of autoantibodies that cross-react with epitopes on specific nervous system structures.

A paraneoplastic antibody syndrome should be suspected in patients with subacute neurologic symptoms that are otherwise unexplained (**Table 40**). Because many of these syndromes are associated with cancers, a first step is to ensure that age-appropriate cancer screening testing is current. Consensus guidelines recommend directing further evaluation on the basis of specific paraneoplastic antibody test results, but this testing may detect only 60% of paraneoplastic antibodies, and it may take several weeks for results to be known. For these reasons, it sometimes may be worthwhile to proceed with whole-body CT and PET scanning or with targeted screening for tumors known to be associated with the patient's constellation of symptoms (such as ovarian ultrasonography or pelvic

TABLE 40. Selected Neuronal Paraneoplastic Antibodies

Paraneoplastic Syndrome	Symptoms	Tumor	Antibody
Cerebellar degeneration	Ataxia, dysarthria, dizziness, vertigo	Breast cancer	ANNA-1 (anti-Hu), ANNA-3, MA, PCA-1 (anti-Yo)
		Hodgkin lymphoma	Tr
		Lung cancer (small-cell)	ANNA-1 (anti-Hu), ANNA-3, CRMP-5, MA, PCA-2, VGCC
		Ovarian cancer	ANNA-1 (anti-Hu), ANNA-3, PCA-1 (anti-Yo)
		Testicular cancer	ANNA-1 (anti-Hu), ANNA-3, CRMP-5, MA
		Thymoma	CRMP-5
Encephalomyelitis	+/− Myelitis (spinal cord syndrome), +/− brainsterm signs (common), +/− limbic encephalitis, +/− neuronopathy, +/− cerebellar degeneration	SCLC	ANNA-1 (anti-Hu)
		Testicular, breast, and lung cancer	Ma2
Lambert-Eaton myasthenic syndrome	Muscle weakness	SCLC	VGCC
Limbic encephalitis	Personality change, psychosis, seizures	SCLC, thymoma	CRMP-5, GABA B receptor
		Tumors of thymus, lung, breast	AMPA receptor
	Personality change, psychosis, seizures, and oral dyskinesias	Ovarian/testicular teratoma	NMDA
	Personality change, psychosis, seizures, and SIADH	Lung cancer, thymoma (although cancer is found in < 20% of patients with limbic encephalitis)	LG1 or CASPR2 (previously known as VGKC)
Opsoclonus-myoclonus	Involuntary eye movements and muscle jerks, ataxia	Breast cancer, lung cancer (small-cell)	ANNA-2 (anti-Ri)
Sensory neuronopathy	Painful sensory neuropathy, sensory ataxia, autonomic dysfunction	Lung cancer (small-cell)	ANNA-1 (anti-Hu)
Stiff-person syndrome	Muscle stiffness and spasms	Breast and lung cancer	Amphiphysin, CRMP-5
		Thymoma	CRMP-5

AMPA = anti-M protein antibody; ANNA = antineuronal nuclear antibody; CASPR2 = contactin-associated protein 2; CRMP-5 = collapsin response mediator protein, GABA B, γ-aminobutyric acid B; MA, mitochondrial antibody, NMDA = N-methyl-D-aspartate; PCA = Purkinje cell antibody; SCLC = small cell lung cancer; SIADH = syndrome of inappropriate antidiuretic hormone secretion, VGCC = voltage-gated calcium channel; VGKC = voltage-gated potassium channel.

H
CONT.

MRI for suspected anti–*N*-methyl-ᴅ-aspartate (NMDA) enceph-alitis and chest radiography or CT for patients with sensory neuronopathy).

Most commercial laboratories offer antibody testing in panels, so it is vital to include the antibodies corresponding to the patient's clinical syndrome (see Table 40). Generally speaking, serum or CSF samples can be sent for antibody testing because serum provides a similar sensitivity to CSF. Exceptions to this are anti-NMDA and anti-Tr antibodies, for which CSF is more sensitive than serum.

Often, PNS presents well before a cancer is detected, even with the most sensitive evaluations for a systemic malignancy. Notably, some of the syndromes previously thought to be "paraneoplastic" are now understood to be primary autoimmune disorders for which an underlying tumor will never manifest. Clinical guidelines suggest serial cancer screening for up to 5 years after presentation with a classic PNS. In most instances (90%), the tumor manifests within the first year.

Most PNSs respond to treatment of the underlying tumor. Intravenous immune globulin and/or glucocorticoid administration may facilitate recovery from or stabilization of the PNS, particularly if no tumor is identified. In certain syndromes that have a more aggressive course and are principally autoimmune (such as NMDA encephalitis), immunotherapy with rituximab or cyclosporine is often necessary if other therapies do not to control symptoms. **H**

KEY POINT

- A paraneoplastic antibody syndrome should be suspected in patients with subacutely progressive neurologic symptoms that are otherwise unexplained.

Bibliography

Headache and Facial Pain

Ashkenazi A, Schwedt T. Cluster headache—acute and prophylactic therapy. Headache. 2011 Feb;51(2):272-86. [PMID: 21284609]

Jackson J, Kuriyama A, Hayashino Y. Botulinum toxin A for prophylactic treatment of migraine and tension headache in adults: a meta-analysis. JAMA. 2012 Apr 25;307(16):1736-45. [PMID: 22535858]

Kennedy F, Lanfranconi S, Hicks C, et al; CADISS Investigators. Antiplatelets vs anticoagulation for dissection: CADISS nonrandomized arm and meta-analysis. Neurology. 2012 Aug 14;79(7):686-9. [PMID: 22855862]

Kurth T, Chabriat H, Bousser MG. Migraine and stroke: a complex association with clinical implications (erratum in Lancet Neurol. 2012 Feb;11(2):125). Lancet Neurol. 2012 Jan;11(1)92-100. [PMID: 22172624]

Loder E, Weizenbaum E, Frishberg B, Silberstein S; American Headache Society Choosing Wisely Task Force. Choosing wisely in headache medicine: The American Headache Society's list of five things physicians and patients should question. Headache. 2013 Nov-Dec;53(10):1651-9. [PMID: 24266337]

MacGregor EA. Contraception and headache. Headache. 2013 Feb;53:247-76. [PMID: 23432442]

Nagy A, Gandhi S, Bhola R, Goadsby P. Intravenous dihydroergotamine for inpatient management of refractory primary headaches. Neurology. 2011 Nov 15;77(20):1827-32. [PMID: 22049203]

Palm-Meinders IH, Koppen H, Terwindt GM, et al. Structural brain changes in migraine. JAMA. 2012 Nov 14;308(18):1889-97. [PMID: 23150008]

Schulman E. Refractory migraine—a review. Headache. 2013 Apr;53(4): 599-613. [PMID: 23405959]

Silberstein SD, Holland S, Freitag F, Dodick DW, Argoff C, Ashman E; Quality Standards Subcommittee of the American Academy of Neurology and the American Headache Society. Evidence-based guideline update: pharmacologic treatment for episodic migraine prevention in adults: report of the Quality Standards Subcommittee of the American Academy of Neurology and the American Headache Society [erratum in Neurology. 2013 Feb26;80(9):871]. Neurology. 2012 Apr 24;78(17):1337-45. [PMID: 22529202]

Head Injury

Giza C, Kutcher J, Ashwal S, et al. Summary of evidence-based guideline update: evaluation and management of concussion in sports: report of the Guideline Development Subcommittee of the American Academy of Neurology. Neurology. 2013 Jun 11;80(24):2250-7. [PMID: 23508730]

Hoge CW, McGurk D, Thomas JL, Cox AL, Engel CC, Castro CA. Mild traumatic brain injury in U.S. soldiers returning from Iraq. N Engl J Med. 2008 Jan 31;358(5):453-63. [PMID: 18234750]

Shively SB, Perl DP. Traumatic brain injury, shell shock, and posttraumatic stress disorder in the military—past, present, and future. J Head Trauma Rehabil. 2012 May-Jun;27(3):234-9. [PMID: 22573042]

Theeler B, Lucas S, Riechers RG 2nd, Ruff RL. Post-traumatic headaches in civilians and military personnel: a comparative, clinical review. Headache. 2013 Jun;53(6):881-900. [PMID: 23721236]

Wilk JE, Herrell RK, Wynn GH, Riviere LA, Hoge CW. Mild traumatic brain injury (concussion), posttraumatic stress disorder, and depression in U.S. soldiers involved in combat deployments: association with postdeployment symptoms. Psychosom Med. 2012 Apr;74(3):249-57. [PMID: 22366583]

Seizures and Epilepsy

Arif H, Buchsbaum R, Pierro J, et al. Comparative effectiveness of 10 antiepileptic drugs in older adults with epilepsy. Arch Neurol. 2010 Apr;67(4): 408-15. [PMID: 20385905]

Brophy GM, Bell R, Claassen J, et al; Neurocritical Care Society Status Epilepticus Guideline Writing Committee. Guidelines for the evaluation and management of status epilepticus. Neurocrit Care. 2012 Aug;17(1):3-23. [PMID: 22528274]

Claassen J, Taccone FS, Horn P, Holtkamp M, Stocchetti N, Oddo M. Recommendations on the use of EEG monitoring in critically ill patients: consensus statement from the neurointensive care section of the ESICM. Intensive Care Med. 2013 Aug;39(8):1337-51. [PMID: 23653183]

Epilepsy Foundation. State Driving Laws Database. Available at: www.epilepsy.com/driving-laws.

French JA, Pedley, TA. Clinical practice. Initial management of epilepsy. N Engl J Med. 2008 Jul 10;359(2):166-76. [18614784]

Glauser T, Ben-Menachem E, Bourgeois B, et al; ILAE Subcommision on AED Guidelines. Updated ILAE evidence review of antiepileptic drug efficacy and effectiveness as initial monotherapy for epileptic seizures and syndromes. Epilepsia. 2013 Mar;54(3):551-63. [PMID: 23350722]

Israni RK, Kasbekar N, Haynes K, Berns JS. Use of antiepileptic drugs in patients with kidney disease. Semin Dial. 2006 Sep-Oct;19(5):408-16. [PMID: 16970741]

Krumholz A, Wiebe S, Gronseth G, et al; Quality Standards Subcommittee of the American Academy of Neurology; American Epilepsy Society. Practice Parameter: evaluating an apparent unprovoked first seizure in adults (an evidence-based review): report of the Quality Standards Subcommittee of the American Academy of Neurology and the American Epilepsy Society. Neurology. 2007 Nov 20;69(21):1996-2007. [PMID: 18025394]

Meador KJ, Baker GA, Browning N, et al; NEAD Study Group. Fetal antiepileptic drug exposure and cognitive outcomes at age 6 years (NEAD study): a prospective observational study. Lancet Neurol. 2013 Mar;12(3):244-52. [PMID: 23352199]

Salinsky M, Spencer D, Boudreau E, Ferguson F. Psychogenic nonepileptic seizures in US veterans. Neurology. 2011 Sep 6;77(10):945-50. [PMID: 21893668]

Stroke

Berkhemer OA, Fransen PS, Beumer D, et al; MR CLEAN Investigators. A randomized trial of intraarterial treatment for acute ischemic stroke. N Engl J Med. 2015 Jan;372(1):11-20. [PMID: 25517348]

Connolly ES Jr, Rabinstein AA, Carhuapoma JR, et al; American Heart Association Stroke Council; Council on Cardiovascular Radiology and Intervention; Council on Cardiovascular Nursing; Council on Cardiovascular Surgery and Anesthesia; Council on Clinical Cardiology. Guidelines for the management of aneurysmal subarachnoid hemorrhage: a guideline for healthcare professionals from the American Heart Association/American Stroke Association. Stroke. 2012 Jun;43(6):1711-37. [PMID: 22556195]

Huttner HB, Schwab S. Malignant middle cerebral artery infarction: clinical characteristics, treatment strategies, and future perspectives. Lancet Neurol. 2009 Oct;8(10):949-58. [PMID: 19747656]

Jauch, EC, Saver JL, Adams HP, et al; American Heart Association Stroke Council, Council on Cardiovascular Nursing, Council on Peripheral Vascular Disease, Council on Clinical Cardiology. Guidelines for the early management of patients with acute ischemic stroke: a guideline for healthcare professionals from the American Heart Association/American Stroke Association. Stroke. 2013 Mar;44(3): 870-947. [PMID: 23370205]

Kernan WN, Ovbiagele B, Black HR, et al; American Heart Association Stroke Council, Council on Cardiovascular Nursing, Council on Clinical Cardiovascular and Stroke Nursing, Council on Clinical Cardiology, and Council on Peripheral Vascular Disease. Guidelines for the prevention of stroke in patients with stroke and transient ischemic attack: a guideline for healthcare professionals From the American Heart Association/American Stroke Association. Stroke. 2014 Jul;45:2160-2236. Epub 2014 May 1 [PMID 24788967]

Kumar S, Selim MH, Caplan LR. Medical complications after stroke. Lancet Neurol. 2010 Jan;9(1):105-18. [PMID: 20083041]

Marquardt L, Geraghty OC, Mehta Z, Rothwell PM. Low risk of ipsilateral stroke in patients with asymptomatic carotid stenosis on best medical treatment: a prospective, population-based study. Stroke. 2010 Jan;41(1): e11-7. [PMID: 19926843]

Morgenstern LB, Hemphill JC 3rd, Anderson C, et al; American Heart Association Stroke Council and Council on Cardiovascular Nursing. Guidelines for the management of spontaneous intracerebral hemorrhage: a guideline for healthcare professionals from the American Heart Association/American Stroke Association. Stroke. 2010 Sep;41(9): 2108-29. [PMID: 20651276]

Stroke Unit Trialists' Collaboration. Organised inpatient (stroke unit) care for stroke. Cochrane Database Syst Rev. 2013 Sep 11;9:CD000197. [PMID: 24026639]

van Gijn J, Kerr RS, Rinkel GJ. Subarachnoid hemorrhage. Lancet. 2007 Jan 27;369(9558):306-18. [PMID: 17258671]

Wiebers DO, Whisnant JP, Huston J 3rd, et al; International Study of Unruptured Intracranial Aneurysms Investigators. Unruptured intracranial aneurysms: natural history, clinical outcome, and risks of surgical and endovascular treatment. Lancet. 2003 Jul 12;362(9378):103-10. [PMID: 12867109]

Cognitive Impairment

Albert MS, DeKosky ST, Dickson D, et al. The diagnosis of mild cognitive impairment due to Alzheimer's disease: recommendations from the National Institute on Aging-Alzheimer Association workgroups on diagnostic guidelines for Alzheimer's disease. Alzheimers Dement. 2011 May;7(3):270-9. [PMID: 21514249]

Barr J, Fraser GL, Puntillo K, et al; American College of Critical Care Medicine. Clinical practice guidelines for the management of pain, agitation, and delirium in adult patients in the intensive care unit. Crit Care Med. 2013 Jan;41(1):263-306. [PMID: 23269131]

Inouye SK, van Dyck CH, Alessi CA, Balkin S, Siegal AP, Horwitz RI. Clarifying confusion: the confusion assessment method. A new method for detection of delirium. Ann Intern Med. 1990 Dec 15;113(12):941-8. [PMID: 2240918]

Knopman DS, DeKosky ST, Cummings JL, et al. Practice parameter: diagnosis of dementia (an evidence-based review). Report of the Quality Standards Subcommittee of the American Academy of Neurology. Neurology. 2001 May 8;56(9):1143-53. [PMID: 11342678]

McKee AC, Stern RA, Nowinski CJ, et al. The spectrum of disease in chronic traumatic encephalopathy. Brain. 2013 Jan;136(Pt 1):43-64. [PMID: 23208308]

McKhann GM, Knopman DS, Chertkow H, et al. The diagnosis of dementia due to Alzheimer disease: recommendations from the National Institute on Aging-Alzheimer Association workgroups on diagnostic guidelines for Alzheimer disease. Alzheimers Dement. 2011 May;7(3):263-9. [PMID: 21514250]

O'Mahony R, Murthy L, Akunne A, Young J. Synopsis of the National Institute for Health and Clinical Excellence guideline for prevention of delirium. Ann Intern Med. 2011 Jun 7;154(11):746-51. [PMID: 21646557]

Petersen RC. Clinical practice. Mild cognitive impairment. N Engl J Med. 2011 Jun 9;364(23):2227-34. [PMID: 21651394]

Rascovsky K, Hodges JR, Knopman D, et al. Sensitivity of revised diagnostic criteria for the behavioural variant of frontotemporal dementia. Brain. 2011 Sep;134(Pt 9):2456-77. [PMID: 21810890]

Movement Disorders

Fox SH, Katzenschlager R, Lim SY, et al. The Movement Disorder Society Evidence-Based Medicine Review Update: Treatments for the motor symptoms of Parkinson's disease. Mov Disord. 2011 Oct;26 Suppl 3:S2-41. [PMID: 22021173]

Ghosh R, Liddle BJ. Emergency presentations of Parkinson's disease: early recognition and treatment are crucial for optimum outcome. Postgrad Med J. 2011 Feb;87(1024):125-31. [PMID: 21106801]

Jankovic J. Treatment of hyperkinetic movement disorders. Lancet Neurol. 2009 Sep;8(9):844-56. [PMID: 19679276]

Merlino G, Gigli GL. Sleep-related movement disorders. Neurol Sci. 2012 Jun;33(3):491-513. [PMID: 22203333]

Okun MS. Deep-brain stimulation for Parkinson's disease. New Engl. J. Med. 2012 Oct 18; 367(16):1529-38. [PMID: 23075179]

Robottom BJ, Weiner WJ, Comella CL. Early-onset primary dystonia. Handb Clin Neurol. 2011;100:465-79. [PMID: 21496603]

Seppi K, Weintraub D, Coelho M, et al. The Movement Disorder Society Evidence-Based Medicine Review Update: Treatments for the non-motor symptoms of Parkinson's disease. Mov Disord. 2011 Oct;26 Suppl 3:S42-80. [PMID: 22021174]

Tarsy D, Simon DK. Dystonia. New Engl J Med. 2006 Aug 24;355(8):818-29. [PMID: 16928997]

Walker RH. Differential diagnosis of chorea. Curr. Neurol. Neurosci. Rep. 2011 Aug;11(4):385-95. [PMID: 21465146]

Zesiewicz, TA, Elble, RJ, Louis, ED, et al. Evidence-based guideline update: treatment of essential tremor: report of the Quality Standards subcommittee of the American Academy of Neurology. Neurology. 2011 Nov 8;77(19): 1752-5. [PMID: 22013182]

Multiple Sclerosis

Burton JM, O'Connor PW, Hohol M, Bevene J. Oral versus intravenous steroids for treatment of relapses in multiple sclerosis. Cochrane Database Syst Rev. 2012 Dec 12;12:CD006921. [PMID: 23235634]

Fox RJ, Miller DH, Phillips JT, et al; CONFIRM Study Investigators. Placebo-controlled phase 3 study of oral BG-12 or glatiramer in multiple sclerosis. N Engl J Med. 2012 Sep 20;367(12):1087-97. [PMID 22992072]

Frohman EM, Goodin DS, Calabresi PA, et al; Therapeutics and Technology Assessment Subcommittee of the American Academy of Neurology. The utility of MRI in suspected MS: report of the Therapeutics and Technology Assessment Subcommittee of the American Academy of Neurology. Neurology. 2003 Sep 9;61(5):602-11. [PMID: 12963748]

Frohman EM, Racke MK, Raine CS. Multiple sclerosis—the plaque and its pathogenesis. N Engl J Med. 2006 Mar 2;354(9):942-55. [PMID: 16510748]

Goodin DS, Cohen BA, O'Connor P, Kappos L, Stevens JC; Therapeutics and Technology Assessment Subcommittee of the American Academy of Neurology. Assessment: the use of natalizumab (Tysabri) for the treatment of multiple sclerosis (an evidence-based review): report of the Therapeutics and Technology Assessment Subcommittee of the American Academy of Neurology. Neurology. 2008 Sep 2;71(10):766-73. [PMID: 18765653]

Goodin DS, Frohman EM, Garmany GP Jr, et al; Therapeutics and Technology Assessment Subcommittee of the American Academy of Neurology and the MS Council for Clinical Practice Guidelines. Disease modifying therapies in multiple sclerosis: report of the Therapeutics and Technology Assessment Subcommittee of the American Academy of Neurology and the MS Council for Clinical Practice Guidelines [erratum in Neurology.2002;59(3):480]. Neurology. 2002 Jan 22;58(2):169-78. [PMID: 11805241]

Kappos L, Radue EW, O'Connor P, et al; FREEDOMS Study Group. A placebo-controlled trial of oral fingolimod in relapsing multiple sclerosis. N Engl J Med. 2010 Feb 4;362(5):387-401. [PMID: 20089952]

Mowry EM, Waubant E, McCulloch CE, et al. Vitamin D status predicts new brain magnetic resonance imaging activity in multiple sclerosis. Ann Neurol. 2012 Aug;72(2):234-40. [PMID: 22926855]

Polman CH, Reingold SC, Banwell B, et al. Diagnostic criteria for multiple sclerosis: 2010 revisions to the McDonald criteria. Ann Neurol. 2011 Feb;69(2):292-302. [PMID: 21387374]

Rutschmann OT, McCrory DC, Matchar DB; Immunization Panel of the Multiple Sclerosis Council for Clinical Practice Guidelines. Immunization and MS: a summary of published evidence and recommendations. Neurology. 2002 Dec 24;59(12):1837-43. [PMID: 12499473]

Disorders of the Spinal Cord

Bracken MB. Steroids for acute spinal cord injury. Cochrane Database Syst Rev. 2012 Jan 18;1:CD001046. [PMID 22258943]

Jung HH, Wimplinger I, Jung S, Landau K, Gal A, Heppner FL. Phenotypes of female adrenoleukodystrophy. Neurology. 2007 Mar 20;68(12):960-1. [PMID: 17372139]

Narvid J, Hetts SW, Larsen D, et al. Spinal dural arteriovenous fistulae: clinical features and long-term results. Neurosurgery. 2008 Jan;62(1):159-66. [PMID: 18300903]

Patchell RA, Tibbs PA, Regine WF, et al. Direct decompressive surgical resection in the treatment of spinal cord compression caused by metastatic cancer: a randomised trial. Lancet. 2005 Aug 20-26;366(9486):643-8. [PMID: 16112300]

Scott TF, Frohman EM, De Seze J, Gronseth GS, Weinshenker BG; Therapeutics and Technology Assessment Subcommittee of the American Academy of Neurology. Evidence-based guideline: clinical evaluation and treatment of transverse myelitis: report of the Therapeutics and Technology Assessment Subcommittee of the American Academy of Neurology. Neurology. 2011 Dec 13;77(24):2128-34. [PMID: 22156988]

Transverse Myelitis Consortium Working Group. Proposed diagnostic criteria and nosology of acute transverse myelitis. Neurology. 2002 Aug 27;59:499-505. [PMID: 12236201]

Neuromuscular Disorders

Barohn RJ, Amato AA. Pattern-recognition approach to neuropathy and neuronopathy. Neurol Clin. 2013 May;31(2):343-61. [PMID: 23642713]

Callaghan BC, Cheng HT, Stables CL, Smith AL, Feldman EL. Diabetic neuropathy: clinical manifestations and current treatments. Lancet Neurol. 2012 Jun;11(6):521-34. [PMID: 22608666]

Chawla J, Gruener G; Management of critical illness polyneuropathy and myopathy. Neurol Clin. 2010 Nov;28(4):961-77. [PMID: 20816273]

Dimachkie MM, Barohn RJ. Idiopathic inflammatory myopathies. Semin Neurol. 2012 Jul;32(3):227-36. Epub 2012 Nov 1. [PMID: 23117947]

England JD, Gronseth GS, Franklin G, et al; American Academy of Neurology. Practice Parameter: evaluation of distal symmetric polyneuropathy: role of autonomic testing, nerve biopsy, and skin biopsy (an evidence-based review). Report of the American Academy of Neurology, American Association of Neuromuscular and Electrodiagnostic Medicine, and American Academy of Physical Medicine and Rehabilitation. Neurology. 2009 Jan 13;72(2):177-84. [PMID: 19056667]

Gronseth GS, Paduga R; American Academy of Neurology. Evidence-based guideline update: steroids and antivirals for Bell palsy: report of the Guideline Development Subcommittee of the American Academy of Neurology. Neurology. 2012 Nov 27;79(22):2209-13. Epub 2012 Nov 7. [PMID: 23136264]

Levine TD, Saperstein DS. Laboratory evaluation of peripheral neuropathy. Neurol Clin. 2013 May;31(2):363-76. [PMID: 23642714]

Radunović, A, Mitsumoto, H, Leigh, P. Clinical care of patients with amyotrophic lateral sclerosis. Lancet Neurol. 2007 Oct;6:913-25. [PMID: 17884681]

Silvestri NJ, Wolfe GI. Myasthenia gravis. Semin Neurol. 2012 Jul;32(3):215-26. [PMID: 23117946]

Zivković SA, Lacomis D, Lentzsch S. Paraproteinemic neuropathy. Leuk Lymphoma. 2009 Sep;50(9):1422-33. [PMID: 19637090]

Neuro-oncology

Call JA, Naik M, Rodriguez FJ, et al. Long-term outcomes and role of chemotherapy in adults with newly diagnosed medulloblastoma. Am J Clin Oncol. 2014 Feb;37(1):1-7 [PMID: 23111362]

Ricard D, Idbaih A, Ducray F, Lahutte M, Hoang-Xuan K, Delattre JY. Primary brain tumours in adults. Lancet. 2012 May 26;379(9830):1984-96. [PMID: 22510398]

Glantz MJ, Cole BF, Forsyth PA, et al. Practice parameter: anticonvulsant prophylaxis in patients with newly diagnosed brain tumors. Report of the Quality Standards Subcommittee of the American Academy of Neurology. Neurology. 2000 May 23;54(10):1886-93. [PMID: 10822423]

Lee AY, Levine MN, Baker RI, et al; Randomized Comparison of Low-Molecular-Weight Heparin versus Oral Anticoagulant Therapy for the Prevention of Recurrent Venous Thromboembolism in Patients with Cancer (CLOT) Investigators. Low-molecular-weight heparin versus a coumarin for the prevention of recurrent venous thromboembolism in patients with cancer. N Engl J Med. 2003 Jul 10;349(2):146-53. [PMID: 12853587]

Smith JS, Chang EF, Lamborn KR, et al. Role of extent of resection in the long-term outcome in low-grade hemispheric gliomas. J Clin Oncol. 2008 Mar 10;26(8):1338-45. [PMID: 18323558]

Strupp R, Hegi ME, Mason WP, et al; European Organisation for Research and Treatment of Cancer Brain Tumour and Radiation Oncology Groups; National Cancer Institute of Canada Clinical Trials Group. Effects of radiotherapy with concomitant and adjuvant temozolomide versus radiotherapy alone on survival in glioblastoma in a randomized phase III study: 5 year analysis of the EORTC-NCIC trial. Lancet Oncol. 2009 May;10(5):459-66. [PMID: 19269895]

Titulaer MJ, Soffietti R, Dalmau J, et al; European Federation of Neurological Societies. Screening for tumours in paraneoplastic syndromes: report of an EFNS task force. Eur J Neurol. 2011 Jan;18(1):19-e3. [PMID: 20880069]

Vedeler CA, Antoine JC, Giometto B, et al; Paraneoplastic Neurological Syndrome Euronetwork. Management of paraneoplastic neurological syndromes: report of an EFNS Task Force. Eur J Neurol. 2006 Jul;13(7):682-90. [PMID: 16834698]

Weller M, Stupp R, Hegi ME, et al. Personalized care in neuro-oncology coming of age: why we need MGMT and 1p/19q testing for malignant glioma patients in clinical practice. Neuro Oncol. 2012 Sep;14 Suppl 4:iv100-8. [PMID: 23095825]

Neurology
Self-Assessment Test

This self-assessment test contains one-best-answer multiple-choice questions. Please read these directions carefully before answering the questions. Answers, critiques, and bibliographies immediately follow these multiple-choice questions. The American College of Physicians is accredited by the Accreditation Council for Continuing Medical Education (ACCME) to provide continuing medical education for physicians.

The American College of Physicians designates MKSAP 17 **Neurology** for a maximum of **16** *AMA PRA Category 1 Credits*™. Physicians should claim only the credit commensurate with the extent of their participation in the activity.

Earn "Instantaneous" CME Credits Online

Print subscribers can enter their answers online to earn Continuing Medical Education (CME) credits instantaneously. You can submit your answers using online answer sheets that are provided at mksap.acponline.org, where a record of your MKSAP 17 credits will be available. To earn CME credits, you need to answer all of the questions in a test and earn a score of at least 50% correct (number of correct answers divided by the total number of questions). Take any of the following approaches:

➤ Use the printed answer sheet at the back of this book to record your answers. Go to mksap.acponline.org, access the appropriate online answer sheet, transcribe your answers, and submit your test for instantaneous CME credits. There is no additional fee for this service.

➤ Go to mksap.acponline.org, access the appropriate online answer sheet, directly enter your answers, and submit your test for instantaneous CME credits. There is no additional fee for this service.

➤ Pay a $15 processing fee per answer sheet and submit the printed answer sheet at the back of this book by mail or fax, as instructed on the answer sheet. Make sure you calculate your score and fax the answer sheet to 215-351-2799 or mail the answer sheet to Member and Customer Service, American College of Physicians, 190 N. Independence Mall West, Philadelphia, PA 19106-1572, using the courtesy envelope provided in your MKSAP 17 slipcase. You will need your 10-digit order number and 8-digit ACP ID number, which are printed on your packing slip. Please allow 4 to 6 weeks for your score report to be emailed back to you. Be sure to include your email address for a response.

If you do not have a 10-digit order number and 8-digit ACP ID number or if you need help creating a user name and password to access the MKSAP 17 online answer sheets, go to mksap.acponline.org or email custserv@acponline.org.

CME credit is available from the publication date of July 31, 2015, until July 31, 2018. You may submit your answer sheets at any time during this period.

Directions

*Each of the numbered items is followed by lettered answers. Select the **ONE** lettered answer that is **BEST** in each case.*

Item 1

A 42-year-old man is evaluated in the emergency department for a 1-week history of bilateral leg weakness and numbness. He has an 8-year history of multiple sclerosis (MS) that is currently well controlled with natalizumab; he has had no MS exacerbations since beginning treatment 2 years ago after unsuccessful trials of interferon beta and glatiramer acetate. The patient also has chronic fatigue and depression. Medications are monthly natalizumab, twice daily amantadine and extended-release bupropion, a daily multivitamin, and a calcium–vitamin D supplement that he rarely takes.

On physical examination, temperature is 36.7 °C (98.1 °F), blood pressure is 124/58 mm Hg, pulse rate is 74/min, and respiration rate is 14/min. Muscle strength is 4/5 in the bilateral hip flexors, knee flexors, and foot dorsiflexors. Decreased pinprick sensation is noted just below the umbilicus.

Laboratory studies performed 3 weeks ago showed no evidence of elevated serum antibody titers against the JC virus. Results of current complete blood count, liver chemistry studies, and a urinalysis show no abnormalities.

An MRI of the brain shows white matter hyperintensities consistent with MS and is unchanged from an MRI obtained 1 year ago.

In addition to a 5-day infusion of intravenous methylprednisolone, which of the following is the most appropriate next step in management?

(A) Discontinuation of natalizumab
(B) Measurement of serum 25-hydroxyvitamin D level
(C) MRI of the lumbar spine
(D) Oral trimethoprim-sulfamethoxazole for 5 days

Item 2

A 67-year-old woman is evaluated for a 1-year history of increasing forgetfulness. She reports greater difficulty keeping track of upcoming appointments, recalling details of recent telephone conversations, and remembering names of new acquaintances. She has completed 16 years of formal education, currently works as a teacher's assistant, and has noticed no change in her ability to perform classroom duties, including carrying out the instructions of the teachers with whom she works. The patient lives alone and is able to care for herself, drive, and manage her finances. She describes her mood as "upbeat," continues to enjoy her life, and has had no other symptoms. She does not take any medication.

On physical examination, vital signs are normal. All other physical examination findings, including those from a neurologic examination, are normal. She scores 24/30 on the Montreal Cognitive Assessment, losing points in the orientation and delayed recall sections.

Which of the following is the most likely diagnosis?

(A) Dementia
(B) Depression
(C) Mild cognitive impairment
(D) Normal aging

Item 3

A 35-year-old man is evaluated in the emergency department for a 7-hour history of midback pain and bilateral leg numbness. He was in a bar fight immediately before symptom onset and sustained forceful kick injuries to the back, head, and limbs; he did not lose consciousness.

On physical examination, temperature is 36.6 °C (97.8 °F), blood pressure is 110/70 mm Hg, pulse rate is 108/min, and respiration rate is 18/min; BMI is 32. The patient is alert without any apparent cognitive deficits. Lacerations on the face, scalp, and extremities are noted, as are hematomas on the midback and chest. No tremors or significant swelling or hematomas on the scalp are detected. Muscle strength is 3/5 in the lower extremities, and muscle tone in the legs is reduced. Muscle tone in the arms is normal, and anal sphincter tone is reduced. Pinprick testing shows a sensory level below T8.

Which of the following is the most appropriate next step in management?

(A) CT of the head
(B) High-dose methylprednisolone
(C) MRI of the thoracic spine
(D) Phenytoin

Item 4

A 55-year-old man is evaluated in the emergency department for a 20-minute episode of left eye visual loss without pain followed by a 5-minute episode of slurred speech. He has no residual symptoms. The patient has hypertension treated with amlodipine. He takes no other medication.

On physical examination, blood pressure is 178/92 mm Hg, pulse rate is 78/min and regular, and respiration rate is 12/min. Carotid upstrokes are normal without bruits. Heart rate is regular, and no murmurs are heard. Other physical examination findings, including those from a neurologic examination, are normal.

Findings on an electrocardiogram and a noncontrast CT scan of the head are normal.

Which of the following is the most appropriate next diagnostic test?

(A) Carotid ultrasonography
(B) CT angiography of the neck
(C) MRI of the brain
(D) Transesophageal echocardiography

Item 5

A 42-year-old man comes to the office to discuss results of imaging studies, which were ordered because of a change in his pattern of chronic migraine. Headache episodes have now improved.

On physical examination, temperature is normal, blood pressure is 110/80 mm Hg, pulse rate is 80/min, and respiration rate is 16/min. All other findings from the general physical and neurologic examinations are normal.

A noncontrast CT scan of the head shows a hyperintense extra-axial lesion located between the frontal lobes (parafalcine), which is confirmed by the axial (*top*) and coronal (*bottom*) MRIs shown.

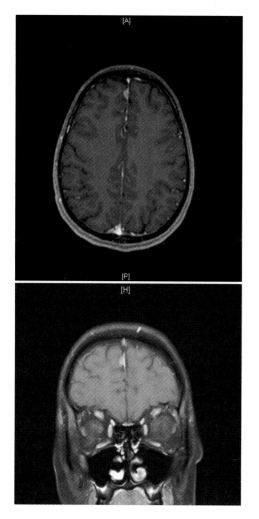

Which of the following is the most appropriate next step in management?

(A) Lumbar puncture
(B) Radiation therapy
(C) Repeat MRI in 3 to 6 months
(D) Surgical resection

Item 6

A 39-year-old woman is evaluated in the emergency department 45 minutes after having a seizure witnessed by her husband. The seizure, which occurred 10 minutes after she awoke this morning, lasted 90 seconds; she reports now being "back to normal." According to her husband, the seizure was characterized by a loud cry and unilateral stiffening and shaking. She has no memory of the seizure but does recall an intense feeling of déjà vu just before losing consciousness; she reports that she has had a similar sensation lasting 5 to 15 seconds several times over the past few years. She had been at a birthday celebration the night before her seizure, had

several alcoholic drinks, and stayed out late, which is unusual for her. She says she fell on ice 1 month ago, striking her head; except for a mild headache that lasted for several days after the fall, she has had no residual symptoms. She has no other significant medical history and takes no medication.

On physical examination, temperature is 37.2 °C (99.0 °F), blood pressure is 120/70 mm Hg, pulse rate is 95/min, and respiration rate is 14/min. All other findings from the general physical and neurologic examinations are unremarkable.

Results of laboratory studies are normal, including a blood ethanol level of 0.

Which of the following is the most likely diagnosis?

(A) Alcohol withdrawal seizure
(B) Focal epilepsy
(C) Generalized epilepsy
(D) Posttraumatic seizure

Item 7

A 48-year-old man is evaluated for increasing depression and suicidal ideation. He reports experiencing feelings of hopelessness, lack of initiative, and general disinterest over the past 5 years that recently have worsened and are now accompanied by mood swings, irritability, impatience, verbal abuse, and physical aggression. Thoughts of death and suicide often have been present in the past month. His gait has become slow and shuffling, and his balance is increasingly impaired. His wife says he is more forgetful than ever and unable to perform home repairs that he previously accomplished easily. He has had no hallucinations or delusions. The patient is retired from a 13-year career playing professional football. Other than minor football injuries, he has no significant medical history and has an unremarkable family history, including no neurologic and psychological disorders. The patient takes no medication.

On physical examination, vital signs are normal. Neurologic examination shows slow processing speed, mild dysarthria, slowed rapid alternating movements bilaterally, and a wide-based gait with decreased foot-floor clearance. The patient scores 20/30 on the Montreal Cognitive Assessment, losing points in the visuospatial/executive function, attention, orientation, and delayed recall sections.

Which of the following is the most likely diagnosis?

(A) Chronic traumatic encephalopathy
(B) Dementia with Lewy bodies
(C) Depression-related cognitive impairment
(D) Parkinson disease

Item 8

A 48-year-old woman is evaluated for a 12-month history of increasingly severe headaches. For the past 25 years, she has had monthly migraine without aura. The headaches have occurred one or two times per month, but over the past year, their severity has increased, with NSAIDs now providing only limited, temporary pain relief. Medications are ibuprofen and naproxen as needed (≤5 days/mo).

On physical examination, blood pressure is 116/70 mm Hg and pulse rate is 80/min. Other physical examination findings, including those from a neurologic examination, are normal.

An MRI of the brain shows several punctate hyperintensities in the bilateral subcortical white matter.

Which of the following is the most appropriate management?

(A) Aspirin
(B) Lumbar puncture
(C) Magnetic resonance angiography
(D) Rizatriptan
(E) Timolol

Item 9

A 26-year-old woman is evaluated for a 10-year history of recurrent episodes of acute-onset feelings of fear and anxiety. These episodes initially occurred approximately four times per year but for the past 3 months have been occurring once or twice per month, especially when she is under stress. She describes the episodes as paroxysmal attacks of fear and anxiety associated with a dry mouth and a consistent "roller coaster" sensation in her stomach that typically last 15 seconds to 1 minute. With more intense attacks, she becomes momentarily confused; her boyfriend says she seems "fidgety" when this occurs. She feels well between episodes. Medical history is otherwise negative, and she takes no medication.

On physical examination, vital signs are normal. All other findings from the general physical and neurologic examinations are unremarkable.

A brain MRI and electroencephalogram are normal.

Which of the following is the most likely diagnosis?

(A) Frontal lobe epilepsy
(B) Juvenile absence epilepsy
(C) Panic disorder
(D) Psychogenic nonepileptic seizures
(E) Temporal lobe epilepsy

Item 10

A 51-year-old woman is evaluated in the emergency department for sudden-onset severe headache and right-sided weakness followed by temporary loss of consciousness that occurred 30 minutes ago. According to her husband, she has hypertension treated with amlodipine and a 20-pack-year smoking history; she stopped smoking 12 years ago.

On physical examination, blood pressure is 158/68 mm Hg, pulse rate is 68/min and regular, and respiration rate is 10/min. Funduscopic examination findings are normal. Nuchal rigidity is noted. On neurologic examination, the patient does not follow commands and has flexor posturing to painful stimuli; pupils are reactive and symmetric in size and shape.

An electrocardiogram shows normal sinus rhythm and no ischemic changes.

Which of the following is the most appropriate next diagnostic test?

(A) Catheter-based cerebral angiography
(B) CT of the head without contrast

(C) Lumbar puncture
(D) MRI of the brain without contrast

Item 11

A 45-year-old man is evaluated for generalized weakness and stiffness. He has had slowly progressive weakness of the lower extremities for the past 5 years. The patient reports that he feels "wobbly" during ambulation, easily becomes fatigued, has bouts of stiffness in the upper and lower extremities, has occasional difficulty holding his hand above his head, and cannot easily stand up from a chair. He has had no diplopia, numbness, or tingling. He says that sometimes it is difficult to release his grip after turning a door knob. Medical history includes cardiomyopathy, first-degree heart block, and cataract surgery 1 year ago. He has a brother with muscle weakness. His only medication is metoprolol.

On physical examination, vital signs are normal. Bilateral ptosis that does not worsen with sustained upward gaze is noted, as is bilateral facial drooping. Speech is dysarthric. Proximal limb muscles are tight, and finger abductors and foot dorsal flexors are weak bilaterally. A delay in releasing his hand grip and slow relaxation of the muscles after percussion are noted. Gait is stiff and unstable.

Which of the following is the most likely diagnosis?

(A) Becker muscular dystrophy
(B) Inclusion body myositis
(C) Lambert-Eaton myasthenic syndrome
(D) Myasthenia gravis
(E) Myotonic dystrophy

Item 12

A 67-year-old man is evaluated in the emergency department for sudden onset of severe headache that has not abated over the past 24 hours.

On physical examination, temperature is 37.4 °C (99.3 °F), blood pressure is 168/78 mm Hg, pulse rate is 68/min and regular, and respiration rate is 12/min. Nuchal rigidity is noted. The left pupil is 5 mm in diameter and unreactive to light, and the right pupil is 3 mm in diameter and reactive to light. A neurologic examination shows normal mental status and motor function.

A CT of the head without contrast is normal.

Which of the following is the most appropriate next diagnostic test?

(A) Lumbar puncture
(B) Magnetic resonance angiography of the brain
(C) Magnetic resonance venography of the brain
(D) MRI of the brain

Item 13

A 69-year-old man is evaluated for a 1-year history of increasing word-finding difficulties. The patient also reports occasional difficulty recalling names of objects and people and has had problems comprehending conversations. His daughter reports sometimes not understanding what her father is saying because of his frequent use of filler words, such as "that thing" and "you know"; she says that otherwise his mind seems sharp, his cognition unimpaired, and his memory excellent. He has no other significant medical history, and he takes no medication. His older brother had onset of dementia at age 56 years, and his father developed dementia at age 60 years.

On physical examination, vital signs are normal. General physical examination results are unremarkable, and a neurologic examination yields no focal findings. However, the patient has trouble answering even simple questions about where he lives or what he had for breakfast and is unable to name simple objects.

Results of laboratory studies, including a complete blood count, comprehensive metabolic profile, and thyroid function studies, are normal.

An MRI of the brain is normal.

Which of the following is the most appropriate next step in management?

(A) Determination of apolipoprotein E (*APOE ε4*) status
(B) Observation with reevaluation in 3 to 6 months
(C) Speech and language therapy
(D) Trial of donepezil

Item 14

A 72-year-old woman is evaluated for a 6-month history of gradually worsening, nonsuppressible involuntary movements. The patient first noticed twitching movements of the lower part of the face, with occasional unintended thrusting of the tongue through the lips and biting of the cheeks inside the mouth. She further reports pressure and a pulling sensation at the back of the neck that causes her head to pull backward suddenly and the occasional tendency to drop objects from her hands secondary to uncontrollable jerking movements. The patient has chronic gastroparesis that is treated with metoclopramide and bipolar disorder that is well controlled with lamotrigine and quetiapine. She has no family history of a movement disorder or any neurologic disease.

On physical examination, temperature is 37.5 °C (99.5 °F), blood pressure is 145/76 mm Hg, and pulse rate is 80/min. Frequent stereotyped pursing movements of the lips, occasional tongue protrusion and forceful jaw closure, continual slow and nonrhythmic movements of the fingers, and recurrent cervical retrocollis are noted. Occasional rapid jerking movements of the arms and infrequent facial grimacing also are present. Gait is slow and marked by short steps and reduced arm swing.

Which of the following is the most appropriate next step in management?

(A) Change quetiapine to risperidone
(B) Discontinue metoclopramide
(C) Start carbidopa-levodopa
(D) Start tetrabenazine

Item 15

A 40-year-old woman is seen for a follow-up evaluation of multiple sclerosis, which was diagnosed 1 month ago.

The patient reports feeling generally well. She has no significant medical history and does not drink or smoke. Her only medication is interferon beta-1a, which she has been taking since diagnosis and tolerates well.

On physical examination, vital signs are normal. Neurologic examination reveals internuclear ophthalmoplegia, right arm weakness, and mild ataxia, which were present at diagnosis and have remained stable. All other physical examination findings are unremarkable.

Which of the following is indicated for periodic monitoring of this patient's disease-modifying therapy?

(A) JC virus antibody measurement
(B) Ophthalmologic evaluation
(C) Serum aminotransferase measurement
(D) Serum amylase and lipase measurement

Item 16

A 68-year-old woman is evaluated 1 month after having an ischemic stroke of the left thalamus. She now has only residual right-sided anesthesia. The patient has hypertension and dyslipidemia, both well controlled by medication, and had been taking a daily aspirin before the stroke. Medications are lisinopril, chlorthalidone, aspirin, and rosuvastatin.

On physical examination, blood pressure is 128/68 mm Hg and pulse rate is 68/min and regular. Findings from the remainder of the general physical examination are normal, including no carotid bruits on cardiac examination. Neurologic examination findings include decreased sensation to light touch and pinprick throughout the right side.

Which of the following is the most appropriate treatment?

(A) Add clopidogrel
(B) Add dipyridamole
(C) Substitute ticlopidine for aspirin
(D) Substitute warfarin for aspirin

Item 17

A 27-year-old woman comes to the office to discuss medications 3 days after experiencing a first seizure. MRI evaluation on the day of the seizure showed left mesial temporal sclerosis, and a subsequent electroencephalogram was significant for temporal sharp waves, findings consistent with temporal lobe epilepsy. She has polycystic ovary syndrome and requires a daily estrogen-progestin combination for symptom management and contraception.

Physical examination findings, including vital signs, are normal.

Which of the following antiepileptic drugs is most appropriate?

(A) Carbamazepine
(B) Lamotrigine
(C) Levetiracetam
(D) Oxcarbazepine
(E) Topiramate

Item 18

An 83-year-old woman is evaluated in the emergency department for a 36-hour history of left-sided weakness. She has noticed no changes in vision or speech. The patient has hypertension and dyslipidemia. Medications are aspirin, losartan, metoprolol, and atorvastatin.

On physical examination, blood pressure is 168/102 mm Hg, pulse rate is 78/min and regular, and respiration rate is 16/min. Other findings from the general medical examination are normal. Neurologic examination shows grade 4/5 weakness of the left face, arm, and leg; dysarthria; and unsteady gait. Her score on the National Institutes of Health Stroke Scale is 8, indicating a moderate stroke; she coughed after attempting to swallow 30 mL of water.

Results of laboratory studies are normal.

An electrocardiogram is normal. A CT scan of the head without contrast shows an infarct in the right pons.

Which of the following is most likely to reduce the 1-year mortality risk in this patient?

(A) Add clopidogrel
(B) Administer labetalol intravenously
(C) Administer recombinant tissue plasminogen activator (rtPA)
(D) Admit to the stroke unit

Item 19

A 24-year-old man is seen for management of seizures. His first seizure occurred 5 years ago, at which time he had a normal MRI and electroencephalogram. Since that time, he has had two additional seizures, one 2 years ago and the other last week. All seizures have been convulsive and occurred without warning. The patient reports being under stress or sleep deprived around the time of the seizures. He has had no paroxysmal symptoms, including staring spells or morning jerks. He takes no medication.

Physical examination findings, including vital signs, are unremarkable.

Laboratory studies, including a complete blood count, a comprehensive metabolic profile, and measurement of serum thyroid-stimulating hormone level, have normal results.

Which of the following treatments is most appropriate?

(A) Carbamazepine
(B) Gabapentin
(C) Phenytoin
(D) Topiramate

Item 20

A 72-year-old man is evaluated for a 1-year history of progressively impaired gait and balance. He reports that he walks more slowly and is not as agile as he used to be, attributing a recently increased number of falls to not paying enough attention before tripping. In the past 6 months, he has had occasional problems recalling details of recent conversations and events, completing tasks around the house in a timely manner, and organizing and balancing his checkbook despite having been an accountant before retiring. The patient also reports some urinary urgency and frequency but otherwise feels well. He has hypertension treated with hydrochlorothiazide and no history of traumatic brain injury, meningitis, or intracranial hemorrhage.

On physical examination, vital signs are normal. General medical examination findings are unremarkable. On neurologic examination, gait is slow, with poor foot clearance, shuffling, multistep turns, and intermittent hesitation. Tandem gait is impaired. The remainder of the physical examination is unremarkable. He scores 23/30 on the Mini-Mental State Examination, with points deducted on the delayed recall and serial 7 calculation sections.

An MRI of the brain is shown.

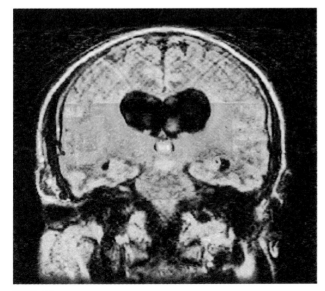
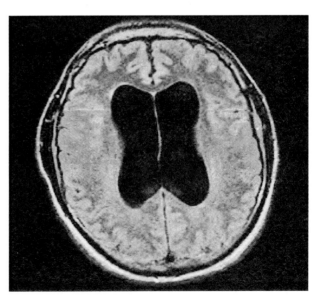

ITEM 20

H CONT.

Which of the following is the most appropriate next step in management?

(A) Brain magnetic resonance angiography
(B) Large-volume lumbar puncture
(C) Trial of donepezil
(D) Trial of levodopa

Item 21

H A 40-year-old man is evaluated in the emergency department for a headache that started 1 day ago while he was lifting weights. He first experienced a severe, sharp, right periorbital pain associated with nausea and ipsilateral neck pain. Although the pain has lessened in intensity, it has persisted, and this morning he had an episode of right monocular visual loss resolving spontaneously after several minutes. The patient has a history of monthly migraine without aura that typically lasts 6 hours and is characterized by bilateral frontotemporal throbbing, pain associated with photophobia, and nausea. He says that his current headache pain is "different" from the pain he experiences during migraine episodes and that the neck pain is new. His only medication is naproxen as needed.

On physical examination, blood pressure is 130/86 mm Hg and pulse rate is 72/min. Palpation of the neck elicits pain. Right ptosis and miosis are noted, but all other physical examination findings are unremarkable.

A CT scan of the head shows normal findings.

Which of the following is the most likely diagnosis?

(A) Carotid artery dissection
(B) Cluster headache
(C) Migraine
(D) Vertebral artery dissection

Item 22

H A 30-year-old man is evaluated in the hospital for hyponatremia and dizziness. He reports a 3-day history of fatigue, headache, and imbalance. The patient has had difficult-to-manage nonlesional epilepsy since age 9 years and has required multiple drugs to maintain a seizure rate of only two or three per month. He has no other significant medical history. Medications are oxcarbazepine, levetiracetam, topiramate, and clonazepam.

On physical examination, mental status is normal. Temperature is 37.3 °C (99.1 °F), blood pressure is 95/60 mm Hg, pulse rate is 100/min, and respiration rate is 14/min. Examination of the eyes reveals end-gaze nystagmus in both directions of gaze; the optic discs are sharp. Gait is ataxic.

Laboratory studies:

Creatinine	0.7 mg/dL (61.9 µmol/L)
Electrolytes	
Sodium	123 mEq/L (123 mmol/L)
Potassium	3.5 mEq/L (3.5 mmol/L)
Chloride	110 mEq/L (110 mmol/L)
Bicarbonate	23 mEq/L (23 mmol/L)

Which of the following medications is most likely responsible for this patient's findings?

(A) Clonazepam
(B) Levetiracetam
(C) Oxcarbazepine
(D) Topiramate

Item 23

A 68-year-old woman is evaluated for memory deficits. She retired from her position as a high school principal 2 years ago. In the past 6 months, she has had increasing forgetfulness, difficulty organizing her belongings, and problems with concentration and indecisiveness; during this period, she also has noticed fatigue, decreased energy, difficulty falling asleep, diminished interest in reading, and decreased appetite, which has caused her to lose 4.5 kg (10.0 lb). The patient has remained independent in activities of daily living, although she has forgotten to pay several monthly bills. She moved closer to her son last year but now has few opportunities to see her friends, which has resulted in feelings of isolation and sadness. The patient had a depressive episode 28 years ago after her husband's death. She takes no medication.

On physical examination, vital signs and general physical examination findings are normal. Neurologic examination reveals psychomotor slowing without decremental response on repetitive finger tapping. The patient scores 27/30 on the Mini–Mental State Examination, losing three points in the attention and calculation section.

Results of a complete blood count, a comprehensive metabolic profile, thyroid function tests, and urinalysis are normal.

Which of the following is the most appropriate next step in management?

(A) Carbidopa-levodopa
(B) Donepezil
(C) Sertraline
(D) Clinical observation

Item 24

A 27-year-old woman is evaluated for a severe migraine with typical aura and right-sided sensory symptoms that occurred 1 day ago. Migraine was diagnosed at age 13 years, is often preceded by 45 minutes of visual loss (which she describes as "losing half my sight"), is only associated with onset of menses, involves hemicranial throbbing pain associated with nausea and vomiting, and lasts 90 minutes if treated and 24 hours if untreated. Yesterday's migraine was again preceded by the typical visual loss and 40 minutes later by numbness and paresthesia in the right upper extremity, starting in her hand and migrating toward her forearm; these sensations eventually involved her right tongue and throat, lasted an additional 50 minutes, and then resolved completely. The patient has experienced no recurrence of symptoms in the past 24 hours. Medications are rizatriptan and a combined estrogen-progesterone oral contraceptive initiated 3 months ago at a family planning clinic.

On physical examination, blood pressure is 122/72 mm Hg and pulse rate is 66/min. All other physical examination findings, including those from a neurologic examination, are unremarkable.

Findings on a brain MRI and magnetic resonance angiogram are normal.

Which of the following is the most appropriate next step in management?

(A) Administer daily aspirin
(B) Administer daily topiramate
(C) Discontinue combined oral contraceptive
(D) Discontinue rizatriptan

Item 25

A 54-year-old man is seen for follow-up evaluation of a tremor in his upper extremities that has been present since age 20 years. The tremor was mild for many years and did not interfere with his work but has become more prominent in recent years. He has difficulty writing and using utensils during meals. He has no associated slowness, stiffness, or change in gait. The patient started a trial of propranolol, which provided better control of the tremor, but after a few months, the tremor again worsened. He has subsequently been taking clonazepam without significant relief of symptoms. Alcohol, which the patient uses infrequently, temporarily diminishes the tremor. He also has kidney stones and glaucoma. His father and two sisters have a similar tremor.

On physical examination, vital signs are normal. A persistent large-amplitude tremor of the upper extremities is noted when the patient holds his arms in an outstretched position and during finger-to-nose testing. The tremor is bilateral and absent at rest. Tandem gait cannot be performed, but gait is otherwise normal.

Which of the following is the most appropriate next step in treating this patient's tremor?

(A) Botulinum toxin
(B) Deep brain stimulation
(C) Levodopa
(D) Primidone
(E) Topiramate

Item 26

A 68-year-old man is evaluated in the hospital for midback pain and right leg weakness. A radiograph of the thoracic spine obtained in the emergency department showed a lytic lesion at T7, and an MRI showed extension of an associated mass lesion into the epidural space, which is causing compression of the spinal cord without spinal instability. His only medication is a daily multivitamin.

High-dose glucocorticoids are administered, and results of a stereotactic biopsy of the mass show a plasmacytoma.

On physical examination, temperature is 37.2 °C (99.0 °F). Other vital signs and findings of a general physical examination are normal. Sensory level is to T8.

Which of the following is the most appropriate next step in treatment?

(A) Chemotherapy
(B) Continued high-dose glucocorticoids only
(C) Radiation therapy
(D) Surgery

Item 27

A 34-year-old man is evaluated in the emergency department for worsening headache, nausea, and two episodes of vomiting 2 hours after hitting his head in a fall from the top of a 6-foot ladder.

On physical examination, temperature is normal, blood pressure is 128/84 mm Hg, pulse rate is 86/min, and respiration rate is 14/min. The patient's Glasgow Coma Scale score is 15/15.

Which of the following is the most appropriate immediate step in management?

(A) Head CT with contrast
(B) Head CT without contrast
(C) Hospital observation
(D) MRI of the brain

Item 28

An 82-year-old woman is seen for follow-up evaluation of Alzheimer disease. Since her last visit 12 weeks ago, she has been taking rivastigmine, with a progressively titrated dosage. The patient's only new symptoms are increasing insomnia, loss of appetite, and occasional diarrhea; she has had no feelings of hopelessness, helplessness, sadness, or guilt. Her only other medication is hydrochlorothiazide for hypertension.

On physical examination, vital signs are normal. The patient has lost 6.8 kg (15.0 lb) since her last visit. She scores 20/30 on a Mini–Mental State Examination, losing points in the recall, orientation to time, complex commands, and attention and calculation sections; her score 12 weeks ago was 21/30. All other findings from the general physical and neurologic examinations are normal.

Results of laboratory studies, including a complete blood count, comprehensive metabolic profile, and thyroid function tests, are normal.

Which of the following is the most appropriate next step in management?

(A) Add donepezil
(B) Add memantine
(C) Add mirtazapine at bedtime
(D) Discontinue rivastigmine

Item 29

A 42-year-old woman is evaluated for progressive difficulty with eyelid closure. She initially noticed frequent blinking 3 years ago; within the past year, she also began having unintended, prolonged, and forceful closure of both eyes that now prevents her driving. Bright light, prolonged conversation, and psychological stress aggravate her symptoms. The severity of symptoms fluctuates from day to day, but she does not have any symptom-free days. She reports occasional blurry vision but has had no visual field loss or diplopia, has no sensory numbness, and has had no other abnormal movements involving the face, head, limbs, or trunk.

On physical examination, vital signs are normal. Examination of the eyes shows repetitive and bilateral clonic eyelid closures that occasionally involve forceful closure of the eyes that the patient cannot resist or suppress. The intensity of these movements varies during the examination. No facial grimacing, asymmetry, or other abnormal movements are noted. Other findings of the general medical and neurologic examinations are normal.

An MRI of the brain is unremarkable.

Which of the following is the most appropriate treatment?

(A) Botulinum toxin
(B) Clonidine
(C) Deep brain stimulation
(D) Risperidone

Item 30

A 44-year-old man is evaluated for a 6-month history of a persistent burning sensation in the feet. He has had no numbness or weakness. Medical history is significant for hyperlipidemia. His only medication is simvastatin.

On physical examination, blood pressure is 145/85 mm Hg sitting and 130/70 mm Hg standing, pulse rate is 75/min sitting and 65/min standing, and respiration rate is 14/min; BMI is 33. Mild red discoloration and sweating of both palms are noted. Cranial nerve examination findings are normal, motor strength is intact, deep tendon reflexes are normal, and no sensory deficit to light touch, pinprick or vibration is noted. Deep tendon reflexes and gait are normal.

Results of laboratory studies include normal fasting plasma glucose, hemoglobin A_{1c}, vitamin B_{12}, and folate levels.

An electromyogram shows no evidence of neuropathy or myopathy.

Which of the following is the most appropriate diagnostic test to perform next?

(A) Glucose tolerance test
(B) MRI of the lumbosacral spine
(C) Serum vitamin D measurement
(D) Sural nerve biopsy

Item 31

A 40-year-old man is reevaluated for a 1-year history of recurrent tonic-clonic seizures that have not responded to treatment with valproic acid and topiramate. When describing the seizures, his wife says that he usually drops to the ground and begins "shaking all over"; the shaking typically lasts 10 to 15 minutes, with the patient's

eyes remaining closed during the event. He subsequently is confused for 30 to 60 minutes. The seizures initially occurred 1 or 2 times per month but recently have been occurring every other day. On several occasions, he has become incontinent. He is a military veteran who sustained a closed head injury in combat 5 years ago and has posttraumatic stress disorder. Medications are twice daily valproic acid and topiramate.

On physical examination, vital signs are normal. General medical examination findings are normal. On neurologic examination, flattening of the nasolabial fold on the right is noted, and right pronator drift is present. Deep tendon reflexes are 3+ in the right upper and lower extremities. A plantar extensor response is noted in the right toe.

Results of laboratory studies are normal, with a serum valproic acid level within the therapeutic range.

An MRI of the brain reveals left frontal lobe encephalomalacia. An electroencephalogram (EEG) shows intermittent left frontal slowing.

Which of the following is the most appropriate management?

(A) Ambulatory EEG monitoring
(B) Carbamazepine
(C) Levetiracetam
(D) Video EEG monitoring

Item 32

A 50-year-old man is evaluated for a 1-year history of increasing urinary frequency and urgency and occasional urge incontinence. He has no symptoms of urinary hesitancy or incomplete emptying. The patient has primary progressive multiple sclerosis. Medications are dalfampridine and vitamin D.

On physical evaluation, temperature is 36.8 °C (98.2 °F), blood pressure is 120/55 mm Hg, and pulse rate is 68/min. Findings of abdominal and digital rectal examinations are normal. Finger-to-nose testing reveals dysmetria bilaterally. Leg tone is increased bilaterally. Muscle strength is 4/5 in both legs. Gait testing reveals spasticity and ataxia.

A urinalysis is negative for infection.

Which of the following is the most appropriate treatment?

(A) Finasteride
(B) Intermittent urinary catheterization
(C) Oxybutynin
(D) Prophylactic antibiotics

Item 33

An 80-year-old man is evaluated for a 5-year history of progressive cognitive decline. According to his daughter, his cognitive difficulties began after a series of "ministrokes" characterized by the acute onset of slurred speech, difficulty ambulating, and weakness; these symptoms typically improved after onset but never resolved entirely. He recently has had difficulty managing his financial affairs, completing tasks, and understanding abstract concepts; other recent symptoms include a slowed reaction time, slowness in speaking and completing tasks, shuffling of gait, urinary incontinence, and sudden involuntary laughing and crying. The patient has hypertension, coronary artery disease, depression, and hyperlipidemia. Medications are lisinopril, aspirin, bupropion, and atorvastatin.

On physical examination, vital signs are normal. Other findings from the general physical examination are unremarkable. Neurologic examination reveals mild right-sided weakness, right-sided hyperreflexia, and difficulty initiating forward movement of the feet ("magnetic gait").

An MRI of the brain shows extensive periventricular white matter lesions and small-vessel disease involving the basal ganglia. The ventricles are normal in size.

Which of the following is the most likely diagnosis?

(A) Alzheimer disease
(B) Normal pressure hydrocephalus
(C) Parkinson disease dementia
(D) Vascular neurocognitive disorder

Item 34

An 80-year-old man is evaluated for a 2-year history of sudden-onset episodes of flashing lights in the right visual field that typically last 10 to 20 seconds. He does not believe that he loses awareness during these events, but his daughter, who accompanied him, reports that he stared and smacked his lips during the two recent episodes she witnessed. Symptoms started 6 months after he had a cryptogenic stroke of the left occipital lobe. The patient also has hypertension. Medications are aspirin, atorvastatin, and lisinopril.

On physical examination, temperature is 36.7 °C (98.0 °F), blood pressure is 140/90 mm Hg, and pulse rate is 67/min and irregular. Visual field testing reveals right homonymous hemianopia. All other findings from the general physical and neurologic examinations are within normal limits.

An MRI reveals a chronic infarct in the territory of the left posterior cerebral artery.

Which of the following is the most appropriate treatment?

(A) Carbamazepine
(B) Lamotrigine
(C) Oxcarbazepine
(D) Phenytoin

Item 35

A 57-year-old man is seen for follow-up evaluation after results of a carotid ultrasound obtained to investigate a left neck bruit show a mixed density plaque at the origin of the left internal carotid artery. Stenosis is estimated to be 60% to 80%. He has had no focal neurologic symptoms or visual loss. The patient has coronary artery disease (CAD) with stable angina, hypertension, dyslipidemia, type 2 diabetes mellitus, and mild kidney failure. He has a 30-pack-year smoking history but stopped smoking 7 years ago when CAD was diagnosed. Medications are aspirin, metoprolol, lisinopril, metformin, and nitroglycerin, as needed. He was taking rosuvastatin but discontinued the medication 2 years ago after developing muscle aches.

On physical examination, blood pressure is 132/78 mm Hg, pulse rate is 78/min and regular, and respiration rate is 16/min. The left neck bruit is unchanged. Cardiopulmonary examination has normal results. All other findings from the general medical and neurologic examinations are unremarkable.

Which of the following is the most appropriate next step in management?

(A) Carotid endarterectomy
(B) Magnetic resonance angiography of the neck
(C) Resumption of statin therapy
(D) Substitution of clopidogrel for aspirin

Item 36

A 47-year-old woman is evaluated in the emergency department for recurrent attacks of severe holocranial pain that began 2 days ago while she was gardening. She first experienced a rapidly progressive, global, explosive headache that lasted 30 minutes and was associated with photophobia and phonophobia. She had identical symptoms 6 hours ago and additionally had 30 minutes of visual blurring and numbness of the left face and left upper extremity. The patient has attention-deficit disorder for which dextroamphetamine was initiated 2 weeks ago. She has no significant headache history.

On physical examination, blood pressure is 130/90 mm Hg and pulse rate is 86/min. Left homonymous hemianopia is noted.

An MRI of the brain shows bilateral occipital areas of acute infarction.

Cerebrospinal fluid analysis shows 10 erythrocytes, 4 leukocytes, and normal protein and glucose levels.

Four hours after entering the emergency department, the patient has a third abrupt-onset headache with worsening visual blurring. Blood pressure is now 190/115 mm Hg, but physical examination and neuroimaging findings are unchanged.

Which of the following is the most appropriate treatment?

(A) Indomethacin
(B) Normalization of blood pressure
(C) Tissue plasminogen activator
(D) Warfarin

Item 37

A 45-year-old man is evaluated in the emergency department for a 3-week history of headache and impaired vision on the right side. He has not previously had frequent headaches, but the current pain has been constant and worsening since onset. The patient thinks that something is wrong with his eyesight because he has been running into or tripping over objects on the right side. He has no significant medical history and takes no medication.

On physical examination, vital signs are normal. No papilledema is noted on funduscopic examination. A slit lamp examination shows no cells in the vitreous humor. Other findings from the general medical examination are

H
CONT.

unremarkable. Neurologic examination reveals the presence of right homonymous hemianopia.

An MRI of the brain shows a lesion in the left occipital lobe that is highly suspicious for central nervous system lymphoma.

Results of laboratory studies include a normal leukocyte count and differential and no evidence of HIV antibodies.

Cytologic analysis of cerebrospinal fluid shows no malignant cells.

Which of the following is the most appropriate next step in management?

(A) Bone marrow biopsy
(B) Surgical biopsy of the brain lesion
(C) Surgical resection of the brain lesion
(D) Treatment with dexamethasone
(E) Treatment with photon-beam radiation

H Item 38

A 57-year-old woman is evaluated in the emergency department 24 hours after new onset of left hemiparesis and left hemineglect. The patient has hypertension and functional class II New York Heart Association nonischemic heart failure. Medications are enalapril, furosemide, and metoprolol.

On physical examination, temperature is normal, blood pressure is 166/78 mm Hg, pulse rate is 68/min and irregular, and respiration rate is 12/min. A cough is noted. Cardiac examination confirms an irregularly irregular heart rhythm. Neurologic examination shows left visual and tactile extinction, left facial weakness, dysarthria, left arm and leg weakness (muscle strength, 4/5), and normal orientation and language function. She is unable to safely swallow water but can swallow thickened liquids.

Results of laboratory studies are notable for an INR of 1.1 and a serum LDL cholesterol level of 54 mg/dL (1.40 mmol/L).

A CT scan of the head shows an acute infarction in the right parietal and frontal lobes involving half of the hemisphere. An electrocardiogram (ECG) shows atrial fibrillation; an ECG obtained 1 year ago was normal. An echocardiogram shows a left ventricular ejection fraction of 50% without valvular disease or wall motion abnormalities. A chest radiograph and a carotid ultrasound show normal findings.

Which of the following is the most appropriate next step in treatment?

(A) Aspirin
(B) Dabigatran
(C) Intravenous heparin
(D) Warfarin

H Item 39

A 65-year-old woman is evaluated in the emergency department for a 2-day history of nausea and vomiting and a 3-week history of increasingly persistent and severe morning headaches. Breast cancer was diagnosed 8 months ago and treated with lumpectomy, radiation therapy, and

chemotherapy, which she recently completed. Her most recently measured functional status was good (Karnofsky Performance Score > 70).

On physical examination, temperature is 36.7 °C (98.1 °F), blood pressure is 110/70 mm Hg, pulse rate is 95/min, and respiration rate is 18/min. The patient is awake, appropriately interactive, and fully oriented. Difficulty with tasks requiring attention, such as stating the months of the year backward, is noted. Mild bilateral papilledema is present. Increased tone of the left upper and lower extremities is noted. Deep tendon reflexes are 3+ on the left and 1+ on the right. The left toe exhibits a plantar extensor response.

Results of laboratory studies, including a complete blood count, are normal.

An MRI of the brain shows a 3- × 2- × 2-cm ring-enhancing lesion at the gray-white junction of the right frontal lobe with surrounding edema.

A recent PET scan of the body showed no evidence of metastatic disease.

Which of the following is the most appropriate next step in management?

(A) Brain PET
(B) Lumbar puncture
(C) Surgical resection of the brain lesion
(D) Whole-brain radiation

Item 40 **H**

A 62-year-old man is evaluated in the emergency department for a 10-day history of progressively worsening shortness of breath, a 3-month history of difficulty with swallowing at dinnertime that resolves by the morning, and a 5-month history of intermittent blurry vision and fatigue. He had a urinary tract infection 2 weeks ago that was treated with ciprofloxacin, after which the fatigue and other symptoms markedly worsened.

On physical examination, temperature, blood pressure, and pulse rate are normal; respiration rate is 24/min. Other notable findings are bilateral ptosis, diplopia with sustained horizontal gaze, nasal speech, a snarling smile, weakness of cervical flexion, and symmetric weakness of shoulder abduction, arm extension, and hip flexion that becomes more severe with repeated effort. Neurologic examination shows an awake and oriented patient with normal sensation and deep tendon reflexes; no atrophy or fasciculation is noted.

Serum magnesium level is 1.5 mg/dL (0.62 mmol/L). Results of other laboratory studies, including a complete blood count and a comprehensive metabolic profile, are normal.

The patient is admitted to the ICU, where serial respiratory measurements reveal declining vital capacity and negative inspiratory force.

Which of the following is the most appropriate emergent treatment?

(A) High-dose intravenous glucocorticoids
(B) Intravenous magnesium
(C) Intravenous pyridostigmine
(D) Plasmapheresis

Item 41

A 44-year-old man is evaluated for a 1-week history of severe, recurrent, left periorbital headaches. The patient has experienced a 10- to 12-week period of similar headaches every spring for the past 3 years. Headaches occur once or twice daily, last 2 to 3 hours if untreated, and are accompanied by nausea, photophobia, and ipsilateral tearing but no aura or vomiting. Resting during headache episodes brings no relief; he instead paces the floor. Simple analgesics and prednisone have been ineffective in treating the headache. Although subcutaneous sumatriptan generally relieves symptoms within 5 to 10 minutes, his headache frequency and dosing limitations preclude his using this drug every time he has symptoms. The patient has a 20-pack-year history of smoking. He takes no other medication.

On physical examination, blood pressure is 134/82 mm Hg and pulse rate is 78/min. All other physical examination findings, including those from a neurologic examination, are unremarkable.

Which of the following is the most appropriate next step?

(A) Amitriptyline
(B) Indomethacin
(C) Propranolol
(D) Topiramate
(E) Verapamil

Item 42

A 50-year-old woman is evaluated for a 4-year history of progressively worsening cognitive function. She now has frequent memory deficits and a decreased ability to concentrate and multitask in her work as a lawyer; she has been reprimanded in recent months by her employer for submitting late and disorganized briefs. She has no other symptoms. The patient has a 15-year history of multiple sclerosis and a 5-year history of depression. She reports that her mood is good, and she is not experiencing her typical symptoms of depression, including anhedonia, depressed mood, and sleep disturbance. Medications are dimethyl fumarate, a vitamin D supplement, fluoxetine, and modafinil.

Physical examination reveals a pleasant, interactive woman. Vital signs are normal. Mild gait ataxia is noted. Mental status examination reveals moderate deficiencies in short-term memory, processing speed, and attention.

An MRI of the brain obtained 2 weeks ago showed multiple white matter lesions consistent with multiple sclerosis, with no significant change from an image obtained 1 year ago.

Which of the following is the most appropriate treatment of this patient's cognitive difficulties?

(A) Amantadine
(B) Counseling and cognitive therapy
(C) Donepezil
(D) High-dose intravenous methylprednisolone for 5 days
(E) Increased fluoxetine dosage

Item 43

A 41-year-old man is evaluated for daily headaches. The patient has had migraine with aura since age 15 years and had a mild traumatic brain injury while playing intramural football at age 22 years. Over the past 10 years, migraine frequency has increased from monthly to several days per week. He describes migraine episodes as global, throbbing, and severe in intensity, noting they are often accompanied by nausea, vomiting, and photophobia and sometimes preceded by 30 minutes of visual scintillations. Migraine duration is typically 2 hours with successful treatment. He takes oral sumatriptan as needed for migraine and typically uses his entire monthly allotment; propranolol was added for migraine prophylaxis 2 months ago with no appreciable effect. Ever since lumbar pain with radiculopathy was diagnosed 6 months ago and treated with hydrocodone 3 or 4 days each week, he also has developed a daily, constant, mild bilateral frontotemporal "squeezing" headache associated with maxillary pressure and neck tightness. He occasionally uses the hydrocodone to treat the headaches.

On physical examination, blood pressure is 120/72 mm Hg and pulse rate is 60/min; BMI is 28. Neurologic examination findings are normal, as are other physical examination findings.

A CT scan of the head is normal.

Which of the following is the most likely diagnosis?

(A) Chronic posttraumatic headache
(B) Chronic tension-type headache
(C) Idiopathic intracranial hypertension
(D) Medication overuse headache

Item 44

A 35-year-old woman is evaluated in the emergency department for a 3-day history of diplopia, vertigo, and gait imbalance that has prevented her going to work. She reports no additional symptoms. The patient has multiple sclerosis, vitamin D deficiency, and depression. Medications are interferon beta-1a, vitamin D, and extended-release venlafaxine.

On physical examination, temperature is 36.5 °C (97.7 °F), blood pressure is 100/55 mm Hg, pulse rate is 72/min, and respiration rate is 14/min. Incomplete abduction of the right eye is noted when the patient looks to the right. Finger-to-nose testing with the right arm reveals dysmetria. Tandem gait testing results in a near fall.

A T2-weighted MRI of the brain shows multiple new lesions, three of which enhance after administration of intravenous contrast.

Which of the following is the most appropriate next step in treatment?

(A) Glatiramer acetate
(B) Intravenous methylprednisolone, 1 g/d
(C) Oral prednisone, 1 mg/kg
(D) Plasmapheresis

Item 45

An 82-year-old man is evaluated in the hospital for right-sided weakness and difficulty speaking. He was found in

CONT.

bed by his son, who last saw him well 18 hours ago. The patient does not seek routine medical care. He takes no medication.

On physical examination, blood pressure is 196/88 mm Hg, pulse rate is 84/min and regular, respiration rate is 12/min, and oxygen saturation is 98% on ambient air. Other general physical examination findings, including those from an evaluation of the fundi, are normal. Neurologic examination reveals right-sided facial weakness, severe dysarthria with an inability to swallow, right-sided arm paralysis, 3/5 muscle strength throughout the right leg, and no aphasia.

Results of laboratory studies show normal serum levels of creatinine and troponin T and I.

An electrocardiogram shows normal sinus rhythm with no ischemic changes, and a chest radiograph is normal. A CT scan of the head without contrast shows a left pontine infarct.

Which of the following is the most appropriate acute blood pressure treatment?

(A) Administer oral captopril
(B) Administer oral metoprolol
(C) Administer sublingual nitroglycerin
(D) No pharmacologic treatment is required

Item 46

A 53-year-old man is evaluated for persistent right-sided facial weakness. Three months ago, he first noticed "droopiness" of the right side of his lower face, difficulty closing the right eye and wrinkling the forehead, increased sensitivity to loud noises, and occasional slurred speech. Bell palsy was diagnosed, and he began a 10-day course of prednisone. He has noted only limited improvement, with continued facial drooping and mildly dysarthric speech; he now uses an eye patch over his right eye at night. The patient takes no medication.

On physical examination, vital signs are normal. Right-sided facial weakness involving the forehead, orbicularis oculi, and lower facial muscles is noted. Taste recognition is impaired on the anterior right side of the tongue. Facial sensation and the muscles of mastication are intact. The corneal reflex is present bilaterally, and the jaw reflex is normal. Hearing is intact bilaterally, as are extraocular reflexes, motor and sensory function, and deep tendon reflexes.

Which of the following is the most appropriate next step in management?

(A) Acyclovir
(B) Clinical observation
(C) MRI of the brain
(D) Physical therapy

Item 47

A 32-year-old man is evaluated in the emergency department 2 hours after having a witnessed tonic-clonic seizure that lasted 2 minutes. After the seizure, he noted transient weakness of the right arm. The weakness has now resolved, and he feels completely normal. The patient reports that

before losing consciousness, he felt a painful numbness in the first and second digits of the right hand, which subsequently assumed a "claw-like" posture. He never has had a similar sensation. He sustained a closed head injury resulting in a brief loss of consciousness 5 years ago in military combat. He takes no medication.

On physical examination, vital signs are normal. The patient's facial features are symmetric. Right pronator drift and difficulty with rapid alternating movements of the right hand are noted. Examination of the right upper extremity shows muscle strength of 4+/5 and 1+ deep tendon reflexes; muscle strength is 5/5 and reflexes are 2+ in all other limbs.

Laboratory studies, including a complete blood count, comprehensive metabolic profile, and urinalysis, have normal results.

An MRI shows encephalomalacia from his previous head trauma in the left parietal lobe and no other acute findings.

Which of the following is the most appropriate next step in management?

(A) Ambulatory electroencephalographic monitoring
(B) Carbamazepine
(C) Clinical observation
(D) Lumbar puncture

Item 48

A 38-year-old man is evaluated for headaches associated with visual changes. He describes intermittent headaches that began 18 years ago, occur three to four times per month, and typically last 12 to 24 hours. The pain is bifrontal, throbbing, occasionally severe, and worsened when he bends forward or ascends stairs. Headaches are accompanied by mild photophobia and phonophobia but no nausea or vomiting. Approximately twice yearly he experiences unilateral visual distortion during a headache attack that he characterizes as "looking through frosted glass"; the visual change typically lasts for only 30 to 40 minutes and then resolves completely. He has taken aspirin, acetaminophen, naproxen, and ibuprofen at various points to relieve his symptoms, but no medication has been effective in relieving either the headaches or visual distortion.

On physical examination, vital signs are normal. All other physical examination findings, including those from a neurologic examination, are unremarkable.

Which of the following is the most appropriate management?

(A) CT of the head
(B) Electroencephalography
(C) Erythrocyte sedimentation rate measurement
(D) MRI of the brain
(E) Sumatriptan administration

Item 49

A 45-year-old man is evaluated for significant fatigue since having a lacunar stroke 6 months ago. He reports not resting well at night and feeling sleepy at work; he does not fall asleep inappropriately during the day. He has been able

Self-Assessment Test

to maintain a daily 20-minute exercise program without difficulty. A recent electrocardiogram and echocardiogram were normal. Since his stroke, the patient has had no depressed mood and has continued to enjoy spending time with family and pursuing his hobbies. He has dyslipidemia, hypertension, and a remote history of depression. Medications are simvastatin, lisinopril, and aspirin.

On physical examination, blood pressure is 146/78 mm Hg, pulse rate is 68/min and regular, and respiration rate is 12/min; BMI is 32. Cardiac examination reveals no carotid bruits or other abnormalities. Neurologic examination shows mild dysarthria and grade 4/5 left-sided weakness throughout.

Which of the following is the most appropriate next step in management?

(A) Cardiovascular stress testing

(B) Citalopram

(C) Dextroamphetamine

(D) Polysomnography

Item 50

A 33-year-old woman is evaluated for a 3-day history of worsening right eye pain and a 1-day history of visual disturbance in the right eye. The pain is aggravated by eye movement. Three years ago, she experienced right arm clumsiness and a mildly unsteady gait but did not seek medical attention; symptoms fully resolved within 1 week. Medical history is otherwise unremarkable, and the patient takes no medication.

On physical examination, temperature is 36.2 °C (97.2 °F), blood pressure is 125/53 mm Hg, pulse rate is 80/min, and respiration rate is 16/min; BMI is 30. Pupillary reactivity is normal when each eye is tested individually; however, when a light is rapidly moved from the left eye to the right, the right pupil dilates by 2 mm. Visual acuity is 20/100 in the right eye and 20/20 in the left. Visual field testing reveals a central scotoma. Slight temporal disc pallor is noted on the right. Other findings from the general medical and neurologic examinations are normal.

Which of the following diagnostic tests is most appropriate to perform next?

(A) Erythrocyte sedimentation rate determination

(B) Lumbar puncture

(C) MRI of the brain

(D) Serum rapid plasma reagin test

Item 51

An 18-year-old man is evaluated for recurrent headaches 1 week after falling on his head during a soccer match at his high school. The patient reports being "dazed" for 15 minutes after the fall but never losing consciousness. Findings from a sideline examination were unremarkable, and the patient was removed from play. Given the temporary alteration in consciousness, a follow-up examination with his internist was recommended. He developed headaches the morning after the injury that for 3 days were severe, global, throbbing, and associated with nausea and dizziness; the

nausea and dizziness have gradually resolved, and for the past 2 days, the headache pain has been controlled with acetaminophen. He has had no cognitive symptoms but has not yet resumed school or sports activities.

Results of physical examination, including vital signs and neurologic examination findings, are unremarkable.

Which of the following is the most appropriate management?

(A) Obtain a CT of the head

(B) Obtain an MRI of the brain

(C) Prohibit contact sports

(D) Restrict classroom participation

Item 52

A 29-year-old woman comes to the office to discuss her plans for pregnancy; she hopes to become pregnant before the end of the year. The patient has juvenile myoclonic epilepsy that was diagnosed 13 years ago. She started taking valproic acid at that time to treat the epilepsy and was seizure free until 1 year ago when she decided to stop taking the valproic acid and had a convulsive seizure. After resuming the medication, she has been otherwise asymptomatic except for occasional brief jerks of her hands that occur in the morning when she is sleep deprived but at no other time. Medications are valproic acid and folic acid.

All physical examination findings, including vital signs and results of a neurologic examination, are normal.

In addition to discontinuing valproic acid, which of the following is the most appropriate next step in treatment?

(A) Begin carbamazepine

(B) Begin levetiracetam

(C) Begin topiramate

(D) Withhold AED therapy until after pregnancy

Item 53

A 56-year-old woman is evaluated for a 1-year history of tremor. The tremor is more prominent on the right side. She also reports increasing problems with balance and numerous falls, especially when arising from a chair or turning. The patient does not have any significant cognitive symptoms. She has occasional urinary incontinence, intermittent constipation, and a history of acting out of dreams during sleep.

On physical examination, blood pressure is 115/75 mm Hg sitting and 85/70 mm Hg standing, pulse rate is 65/min sitting and 75/min standing, and respiration rate is 22/min. Bruises over the upper and lower extremities secondary to falls are present. On cranial nerve examination, dysmetric saccades, decreased facial expression, and hypophonic speech are noted. Vertical eye movements are normal. A low-amplitude tremor at rest that is more prominent on the right side is present. Repetitive finger tapping movements are bradykinetic. On finger-to-nose testing, mild dysmetria is present. Gait is ataxic with a wide base and frequent veering to both sides; she is unsteady on turning. Gait speed is normal, but arm swing is decreased. A pull test confirms postural instability. No sensory deficits are noted.

Which of the following is the most likely diagnosis?

(A) Multiple system atrophy

(B) Parkinson disease

(C) Progressive supranuclear palsy

(D) Vascular parkinsonism

Item 54

A 52-year-old woman is evaluated for a 3-year history of progressively worsening bilateral hand tingling and numbness that are more prominent in the right hand. The numbness involves the thumb and index finger and part of the palm adjacent to the thumb. She says that symptoms are aggravated when she types on a computer keyboard at work, where she is employed as a secretary. She also reports persistent burning and tingling paresthesia over the palmar side of the right thumb and index finger and says she occasionally drops objects with her right hand. The patient has type 2 diabetes mellitus managed by diet and exercise. She takes no medication.

On physical examination, vital signs are normal. Right thumb abductor strength is 4/5; strength in the other muscles of the right hand and right hand grip are normal. Mild atrophy of right thenar eminence in noted. Muscles of the left hand have full strength. Tapping of the right wrist reproduces the symptoms.

Results of nerve conduction studies show ongoing sensorimotor denervation isolated to the right median nerve.

Which of the following is the most appropriate next step in management?

(A) Decompression surgery

(B) Glucocorticoid injection

(C) Nocturnal neutral position wrist splint

(D) Occupational therapy

Item 55

A 58-year-old man is evaluated in the emergency department for a 2-hour history of right-sided weakness. He has hypertension and chronic kidney disease. Medications are amlodipine, lisinopril, and aspirin.

On physical examination, the patient is awake and interactive. Blood pressure is 190/88 mm Hg, pulse rate is 72/min and regular, respiration rate is 16/min, and oxygen saturation is 97% on ambient air. Papilledema is noted. Neurologic examination shows right-sided facial weakness, slurred speech, and absent movement and pinprick sensation in the right arm and leg, but no aphasia.

A CT scan of the head without contrast shows a left thalamic intracerebral hemorrhage.

Results of laboratory studies include a platelet count of 170,000/µL (170×10^9/L), an INR of 0.9, and a serum creatinine level of 1.8 mg/dL (159 µmol/L).

Which of the following is the most appropriate treatment?

(A) Intravenous labetalol

(B) Intravenous nitroprusside

(C) Platelet transfusion

(D) Recombinant factor VIIa

Item 56

A 45-year-old woman is evaluated in the emergency department (ED) 5 minutes after having a witnessed convulsive seizure in the parking lot of the hospital, where she recently started working in the cafeteria. On arrival at the ED, she is obtunded and soon begins to convulse again, exhibiting tonic-clonic movements of both upper extremities. The patient is positioned on her side, and intravenous access is obtained. Medical history cannot be immediately obtained.

On physical examination, temperature is 37.7 °C (99.9 °F), blood pressure is 110/70 mm Hg, pulse rate is 130/min, and oxygen saturation is 93% on ambient air; respiration rate cannot be assessed. This latest seizure has already lasted 6 minutes. Her eyes are open and rolled upward, and the patient is actively convulsing. Initial inspection reveals no evidence of trauma.

Fingerstick blood glucose level is 90 mg/dL (5.0 mmol/L).

Which of the following is the most appropriate intravenous treatment?

(A) Diazepam followed by levetiracetam

(B) Diazepam followed by phenytoin

(C) Lorazepam followed by levetiracetam

(D) Lorazepam followed by phenytoin

Item 57

A 49-year-old man is evaluated for persistent sensorimotor symptoms. Five months ago, he developed tingling and mild bilateral pain in the thighs followed by mild weakness and hand numbness. Over the next 3 months, his lower extremity weakness progressively worsened, and his gait became unstable. He began having difficulty going up stairs and opening jars and had several episodes of presyncopal symptoms on standing; his speech, swallowing, and vision were unaffected. His weakness has plateaued within the past 2 months without any improvement. He continues to have tingling in the lower extremities, but the pain has dissipated. The patient has diabetes mellitus treated with metformin. Family history is noncontributory.

On physical examination, blood pressure is 130/75 mm Hg sitting and 95/60 mm Hg standing; other vital signs are normal. Extraocular movements and muscle tone are normal; no fasciculations are present. Diffuse areflexia is noted, with moderate bilateral symmetric weakness in the distal upper extremities and proximal and distal lower extremities. Decreased sensation to pinprick and vibration is noted in both feet; no evidence of high arches or hammertoes is found.

Results of nerve conduction studies show diffuse and severe slowing of motor nerve conduction velocities and the presence of conduction blocks.

Which of the following is the most likely diagnosis?

(A) Charcot-Marie-Tooth disease type 1

(B) Chronic inflammatory demyelinating polyradiculoneuropathy

(C) Diabetic amyotrophy

(D) Guillain-Barré syndrome

Item 58

A 26-year-old woman is evaluated for progressively worsening headaches that began intermittently 6 months ago and became daily 3 months ago. The patient describes bilateral "vise-like" pain that is steady, moderate in intensity, and unaffected by physical activity. She also has experienced brief, temporal, sharp pains and a few episodes of transient binocular visual dimming. The headaches are accompanied by moderate neck stiffness and mild photophobia but no nausea, phonophobia, or focal neurologic symptoms. She has polycystic ovary syndrome diagnosed 2 years ago and treated with metformin and a combined oral contraceptive but no personal or family history of headache. The patient takes no other medication or supplement.

On physical examination, blood pressure is 124/80 mm Hg and pulse rate is 72/min; BMI is 30. Partial left palsy of the abducens nerve (cranial nerve VI) is noted. A funduscopic photograph is shown.

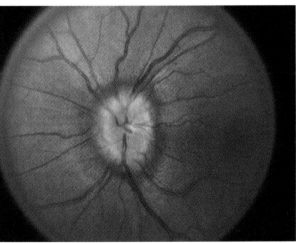

An MRI is normal. Analysis of cerebrospinal fluid obtained on lumbar puncture shows an opening pressure of 350 mm H$_2$O.

Which of the following is the most appropriate treatment?

(A) Acetazolamide
(B) Amitriptyline
(C) Epidural blood patch
(D) Optic nerve sheath fenestration
(E) Spironolactone

Item 59

A 71-year-old man is seen for follow-up evaluation 2 weeks after having an ischemic stroke. The patient has hypertension and type 2 diabetes mellitus. Medications are enalapril, chlorthalidone, atorvastatin, metformin, and aspirin.

An MRI of the brain obtained during hospitalization showed a right paramedian frontal lobe acute infarction. A magnetic resonance angiogram of the head and neck showed abrupt termination of the distal right anterior cerebral artery but was otherwise normal. An electrocardiogram was normal, and a transthoracic echocardiogram

showed a patent foramen ovale, normal systolic and diastolic function, and no valvular disease. Telemetry findings revealed occasional premature atrial contractions.

On current physical examination, vital signs are normal. On neurologic examination, increased tone in the left leg and weakness below the left knee (muscle strength, 4+/5) are noted; the patient ambulates with a cane.

Which of the following is the most appropriate next step in management?

(A) Addition of clopidogrel
(B) Addition of dabigatran
(C) Cardiac rhythm monitoring
(D) Percutaneous device closure of the patent foramen ovale

Item 60

A 68-year-old man is seen for follow-up evaluation of Parkinson disease, which was diagnosed 10 years ago. Although his symptoms initially were well controlled with medications, he has experienced increasing fluctuations in motor symptoms, specifically tremor at rest and slowness, within the past 3 years. Medications are carbidopa-levodopa, entacapone, and amantadine. He notes marked symptom improvement after taking these medications, but the benefit lasts only for 2 hours. Increased dosing of carbidopa-levodopa causes visual hallucinations.

On physical examination performed 3 hours after the patient took carbidopa-levodopa, blood pressure is 130/65 mm Hg and pulse rate is 85/min. Masked facies, an asymmetric upper extremity tremor at rest, marked bradykinesia, and cogwheel rigidity are noted. Gait is slow, but cognitive assessment findings are normal. Repeat examination performed 1 hour after the patient took carbidopa-levodopa reveals notable improvement in bradykinesia, rigidity, and gait and the emergence of prominent dyskinesia.

Which of the following is the most appropriate treatment of this patient's motor complications?

(A) Deep brain stimulation
(B) Discontinuation of entacapone
(C) Increased amantadine dosage
(D) Ropinirole
(E) Selegiline

Item 61

An 84-year-old woman is evaluated for rapidly increasing confusion and behavioral problems. Alzheimer disease was diagnosed 2 years ago, and she was started on donepezil at that time; symptoms have slowly progressed since diagnosis. Her husband, who is her caregiver, reports that 5 days ago, she began having greater difficulty locating the bathroom in their home, has not recognized members of her immediate family on several occasions, has experienced greater nighttime confusion, has become verbally abusive, and has frequently attempted to leave the house unaccompanied. The patient also has hypertension. Medications are donepezil and enalapril.

On physical examination, temperature is 37.2 °C (99.0 °F), blood pressure is 110/70 mm Hg, pulse rate is 84/min and regular, respiration rate is 14/min, and oxygen saturation is 99% on ambient air. Neurologic examination shows a drowsy but easily arousable patient who is oriented to neither time nor place. Her attention is poor, and she has difficulty following even simple commands. Other physical examination findings are unremarkable.

Which of the following is the most appropriate next step in management?

(A) Add quetiapine
(B) Discontinue donepezil
(C) Evaluate for concurrent illness
(D) Order head CT

Item 62

A 49-year-old man has a follow-up evaluation 3 months after an exacerbation of multiple sclerosis (MS) that resulted in bilateral leg weakness. He has had MS for 15 years. The patient reports that for the past 10 weeks, he has had bilateral muscle cramps in the thighs and calves and frequent nighttime episodes of right leg stiffening and spasms that can last from seconds to hours and impair his sleep. He has no other symptoms and no significant family history. Medications are fingolimod and vitamin D supplements.

On physical examination, temperature is 36.4 °C (97.5 °F), blood pressure is 130/50 mm Hg, and pulse rate is 88/min. Increased tone is noted in both legs. Palpation of the leg muscles elicits no pain or fasciculations. Muscle strength is 4/5 in both legs. Patellar and ankle reflexes are 3+. An extensor plantar response is noted on the right. Gait requires the assistance of a cane, and both legs appear stiff when walking.

Results of laboratory studies show a normal serum creatine kinase level.

Which of the following is the most appropriate management?

(A) Electroencephalography
(B) Electromyography
(C) Oral baclofen
(D) Oral pramipexole

Item 63

A 24-year-old woman is seen for a follow-up evaluation of epilepsy first diagnosed 4 years ago. The patient has five or six simple or complex partial seizures annually that have been difficult to control. The epilepsy was first treated with lamotrigine, to which levetiracetam was added 2 years ago. Although both medications decreased the frequency and intensity of the seizures when initiated, the episodes returned to their former state after several months. She cannot drive because the seizures often cause loss of consciousness. She has a history of febrile seizure as an infant. She otherwise has no significant medical history, and her only medications are lamotrigine, levetiracetam, and folic acid.

All physical examination findings are within normal limits.

An MRI shows right mesial temporal sclerosis. Video electroencephalographic monitoring records three complex partial seizures, all originating from the right temporal lobe, and interictal right anterior temporal sharp waves.

Which of the following is the most effective treatment?

(A) Addition of carbamazepine
(B) Ketogenic diet
(C) Right temporal lobectomy
(D) Vagal nerve stimulation

Item 64

A 66-year-old man is evaluated in the hospital 3 days after fracturing his hip in a fall. He underwent surgical repair 1 day after admission and had an unremarkable initial postoperative course but now is confused and agitated. Medical history includes anxiety disorder and a 10-year history of Parkinson disease. Medications before hospitalization were levodopa, amantadine, and citalopram. All medications have been withheld since admission.

On physical examination, temperature is 39.5 °C (103.1 °F), blood pressure is 168/80 mm Hg (baseline, 118/70 mm Hg), pulse rate is 90/min, and respiration rate is 28/min. The patient appears rigid, does not follow commands, and is agitated. Deep tendon reflexes are normal, but muscle tone is markedly increased. A resting tremor is present bilaterally but is more pronounced on the right side. No spontaneous or stimulus-induced myoclonus is noted. Dystonic posturing is noted in the right foot.

In addition to continuing supportive care, which of the following is the most appropriate treatment?

(A) Administer baclofen
(B) Administer dantrolene
(C) Restart citalopram
(D) Restart levodopa

Item 65

A 23-year-old woman is evaluated in the hospital for a 3-day history of a severe right hemicranial headache that has not responded to medication. She has had recurrent migraine for 17 years that typically involves severe right hemicranial throbbing pain associated with nausea and vomiting. Once or twice annually, the headaches are preceded by visual aura. Since age 13 years, migraine attacks have occurred twice monthly, with menses and ovulation as triggers. Typical duration is 24 hours, although occasionally episodes linger for 4 to 5 days. The patient also has anxiety. Medications are zolmitriptan for acute treatment of headache and alprazolam for anxiety. An infusion of fluids, intravenous prochlorperazine, and ketorolac in the emergency department brought no relief of symptoms.

On physical examination, blood pressure is 108/68 mm Hg and pulse rate is 86/min. All other physical examination findings, including those from a neurologic examination, are normal.

Which of the following is the most appropriate next step in management?

(A) Brain MRI

(B) Combined oral contraceptives

(C) Dihydroergotamine

(D) Hydromorphone

(E) Sertraline

Item 66

A 29-year-old woman is evaluated during a routine follow-up examination of multiple sclerosis, which was diagnosed 3 years ago. The patient says she wishes to discontinue her oral contraceptive and attempt to become pregnant. She has no other personal or family medical history of note. Medications are fingolimod, vitamin D, and an oral contraceptive.

On physical examination, temperature is 36.9 °C (98.5 °F), blood pressure is 100/50 mm Hg, pulse rate is 66/min, and respiration rate is 14/min; BMI is 27. A right afferent pupillary defect is noted. All other physical examination findings are normal.

Besides discontinuing the oral contraceptive, which of the following is the most appropriate next step in management?

(A) Advise against pregnancy

(B) Discontinue fingolimod

(C) Substitute mitoxantrone for fingolimod

(D) Substitute teriflunomide for fingolimod

Item 67

A 37-year-old woman is admitted to the ICU after a CT scan of the head without contrast obtained in the emergency department showed a thin, diffuse subarachnoid hemorrhage without hydrocephalus or cerebral edema and a subsequent angiogram revealed a 10-mm anterior communicating artery aneurysm. The patient is treated with a coiling procedure without complications.

One day after the procedure, physical examination shows a blood pressure of 134/68 mm Hg, a pulse rate of 96/min, and a respiration rate of 12/min. Nuchal rigidity is noted. The patient has difficulty remaining awake unless spoken to loudly, but no other abnormalities are seen on neurologic examination.

A transcranial ultrasound obtained the same day is normal. Fingerstick blood glucose readings over the next 24 hours range between 120 and 150 mg/dL (6.7-8.3 mmol/L).

Which of the following is the most appropriate next step in treatment?

(A) Intravenous dopamine

(B) Intravenous insulin

(C) Oral nimodipine

(D) Oral simvastatin

Item 68

A 29-year-old woman is seen for a routine follow-up evaluation. Multiple sclerosis (MS) was diagnosed 2 months

ago. She has no current symptoms. The patient does not smoke, drinks a glass of wine with dinner three or four times weekly, and exercises at least 3 hours weekly. Her father has hypertension, but she has no other significant family history. Daily medications are glatiramer acetate, a multivitamin, and a calcium–vitamin D supplement.

On physical examination, temperature is 37.3 °C (99.1 °F), blood pressure is 108/48 mm Hg, pulse rate is 62/min, and respiration rate is 12/min; BMI is 20. All other physical examination findings, including those from a neurologic examination, are normal.

Which of the following is the most appropriate preventive or screening strategy for this patient?

(A) Alcohol cessation

(B) Annual influenza vaccination

(C) Urinalysis

(D) Use of an oral contraceptive

Item 69

A 35-year-old man is evaluated for recurrent headaches. For the past 5 years, he has had weekly episodes of headache lasting 6 to 8 hours. The patient describes the pain as a steady pressure affecting the frontal and maxillary regions that is exacerbated by physical activity. When severe, the pain radiates to the temples and occiput. He also experiences nasal congestion and sensitivity to light, noise, and odors with the headaches but has had no gastrointestinal or other neurologic symptoms. Potential headache triggers include drastic weather changes, strong odors, and stress. The patient also has allergic rhinitis. Medications are acetaminophen and fexofenadine, which have been ineffective in relieving the headaches and their associated symptoms.

On physical examination, blood pressure is 114/72 mm Hg and pulse rate is 66/min. Other physical examination findings, including those from a neurologic examination, are normal.

Which of the following is the most appropriate next step in management?

(A) CT of the head

(B) CT of the sinuses

(C) Naproxen

(D) Pseudoephedrine

(E) Sumatriptan

Item 70

A 48-year-old man is evaluated for right upper extremity weakness. For the past 8 months, he has noticed progressive weakness in the right arm that is more prominent in the fingers; proximal strength is preserved. He also has noted frequent, painful muscle cramping in the right arm, lower back, and left lower extremity that recently has been accompanied by muscle twitching. He has had no sensory deficit or significant medical history. The patient takes no medication.

On physical examination, vital signs are normal. The patient's speech is dysarthric. Muscle strength testing shows weakness with atrophy in the distal right upper extremity and mild weakness without atrophy in the left lower extremity. Fasciculations are present in the bilateral upper and lower extremities and the paraspinal muscles. Deep tendon reflexes are brisk in all extremities, and the plantar response is extensor. Results of sensory and motor examinations are normal.

Results of laboratory studies—including a complete metabolic profile; serum lead, copper, vitamin B_{12}, and parathyroid hormone levels; and Lyme antibody titers—are unremarkable.

MRIs of the cervical and lumbar spines are normal. Results of needle electrode examination show evidence of lower motoneuron abnormalities in multiple body regions, including the limbs, trunk, and face.

Which of the following is the most appropriate treatment?

(A) Bilevel positive airway pressure
(B) Intravenous immune globulin
(C) Percutaneous endoscopic gastrostomy
(D) Riluzole

Item 71

A 59-year-old woman is evaluated for headaches and occasional double vision. The patient has had episodes of migraine with aura since age 12 years. Aura symptoms include visual blurring and ipsilateral facial numbness lasting approximately 15 minutes. After menopause, migraine attacks became less frequent and intense, declining from 12 to 5 days per month, but over the past 4 months have again become more frequent, increasing to 15 days per month. She describes these recent headaches, which are not associated with her typical aura, as more bilateral and "squeezing" in nature than previous ones and reports intermittent visual blurring and two instances of horizontal diplopia lasting 2 hours. The patient has had no other neurologic symptoms. The recent headaches respond to neither ibuprofen nor to the naratriptan she uses to treat acute migraine episodes. Her only other medication is amitriptyline for migraine prophylaxis.

On physical examination, blood pressure is 128/86 mm Hg and pulse rate is 78/min; BMI is 27. Other results of the general medical and neurologic examinations are normal.

Which of the following is the most appropriate management?

(A) Brain MRI
(B) Discontinuation of ibuprofen
(C) Lumbar puncture
(D) Substitution of sumatriptan for naratriptan
(E) Substitution of topiramate for amitriptyline

Item 72

A 46-year-old woman is evaluated for intermittent left-sided tingling and a subsequent headache. She was seen in an emergency department 3 weeks ago for similar symptoms. At that time, a noncontrast CT scan of the head and

an MRI of the brain were normal, but a magnetic resonance angiogram showed a 5-mm left middle cerebral artery aneurysm. Results of cerebrospinal fluid analysis were normal. The patient has hypertension and migraine, but she has no other medical history of note. She has a 15-pack-year smoking history, currently smoking approximately ten cigarettes daily, and does not drink alcoholic beverages. Her only medication is amlodipine.

On physical examination, vital signs are normal. Other results of the general and neurologic examinations are normal.

Which of the following is the most appropriate next step?

(A) Aneurysmal clipping
(B) Endovascular coiling
(C) Smoking cessation counseling
(D) Substitution of nimodipine for amlodipine

Item 73

A 59-year-old man is evaluated for a 10-month history of hand tremor. The tremor is more prominent when he is tired, anxious, or walking. He also reports occasional difficulty with fine-motor movements, a deterioration of his handwriting, and a softening of his voice. His gait is not magnetic, and he has had no problem with balance or falls. The patient does not have urinary incontinence or dementia. His paternal grandfather had essential tremor and his paternal aunt had Parkinson disease.

On physical examination, vital signs are normal. Facial expression is normal, and his voice is low in volume but not tremulous. With the patient at rest, a low-frequency tremor is noted in the right hand and chin. With the arms in an outstretched position, a bilateral tremor emerges after a delay of several seconds that is more prominent on the right side. Finger-to-nose testing reveals a mild bilateral tremor that does not worsen near the target. Rapid alternating movements of the right upper and lower extremities become slower and shorter in amplitude with repetition. Muscle tone is increased bilaterally, with stepwise resistance to passive movements. Gait is normal, but arm swing is decreased and a tremor emerges on the right side during ambulation.

Which of the following is the most appropriate next step in confirming the diagnosis?

(A) Dopamine transporter scan
(B) MRI of the brain
(C) Needle electrode electromyography
(D) No further testing

Item 74

A 52-year-old man is evaluated for worsening leg stiffness and pain. He has secondary progressive multiple sclerosis with associated chronic gait instability, leg weakness, spasticity, and urinary frequency. The patient reports an upper respiratory tract infection over the past week with nasal congestion and rhinorrhea and a mild, nonproductive cough. His leg stiffness and urinary frequency worsened shortly after the onset of respiratory symptoms but have persisted despite improvement in his congestion, rhinorrhea, and cough. Medications are interferon beta-1b, a vitamin D supplement, dalfampridine, tizanidine, and oxybutynin.

On physical examination, temperature is 37.8 °C (100.0 °F), blood pressure is 139/58 mm Hg, and pulse rate is 98/min. The nasal passages show moderate edema, and postnasal drip is present in the posterior oropharynx. The lungs are clear. Lower extremity spasticity and weakness are noted. All other physical examination findings are unremarkable.

Urinalysis is negative for leukocyte esterase and nitrite.

Bladder ultrasonography shows a postvoid residual urine volume of 180 mL.

Which of the following is the most appropriate treatment?

(A) Amoxicillin-clavulanate
(B) Increased dosage of oxybutynin
(C) Methylprednisolone
(D) Supportive care and clinical observation

Item 75

A 57-year-old man is evaluated in the ICU 7 days after admission for a subarachnoid hemorrhage. An initial noncontrast head CT scan obtained in the emergency department showed a diffuse subarachnoid hemorrhage at the base of the brain that was thickest over the left hemisphere and accompanied by hydrocephalus. An external ventricular drain was placed to treat the hydrocephalus, and he subsequently underwent successful clipping of a 9-mm aneurysm of the left posterior communicating artery. Oral nimodipine was initiated.

On physical examination, temperature is 37.8 °C (100.1 °F), blood pressure is 138/78 mm Hg, pulse rate is 78/min, and respiration rate is 12/min. Neurologic examination shows an extremely somnolent patient who cannot follow commands and is unable to move the right arm and leg; on initial neurologic examination in the emergency department, the patient responded to loud noises, was able to follow simple commands, was oriented to time and place, and exhibited briskly reactive pupils and right arm drift. Results of standard laboratory studies are normal.

Which of the following is the most appropriate next diagnostic test?

(A) CT angiography of the brain
(B) Electroencephalography
(C) Lumbar puncture
(D) MRI of the brain

Item 76

A 42-year-old man is evaluated for nighttime cramping and crawling sensations in his calves. He experiences these symptoms in the late evening, especially when watching television or getting ready for bed. At times, he feels an urge to stand up and pace around the room, which provides brief relief of symptoms. He has had no pain,

weakness, or excessive daytime sleepiness. His mother has similar symptoms. His only medication is loratadine for seasonal allergies.

On physical examination, vital signs are normal. No abnormal movements are noted, and testing of deep tendon reflexes and sensation shows no anomalies.

Results of standard laboratory testing include a normal complete blood count and a serum ferritin level of 120 ng/mL (120 µg/L).

Which of the following is the most appropriate treatment?

(A) Iron supplementation
(B) Pentoxifylline
(C) Ropinirole
(D) Zolpidem

Item 77

A 71-year-old man is evaluated for progressive memory decline. In the past 3 years, he has noticed increasing word-finding difficulties and forgetfulness; he now requires frequent reminders to keep track of appointments. He has remained independent in activities of daily living, except for having to hire an accountant this year to file his taxes. His wife, who accompanied him to the appointment, reports that he is more irritable and impatient than before. The patient describes his mood as upbeat and says he has had no feelings of sadness or hopelessness. He has hyperlipidemia controlled with atorvastatin. His paternal uncle died of Alzheimer disease in his 80s.

On physical examination, vital signs are normal. The patient scores 27/30 on a Mini–Mental State Examination, losing points in the recall section. All other physical examination findings, including those from a neurologic examination, are normal.

Results of laboratory studies, including a complete blood count, a comprehensive metabolic profile, thyroid function tests, and measurement of serum vitamin B_{12} level, are normal.

Which of the following is the most appropriate next step in management?

(A) Amyloid PET imaging
(B) Brain MRI
(C) Carotid Doppler ultrasonography
(D) Determination of apolipoprotein E (*APOE ε4*) status
(E) Fluorodeoxyglucose-PET imaging of the brain

Item 78

A 75-year-old woman is evaluated in the emergency department 90 minutes after onset of right arm weakness and an inability to speak. The patient has atrial fibrillation, hypertension, and dyslipidemia. Medications are warfarin, nifedipine, hydrochlorothiazide, and simvastatin.

On physical examination, blood pressure is 148/78 mm Hg and pulse rate is 86/min and irregular. On neurologic examination, global aphasia, right arm paralysis, antigravity movement in the right leg, left gaze preference, and decreased blink response to threat from the right side are

CONT.

noted. Her score on the National Institutes of Health Stroke Scale is high at 22, indicating a severe stroke.

Results of standard laboratory studies include an INR of 1.4 but are otherwise normal.

A noncontrast CT scan of the head shows hyperdensity in the territory of the left middle cerebral artery but is otherwise normal.

After exclusion criteria are ruled out, treatment with intravenous recombinant tissue plasminogen activator (rtPA) is begun 40 minutes after arrival at the emergency department; 60 minutes into the infusion, blood pressure is 168/78 mm Hg, pulse rate is 84/min and irregular, and repeat neurologic examination shows paralysis of the right leg.

Which of the following is the most appropriate next step in management?

(A) Intra-arterial thrombectomy
(B) Intravenous labetalol
(C) Rectal aspirin
(D) Repeat noncontrast CT of the head

Item 79

A 30-year-old woman is evaluated for difficult-to-treat migraine. She has had severe headaches, usually on the first day of menses, since menarche. The pain is hemicranial, pulsatile, and associated with severe nausea and vomiting but no aura. She frequently awakens with the attack already in progress. Ibuprofen was helpful in controlling migraine pain during her teenage years and early 20s but was replaced 5 years ago by oral eletriptan after the pain was no longer controlled; this drug now also is ineffective in relieving symptoms. A trial of oral frovatriptan for menstrual migraine relief also has been unsuccessful. The patient reports receiving intravenous dihydroergotamine and magnesium at an urgent care facility twice in the past 3 months as treatment of refractory headaches.

On physical examination, blood pressure is 98/60 mm Hg and pulse rate is 72/min. All other physical examination findings, including those from a neurologic examination, are normal.

Which of the following is the most appropriate next step in treatment?

(A) Butalbital
(B) Hydrocodone
(C) Naproxen
(D) Orally dissolvable rizatriptan
(E) Subcutaneous sumatriptan

Item 80

A 44-year-old man is evaluated in the emergency department for a severe global headache and blurred vision. Two hours ago, he was struck with a pipe in the right frontotemporal region and anterior neck and knocked to the ground but did not lose consciousness. While describing the assault, the patient becomes stuporous.

On physical examination, blood pressure is 150/100 mm Hg, pulse rate is 50/min, and respiration rate is 10/min.

Continued stupor is noted, as are right pupillary dilation, palsy of the oculomotor nerve (cranial nerve III), and an extensor plantar response on the left. The patient withdraws from pain more weakly on the left than the right. No other cranial nerve abnormalities are detected.

Which of the following is the most likely diagnosis?

(A) Epidural hematoma
(B) Left internal carotid artery dissection
(C) Postconcussion syndrome
(D) Posttraumatic seizure

Item 81

A 22-year-old woman is evaluated for a 2-year-history of abnormal involuntary movements. She describes these movements as a quick elevation of the left shoulder followed by a rolling movement of the neck from side to side. The patient is able to suppress the movements completely for brief periods but then feels pressure building at the left shoulder and the urge to release it. She has experienced no other abnormal movements recently but reports uncontrollable blinking 5 years ago and occasional facial grimacing 3 years ago, both of which resolved after 2 years. She also recently has exhibited obsessive-compulsive behavior, such as repeatedly checking that the oven is turned off and all the doors are locked. The patient has anxiety disorder treated with cognitive behavioral therapy. Her father and brother have facial twitching. She takes no medication.

On physical examination, vital signs are normal. The patient is asked to relax and not suppress any movement, after which the left shoulder quickly elevates, followed by the described repeated slower rolling movement of the neck. In the interval between movements, the neck is at midline with no evidence of pulling, tilting, or turning. The movements are more frequent initially but completely disappear during the second half of the visit. She often clears her throat, even during conversation, and frequently blinks. Neurologic examination findings are otherwise unremarkable.

Which of the following is the most likely diagnosis?

(A) Chorea
(B) Dystonia
(C) Myoclonus
(D) Tic disorder

Item 82

A 55-year-old man is evaluated in the hospital for an episode of painful tingling in the right arm followed by clonic jerking of that arm lasting 3 minutes. Medical history is significant for non–small cell lung cancer diagnosed 1 year ago and treated with surgical resection. He was evaluated in the emergency department 1 week ago for a new-onset headache, at which time an isolated brain metastasis in the left parietal area was identified. He subsequently was admitted for planned surgical resection of this lesion, adjuvant local radiation, and systemic chemotherapy.

On physical examination, temperature is 36.6 °C (97.9 °F), blood pressure is 120/92 mm Hg, pulse rate is

CONT. 105/min, and respiration rate is 16/min. Right inferior quad-rantanopia, right neglect, increased tone in the right arm and leg, and a plantar extensor response in the right toe are noted.

An MRI of the brain shows a stable contrast-enhancing lesion in the left parietal lobe consistent with the patient's known metastasis.

An electroencephalogram shows left hemispheric slowing with no evidence of epileptiform discharges.

Which of the following is the most appropriate management?

(A) Carbamazepine
(B) Phenytoin
(C) Valproic acid
(D) Deferral of antiepileptic drug therapy

Item 83

A 66-year-old man is evaluated in the emergency department for increasingly difficult-to-manage behaviors. According to his son with whom he lives, he has exhibited intermittent forgetfulness, gotten lost while driving on familiar routes, and had brief but frequent periods of nonsensical speech, excessive daytime sleepiness, and an inability to use familiar objects during the past year. Over the past 3 months, the patient has had increasing visual hallucinations and paranoia accompanied by agitation and restlessness. Medical history is significant for mild depression. His only medication is sertraline. A depression screen is negative for a depressed mood.

On physical examination, temperature is 36.8 °C (98.2 °F), blood pressure is 135/70 mm Hg, pulse rate is 80/min, respiration rate is 16/min, and oxygen saturation is 98% on ambient air. General physical examination findings are normal. Neurologic examination shows an agitated man with masked facies, a soft voice, postural instability, and a slow gait. He scores 24/30 on the Mini-Mental State Examination, missing points on orientation to time and place, delayed recall, and figure drawing.

The patient is given haloperidol in the emergency department to treat the agitation, which results in worsening agitation and limb and neck stiffness.

Which of the following is the most likely diagnosis?

(A) Alzheimer disease
(B) Delirium
(C) Dementia with Lewy bodies
(D) Major depression with psychotic features

Item 84

A 36-year-old woman is evaluated for a 1-week history of recurrent episodes of facial pain that are 1 to 3 seconds in duration and occur spontaneously dozens of times throughout the day. The pain is sharp, severe, and located in the right infraorbital area. During this same period, she has developed worsening bilateral lower extremity weakness and urinary incontinence. The patient has an 18-year history of relapsing-remitting multiple sclerosis treated with interferon beta-1a; she also takes baclofen to control spasticity. She has had no nausea, photophobia,

phonophobia, nasal congestion, nasal drainage, or ocular/visual changes.

On physical examination, blood pressure is 100/64 mm Hg and pulse rate is 80/min. Moderate bilateral lower extremity weakness and hyperreflexia are noted. Sensory spinal cord level for pain and temperature is T6. Plantar responses are extensor bilaterally. Internuclear ophthalmoplegia is noted, but other findings from an examination of the cranial nerves are unremarkable.

Results of laboratory studies, including a comprehensive metabolic profile, a complete blood count, and urinalysis, are normal.

Which of the following is the most likely cause of the facial pain?

(A) Chronic paroxysmal hemicrania
(B) Herpes zoster
(C) Primary stabbing headache
(D) Trigeminal neuralgia

Item 85

A 64-year-old woman is evaluated for persistent myopathy. Polymyositis was confirmed by muscle biopsy 6 months ago. High-dose prednisone was started, with almost full recovery within 4 months; the glucocorticoid was subsequently tapered to daily low-dose prednisone. For the past month, she has experienced a recurrence of weakness in the deltoid and hip flexor muscle groups. Her only medication is prednisone, 20 mg.

On physical examination, blood pressure is 132/80 mm Hg and pulse rate is 80/min; BMI is 35. Neck extensor, arm abductor, elbow extensor, hip flexor, and knee extensor muscles are moderately weak; distal muscle strength is normal. Muscle tone is flaccid, but sensory examination findings are normal. Deep tendon reflexes are absent at the triceps muscle and patella but normal elsewhere. The plantar response is flexor. Assessment of cranial nerves and mental status shows no abnormalities.

Results of laboratory studies show a serum creatine kinase level of 80 U/L.

Which of the following is the most appropriate management?

(A) Add intravenous immune globulin
(B) Increase prednisone dosage
(C) Taper prednisone dosage
(D) Repeat muscle biopsy

Item 86

A 49-year-old woman is evaluated in the emergency department 45 minutes after onset of right-sided weakness and loss of vision. She has dyslipidemia and hypertension. Medications are simvastatin and hydrochlorothiazide.

On physical examination, blood pressure is 160/88 mm Hg, pulse rate is 78/min and irregular, and respiration rate is 12/min. No carotid bruits are heard on cardiac examination. On neurologic examination, speech is fluent with occasional word-finding difficulties. A right inferior visual field deficit, right facial weakness, mild dysarthria, right arm pronator drift, and loss of pinprick sensation on the right arm and face are noted. No right leg weakness is detected. The National Institutes of Health Stroke Scale score is 7 (moderate stroke).

An electrocardiogram shows atrial fibrillation with no ST-segment or T-wave changes. A noncontrast CT scan of the head is normal.

The patient receives intravenous recombinant tissue plasminogen activator 50 minutes after arrival in the emergency department. Three hours after the infusion is completed, her blood pressure is 188/110 mm Hg and pulse rate is 68/min. Other physical examination findings are unchanged.

Which of the following is the most appropriate treatment?

(A) Intravenous nicardipine
(B) Oral aspirin
(C) Subcutaneous heparin
(D) Sublingual nitroglycerin

Item 87

A 39-year-old woman is evaluated for worsening headaches. Headache episodes initially developed while she was in high school but have become increasingly severe and frequent over the past 3 years. She describes these recent headaches as an intense, hemicranial, throbbing pain that occurs two or three times per week and is associated with nausea and photophobia. For the past year, she has experienced additional daily episodes of dull, mild, global head pressure without associated features. The patient also has asthma and mild depression. She stopped taking over-the-counter analgesics 6 months ago when they became ineffective; other medications are albuterol and fluticasone.

On physical examination, blood pressure is 122/78 and pulse rate is 74/min; BMI is 22. Other physical examination findings, including those from a neurologic examination, are unremarkable.

An MRI of the brain is normal.

Which of the following is the most appropriate treatment?

(A) Carbamazepine
(B) Duloxetine
(C) Propranolol
(D) Topiramate
(E) Verapamil

Item 88

A 51-year-old woman is evaluated in the emergency department (ED) for increasingly agitated and paranoid behavior. Over the past 4 weeks, she has exhibited short-term memory loss and has been less organized and more confused, which necessitated her taking a leave from work. Her son also has noticed her occasionally sitting motionless, staring at nothing and smacking her lips. She was brought to the ED after she stopped eating because of a belief that someone was trying to poison her. The patient has no other personal medical history and no family history of dementia or psychiatric disorders. She takes no medication.

On physical examination, temperature is 36.1 °C (97.0 °F), blood pressure is 100/70 mm Hg, pulse rate is 70/min, and respiration rate is 16/min. The patient is agitated, with wandering attention. She does not know the date, often missing it by a decade. She can repeat three of three words but 5 minutes later does not recall any of them. Findings of cranial nerve examination are normal, as are muscle strength, coordination, and reflexes.

Serum sodium level is 128 mEq/L (128 mmol/L). All other results of laboratory studies, including a comprehensive metabolic profile and complete blood count, are normal.

An MRI shows increased flair signal in both mesial temporal regions. Continuous EEG monitoring reveals frequent temporal lobe seizures (8/day) occurring from both the left and right temporal lobes.

Which of the following is the most likely diagnosis?

(A) Alzheimer disease
(B) Human herpesvirus 1 encephalitis
(C) Lewy body dementia
(D) Paraneoplastic limbic encephalitis

Item 89

A 90-year-old man is evaluated in the hospital for disorientation. He was admitted 5 days ago after having a myocardial infarction. Before hospitalization, he was living alone and functioning independently. Since hospitalization, the patient has had periods of daytime sleepiness alternating with periods of agitation. Medications are aspirin, clopidogrel, metoprolol, lisinopril, and atorvastatin.

On physical examination, temperature is normal, blood pressure is 130/82 mm Hg, pulse rate is 70/min, and respiration rate is 16/min. Cardiac examination shows an early systolic murmur and normal heart sounds. Neurologic evaluation shows sudden involuntary jerks of the upper extremities that increase in frequency when the arms are outstretched and wrists are extended. The patient is oriented to self and location but not to date and believes he has been hospitalized for only 1 day. He cannot spell the word "world" backwards, and his responses to questions are at times inappropriate or tangential. He requires frequent redirection during the interview and appears to be distracted by something on the wall. Findings from the rest of the physical examination are otherwise unremarkable.

Laboratory studies:

Complete blood count	Normal
Liver chemistry studies	Normal
Glucose, fasting	Normal
Creatine kinase	Normal
Creatinine	2.9 mg/dL (256 µmol/L) (2.0 mg/dL [177 µmol/L] on admission)

Which of the following is the most likely diagnosis?

(A) Delirium
(B) Dementia
(C) Nonconvulsive status epilepticus
(D) Stroke

Item 90

A 49-year-old woman is evaluated for a 1-year history of severe fatigue. She often requires a nap in the middle of the day to continue to function and notes that her work productivity is reduced. The patient has multiple sclerosis (MS), which was diagnosed 2 years ago and is well controlled with daily teriflunomide. Other medications are nightly amitriptyline and weekly vitamin D supplementation.

On physical examination, temperature is 36.9 °C (98.4 °F), blood pressure is 105/64 mm Hg, pulse rate is 68/min, and respiration rate is 14/min; BMI is 21. All other physical examination findings are normal, and neurologic examination findings are unchanged from those obtained at her baseline examination.

Results of laboratory studies show a hemoglobin level of 13.1 g/dL (131 g/L), a mean corpuscular volume of 90 fL, and a serum thyroid-stimulating hormone level of 1.4 µU/mL (1.4 mU/L).

An MRI of the brain obtained 1 month ago as part of routine surveillance showed white matter lesions consistent with MS and unchanged from their appearance 1 year ago.

Which of the following is the most appropriate treatment for this patient?

(A) Iron supplementation
(B) Levothyroxine
(C) Modafinil
(D) Nocturnal continuous positive airway pressure
(E) Substitution of dimethyl fumarate for teriflunomide

Item 91

A 74-year-old woman is seen for a follow-up evaluation of generalized muscle pain. She first noticed diffuse myalgia 6 months ago; the pain became more severe over the next 2 months, and she began experiencing mild proximal weakness in both upper and lower extremities. Her serum creatine kinase level at that time was 2200 U/L. She was instructed to discontinue the simvastatin she took for hyperlipidemia, and the muscle pain and weakness resolved. The patient also has coronary artery disease treated with aspirin, metoprolol, and isosorbide dinitrate.

On physical examination, blood pressure is 130/80 mm Hg; other vital signs also are normal. No muscle tenderness is noted. All other findings of the general physical and neurologic examinations are normal.

Laboratory studies show a serum creatine kinase level of 250 U/L.

Which of the following is the most appropriate treatment?

(A) Atorvastatin
(B) Gemfibrozil
(C) Rosuvastatin
(D) Selenium

Item 92

A 56-year-old man is evaluated for a 5-year history of gradually worsening behavioral problems. During this period, the patient has lost four different jobs because of argumentativeness with his bosses and rudeness toward coworkers and customers. According to his wife, he has become increasingly indifferent toward most things, including his family about whom he used to care deeply; has lost all interest in socializing with friends; and has started to drink excessively. He has become preoccupied with counting change and other belongings and has developed compulsive rituals from which he does not diverge. The patient also has begun collecting scrap metals, an activity he greatly enjoys. He says he does not feel down or hopeless and has not had periods of elation, euphoria, or irritability accompanied by an increased energy level. His memory has remained good. During the interview, the patient states that he has not noticed any change in his behavior and contributes little else to the history. His father was institutionalized for an unknown psychiatric illness at age 55 years.

On physical examination, vital signs are normal. The general physical and neurologic examinations are normal. His score on the Mini–Mental State Examination is 29/30, with one point deducted for orientation to date.

Which of the following is the most likely diagnosis?

(A) Alzheimer disease
(B) Dementia with Lewy bodies
(C) Depression
(D) Frontotemporal dementia

Item 93

A 58-year-old woman is evaluated for cognitive impairment. The patient was brought to the office by her daughter because of a progressive inability to care for herself and manage her finances over the past 2 months. She also has become more withdrawn, emotionally blunted, and disinterested in former social activities and hobbies. She previously was successfully employed as a substitute teacher. She has no significant medical history and no family history of a neurologic or psychiatric disorder.

On physical examination, vital signs are normal. Neurologic examination shows generalized slowness, but findings are otherwise normal. She scores 10/30 on the Montreal Cognitive Assessment, losing points in all eight sections.

Results of laboratory studies, including a complete blood count, comprehensive metabolic profile, thyroid function tests, vitamin B_{12} level, erythrocyte sedimentation rate, rapid plasma reagin test, HIV antibody titer, and urinalysis, are normal.

A diffusion-weighted MRI of the brain is shown on page 114.

Which of the following is the most likely diagnosis?

(A) Alzheimer disease
(B) Creutzfeldt-Jakob disease
(C) Herpes simplex virus 1 encephalitis
(D) Vascular neurocognitive disorder

Item 94

A 57-year-old man is evaluated in the emergency department 45 minutes after developing acute-onset left arm

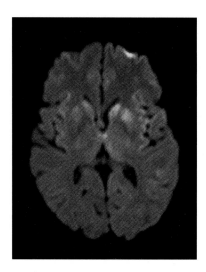

ITEM 93

confused 30 minutes after treatment. According to his wife who accompanied him, a left temporal cavernous malformation was detected 3 years ago and has been managed conservatively. He has no significant family medical history and takes no chronic medication.

On physical examination, temperature is 36.8 °C (98.2 °F), blood pressure is 130/90 mm Hg, pulse rate is 115/min, and respiration rate is 12/min. The patient is generally stuporous but intermittently alert to voice or sternal rub. He occasionally utters nonsensical phrases, mostly consisting of syllables that are not real words, and inconsistently follows some one-step commands. Cranial nerves are intact, and pupils are symmetric and reactive. No weakness is detected in the face or limbs.

A CT of the head shows an acute hemorrhage in the region of the patient's cavernous malformation. The hemorrhage measures $0.5 \times 0.5 \times 1.0$ cm. No significant mass effect or midline shift is noted.

Which of the following is the most appropriate next step in management?

(A) Continuous electroencephalographic monitoring

(B) Intravenous flumazenil

(C) Urgent surgical resection of the vascular malformation

(D) Withholding of further doses of antiepileptic drugs

Item 96

A 65-year-old woman is admitted to the hospital for evaluation of acute kidney injury secondary to dehydration after an episode of severe gastroenteritis. She has type 1 diabetes mellitus, secondary progressive multiple sclerosis, and osteopenia. Medications are irbesartan, insulin glargine, insulin lispro, glatiramer acetate, dalfampridine, baclofen, vitamin D, and calcium.

On physical examination, temperature is normal, blood pressure is 110/60 mm Hg, pulse rate is 108/min, and respiration rate is 14/min. She appears weak and tired. Neck veins are flat. The remainder of the physical examination is normal.

Results of laboratory studies show a serum creatinine level of 3.9 mg/dL (345 µmol/L), which is increased from her baseline level of 1.4 mg/dL (124 µmol/L).

Intravenous fluids are initiated.

In addition to irbesartan, which of the following medications must be discontinued?

(A) Baclofen

(B) Dalfampridine

(C) Glatiramer acetate

(D) Vitamin D

CONT.

weakness. He has type 2 diabetes mellitus and a 50-pack-year smoking history. He has no history of stroke, trauma, bleeding, cardiac disease, or surgery. His only medications are atorvastatin and metformin.

On physical examination, blood pressure is 168/98 mm Hg and pulse rate is 86/min and irregular. Neurologic examination reveals left hemineglect, an inferior left visual field deficit, left facial weakness, mild dysarthria, and left arm and leg drift. He scores 6 on the National Institutes of Health Stroke Scale, indicating a moderate stroke.

Laboratory study findings include a plasma glucose level of 162 mg/dL (9.0 mmol/L); results of a complete blood count, a comprehensive metabolic profile, and coagulation studies are normal.

An electrocardiogram shows atrial fibrillation. A noncontrast CT scan of the head shows no acute infarct or hemorrhage.

Which of the following is the most appropriate next step in treatment?

(A) High-dose aspirin

(B) Insulin

(C) Intravenous heparin

(D) Intravenous recombinant tissue plasminogen activator

Item 95

A 55-year-old man is treated in the emergency department for convulsive status epilepticus. He stops convulsing after receiving intravenous lorazepam and phenytoin but is still

Answers and Critiques

Item 1   Answer: B

Educational Objective: Diagnose vitamin D deficiency in a patient with multiple sclerosis.

This patient's serum 25-hydroxyvitamin D level should be measured. He most likely has experienced a breakthrough relapse of multiple sclerosis (MS), which should be treated with intravenous methylprednisolone. Given his 2 years without relapses, the MS is relatively well-controlled. However, his care is not fully optimized because he rarely takes the vitamin D supplement. Accumulating evidence suggests that disease activity in MS is highly linked with serum vitamin D levels, with less frequent relapses and fewer new MRI lesions in patients with higher levels. This patient's serum 25-hydroxyvitamin D level should thus be measured to determine if he is vitamin D deficient. Vitamin D supplementation as an adjunctive treatment in MS has been shown to be superior to disease-modifying therapy alone and has become a standard of care for MS patients, especially those who are vitamin D deficient, although the ideal dosing regimen and serum 25-hydroxyvitamin D level are still unknown. Pharmacodynamic studies are under way that may help inform dosing regimens. Vitamin D supplementation also protects against osteoporosis, for which patients with MS are at higher risk.

This patient has no clear indications supporting discontinuation of natalizumab at this time. Natalizumab is the most highly effective drug for MS currently available, which is borne out by his relapse-free status for 2 years and stable brain MRI results. Although this drug is sometimes associated with progressive multifocal leukoencephalopathy (PML), his recent negative result on JC virus antibody testing place him at a very low risk for development of PML, and the spinal cord localization of this current relapse also argues against PML, which does not affect the spinal cord.

The bilateral leg weakness and sensory level around the umbilicus (T10) are consistent with localization to the thoracic spinal cord. Therefore, an MRI of the lumbar spine would not be appropriate.

This patient has no indication for antibiotic therapy, which makes a 5-day course of trimethoprim-sulfamethoxazole inappropriate.

KEY POINT

- Vitamin D supplementation as an adjunctive treatment in multiple sclerosis (MS) has been shown to be superior to disease-modifying therapy alone and has become a standard of care for patients with MS, especially those who are vitamin D deficient.

Bibliography

Golan D, Halhal B, Glass-Marmor L, et al. Vitamin D supplementation for patients with multiple sclerosis treated with interferon-beta: a randomized controlled trial assessing the effect on flu-like symptoms and immunomodulatory properties. BMC Neurol. 2013 Jun 14;13:60. [PMID: 23767916]

Item 2   Answer: C

Educational Objective: Diagnose mild cognitive impairment.

The most likely underlying cause of this patient's symptoms is mild cognitive impairment (MCI). MCI is a cognitive state between normal aging and dementia characterized by a decline in cognitive functioning that is greater than what is expected with normal aging but has not resulted in significant functional disability. For most patients, the onset is insidious, and for some, the course may be progressive; 10% to 15% of patients with MCI transition to dementia per year, compared with 1% to 2% per year of the general population. The Montreal Cognitive Assessment is a screening tool that is more sensitive than the Mini–Mental State Examination in the detection of MCI because it has more cognitively challenging tests of memory/recall and executive function. A score lower than 26/30 generally suggests cognitive impairment, especially in patients with 16 years of formal education. In clinical practice, a careful history and results of a standard mental examination are often sufficient to make a diagnosis of MCI, and extensive cognitive testing is not routinely required. Occasionally, a formal battery of neuropsychological testing beyond the standard mental examination is needed to distinguish particularly mild cases of cognitive impairment from normal aging.

In order to meet criteria for dementia, a patient's cognitive deficits must interfere with daily functioning and result in some loss of independence. A detailed history of the patient's abilities to perform activities of daily living, such as paying bills, managing financial records, assembling tax records, shopping alone, working on hobbies, taking medications, driving, and remembering recent holidays or family events, should be obtained to elicit any change in function. This patient does not meet the criteria for dementia.

The diagnosis of clinical depression is based on patient history and exclusion of alternative diagnoses; no additional tests can confirm the diagnosis. The evaluation must establish whether the patient meets established criteria for major depression, dysthymia, or a different psychiatric condition and also assess for substance abuse. Depressed mood and anhedonia are cardinal symptoms, and the presence of either is highly sensitive but not specific for major depression. Using a two-item questionnaire that assesses for the presence of depressed mood or anhedonia is a quick way to screen for depression. If either depressed mood or anhedonia is present, further inquiry or employing a second tool to diagnose depression should be pursued. This patient, who describes her mood as upbeat and says she enjoys her life, has neither depressed mood nor anhedonia. Therefore, depression is unlikely to be the cause of her symptoms.

Patients with memory problems due to normal aging have symptoms, most notably memory loss, that are commonly associated with cognitive impairment, but cognitive testing shows functioning within the normal range. This patient's memory difficulties are greater than what is expected with normal aging, and her score on the Montreal Cognitive Assessment is not in the normal range.

KEY POINT

- A score lower than 26/30 on the Montreal Cognitive Assessment generally suggests cognitive impairment, especially in patients with many years of formal education.

Bibliography
Petersen RC. Clinical practice. Mild cognitive impairment. N Engl J Med. 2011 Jun 9;364(23):2227-34. [PMID: 21651394]

Item 3   Answer: B

Educational Objective: Treat acute spinal cord injury.

This patient should receive high-dose methylprednisolone as the next step in management. He has an acute spinal cord injury most likely due to traumatic fracture of a thoracic vertebra and subsequent spinal cord compression. The localization of the injury at approximately the T8 level of the spinal cord is clear, given the bilateral leg weakness and reduced tone, reduced anal sphincter tone, and the sensory level on pinprick testing. Large clinical trials have shown improved motor function recovery up to 1 year after administration of an intravenous bolus of methylprednisolone, 30 mg/kg, within the first 8 hours of traumatic spinal cord injury followed by a 5.4-mg/kg infusion over the next 23 hours. A recent trial has shown that extending this infusion for an additional 24 hours further increases recovery. Because of these studies, immediate administration of high-dose methylprednisolone for suspected traumatic spinal cord injury has become standard of care.

Diagnostic studies are not appropriate because of the acuity of the situation. Given that the patient experienced the trauma 7 hours before he was seen in the emergency department, ordering CT or MRI would delay initiation of treatment, which is necessary within the first 8 hours of the traumatic event. Obtaining a confirmatory MRI of the thoracic spine at a later time is appropriate. However, CT of the head is not needed because the injury localizes to the thoracic spine on examination. Although the patient received some trauma to the head, CT is likely unnecessary, given that he had no loss of (or impaired) consciousness, no evidence of significant external head trauma, and no other signs or symptoms of traumatic brain injury.

Phenytoin would not treat this patient's spinal cord injury. Administration of phenytoin after significant head trauma may be indicated to prevent seizures, but this patient does not appear to have significant head trauma, nor is this the most acute issue at this time.

KEY POINT

- High-dose methylprednisolone administered within 8 hours of a traumatic spinal cord injury has been shown to improve motor function recovery.

Bibliography
Bracken MB. Steroids for acute spinal cord injury. Cochrane Database Syst Rev. 2012 Jan 18;1:CD001046. [PMID: 22258943]

Item 4   Answer: A

Educational Objective: Evaluate transient ischemic attack.

The patient should undergo carotid ultrasonography. He most likely has experienced a transient ischemic attack (TIA), which implies the absence of retinal or cerebral infarction. His ABCD^2 score, which is based on a patient's Age, Blood pressure, Clinical presentation, Duration of symptoms, and the presence of Diabetes mellitus, is 2 (one point for elevated blood pressure and one point for the symptom of slurred speech), which indicates a 2-day stroke risk of 1.3%. The antecedent transient monocular blindness in the left eye is concerning for extracranial atherosclerosis of the internal carotid artery. Hospital admission is recommended for all patients with TIAs who have an ABCD^2 score of 3 or greater to expedite diagnostic testing and stroke subtyping; admission is also recommended for patients with a score of 0 to 2 if rapid outpatient evaluation cannot be performed.

Carotid ultrasonography to evaluate for symptomatic extracranial internal carotid artery stenosis is the most appropriate next diagnostic test in this patient with a TIA, given the high risk of early recurrence. Patients with greater than 70% extracranial internal carotid artery atherosclerotic stenosis have the highest risk of stroke in the 2 weeks after a TIA. Carotid Duplex ultrasonography is noninvasive and can effectively rule out significant atherosclerotic disease. If the ultrasound suggests greater than 50% stenosis, hospital admission and a confirmatory test with magnetic resonance or CT angiography is appropriate, with plans for early revascularization. Rapid cardiac testing with transthoracic echocardiography and cardiac rhythm evaluation also is advised within 24 hours for all patients with suspected TIA, as is vascular imaging of the extracranial carotid arteries.

CT angiography of the neck is inappropriate at this point because extracranial internal carotid artery stenosis can be excluded without exposing the patient to a highly invasive procedure with contrast and radiation.

Although an MRI of the brain can distinguish a TIA from an ischemic stroke and reveal infarcts in other arterial territories, it is inappropriate as the next diagnostic test in this patient because results are unlikely to affect immediate management. In addition, MRI may not be readily available and may be contraindicated in some patients.

Transesophageal echocardiography may be indicated to identify embolic sources of a TIA or stroke in patients in whom noninvasive diagnostic testing has been unrevealing. However, the yield of transesophageal echocardiography is

Answers and Critiques

CONT. low (approximately 1%) in patients who are in sinus rhythm, particularly among those older than age 45 years. Although MRI ultimately may be indicated for this patient, appropriate noninvasive testing should be performed first, including cardiac rhythm evaluation and vascular imaging of the carotid arteries.

KEY POINT

- In a patient with a suspected transient ischemic attack, noninvasive carotid ultrasonography is the most appropriate test to exclude significant athero-sclerotic disease.

Bibliography

Easton JD, Saver JL, Albers GW, et al; American Heart Association; American Stroke Association Stroke Council; Council on Cardiovascular Surgery and Anesthesia; Council on Cardiovascular Radiology and Intervention; Council on Cardiovascular Nursing; Interdisciplinary Council on Peripheral Vascular Disease. Definition and evaluation of transient ischemic attack: a scientific statement for healthcare professionals from the American Heart Association/American Stroke Association Stroke Council; Council on Cardiovascular Surgery and Anesthesia; Council on Cardiovascular Radiology and Intervention; Council on Cardiovascular Nursing; and the Interdisciplinary Council on Peripheral Vascular Disease. The American Academy of Neurology affirms the value of this statement as an educational tool for neurologists. Stroke. 2009 Jun;40(6):2276-93. Epub 2009 May 7. [PMID: 19423857]

Item 5   Answer: C

Educational Objective: Monitor an incidentally discovered meningioma.

Repeat MRI in 3 to 6 months is the most appropriate next step in management. The radiographic features associated with this patient are most consistent with a meningioma, which may be unrelated to his previous headaches, given the tumor's small size and lack of other symptoms. Meningiomas are benign tumors that arise from the meningeal coverings of the brain. They are the most common extra-axial (not in the brain parenchyma) intracranial lesion in adults. Meningiomas are typically slow-growing tumors, and clinical signs tend to be subtle. They also are often discovered incidentally, as in this patient. Meningiomas have characteristic imaging features, including intense homogeneous contrast enhancement ("lightbulb sign"), areas of calcification, and a dural tail, which is thickening of the dura adjacent to the mass. Patients with small, asymptomatic meningiomas without evidence of invasion of other intracranial structures and without surrounding edema are usually followed clinically and radiographically. Meningiomas should be monitored for growth, with a first follow-up scan performed 3 to 6 months after they are identified.

Lumbar puncture is not indicated in this patient whose imaging findings are characteristic of a meningioma. Lumbar puncture may be indicated in patients with suspicious imaging findings (such as partial enhancement or ring enhancement) suggestive of an infectious or inflammatory process. Lumbar puncture is only appropriate in these patients if they also have evidence of increased intracranial pressure, such as papilledema.

Patients with symptomatic tumors, tumors that invade surrounding parenchyma, or tumors that grow over time may be considered for surgery and/or radiation therapy. If intervention is indicated, surgical intervention is usually the first-line therapy, followed by radiation for higher grade tumors or tumors that could not be resected completely. These treatments are not appropriate at this time in this patient who has none of these indications.

KEY POINT

- Meningiomas have characteristic imaging features, including intense homogeneous contrast enhancement ("lightbulb sign") and a dural tail.

Bibliography

Yano S, Kuratsu J; Kumamoto Brain Tumor Research Group. Indications for surgery in patients with asymptomatic meningiomas based on an extensive experience. J Neurosurg. 2006 Oct;105(4):538-43. [PMID: 17044555]

Item 6   Answer: B

Educational Objective: Diagnose focal epilepsy.

This patient most likely has a focal epilepsy syndrome. It is crucial to ask a patient being evaluated for a first seizure about previous more subtle events, such as auras, changes in awareness, and periods of inattention, that may indicate the presence of an as yet unrecognized epilepsy syndrome. The difficult-to-describe sensation of déjà vu that occurred just before this patient's seizure most likely represents an epileptic aura, which is actually a simple partial seizure. The fact that she had the same sensation previously over the past several years suggests that she has had partial seizures before. The features of her current seizure (unilateral shaking and a subjective aura before the onset of convulsion) suggest progression to a secondarily generalized seizure typical of focal epilepsy, although these features are not always present in secondarily generalized seizures.

Alcohol withdrawal is among the many metabolic stressors that can lead to a provoked seizure. Alcohol withdrawal seizures typically occur with other symptoms of withdrawal (behavioral changes and autonomic symptoms) but can sometimes occur in isolation before other withdrawal symptoms. This type of seizure typically does not have the focal features described in this patient, whose previous, recurrent seizures support a diagnosis of epilepsy. In patients with epilepsy, similar triggers, particularly alcohol ingestion and sleep deprivation (as in this patient), can precipitate a seizure or a more serious seizure. However, these seizures are not considered "provoked"; this term is reserved for isolated events in patients without epilepsy.

Distinguishing between focal and generalized epilepsy syndromes may not be possible if a patient has convulsions only. This patient's seizure was preceded by an aura, which is associated with focal epilepsy. The age of onset in this patient (between 30 and 40 years) is also atypical for generalized epilepsy, which usually begins in adolescence or early adulthood.

A posttraumatic seizure can occur within a week of significant head trauma. This patient had head trauma without loss of consciousness 1 month before onset of her first recognized seizure. Her mild head trauma most likely is not

H CONT. related to her convulsive seizure or the diagnosis of epilepsy, particularly because her auras began before she hit her head.

KEY POINT

- Evaluating a patent with an apparent first seizure should include direct questioning about previous subtle events, such as auras, changes in awareness, and periods of inattention, that may indicate the presence of an as yet unrecognized epilepsy syndrome.

Bibliography

French JA, Pedley TA. Clinical practice. Initial management of epilepsy. N Engl J Med. 2008 Jul 10;359(2):166–76. [PMID: 18614784]

Item 7   Answer: A

Educational Objective: Diagnose chronic traumatic encephalopathy.

The most likely diagnosis for this patient is chronic traumatic encephalopathy. Chronic traumatic encephalopathy is a progressive neurodegenerative disorder triggered by repetitive mild head injury that has most often been described in military combat veterans and athletes with a history of multiple concussions and subconcussions. This patient's career as a professional football player would have made him particularly susceptible to this type of injury. Clinical symptoms typically manifest years or decades after repeated head trauma and present insidiously. Behavioral symptoms are common and include depression, suicidal ideation, apathy, and irritability. Disinhibition, impulsivity, and aggression can also occur in the later stages. Cognitive symptoms include problems with memory, attention, concentration, and executive function. With disease progression, poor judgment and poor insight become more prominent. Parkinsonism, disturbance of gait, and speech abnormalities often occur later in the disease course.

Although this patient exhibits mild parkinsonism on clinical examination, he lacks other features to support a diagnosis of dementia with Lewy bodies, such as fluctuating cognition, visual hallucinations, rapid eye movement sleep behavior disorder, and autonomic dysfunction. In addition, his age at symptom onset is unusual for dementia with Lewy bodies, which typically presents in the sixth decade of life or later.

Depression-related cognitive impairment refers to the cognitive deficits associated with depression and most often is characterized by frontal-subcortical dysfunction and slowed processing speed. Cognitive symptoms improve with treatment of depression. The patient has depression accompanied by suicidal ideation, but his history and constellation of additional neurologic and behavioral symptoms are more suggestive of chronic traumatic encephalopathy.

Parkinsonism tends to occur in chronic traumatic encephalopathy during the later stages of the disease. Comorbid neurodegenerative disease, such as Alzheimer disease, Lewy body disease, and Parkinson disease, can be seen in a percentage of patients with chronic traumatic encephalopathy at autopsy, and some evidence suggests that repetitive head injury is associated with increased risk of

these disorders. This patient has slow and shuffling gait and bradykinesia but lacks the cardinal signs of idiopathic Parkinson disease, including resting tremor or rigidity, a unilateral onset, and asymmetric parkinsonism. The most likely diagnosis for his clinical syndrome of cognitive, behavioral, and motor decline is chronic traumatic encephalopathy.

KEY POINT

- Chronic traumatic encephalopathy is a progressive neurodegenerative disorder triggered by repetitive mild head injury as occurs in military combat veterans and athletes with a history of multiple concussions and subconcussions.

Bibliography

McKee AC, Stern RA, Nowinski CJ, et al. The spectrum of disease in chronic traumatic encephalopathy [erratum in Brain.2013 Oct;136(Pt 10):e255]. Brain. 2013 Jan;136(Pt 1):43–64. Epub 2012 Dec 2. [PMID: 23208308]

Item 8   Answer: D

Educational Objective: Treat migraine in a patient with nonspecific MRI abnormalities.

This patient should receive rizatriptan to treat migraine, which is no longer adequately controlled by NSAIDs. Other than increased intensity, the headache pattern has been stable for 25 years. Her history, physical examination findings, and MRI provide no evidence of a secondary headache disorder. The white matter signal abnormalities evident on the MRI are typical of those seen with migraine, specifically in the posterior circulation and particularly in women, as documented in several population-based studies. Data suggest that these lesions are benign and have no correlation with migraine frequency or the appearance of neurologic or cognitive anomalies or deficits. Initiation of a triptan is appropriate in patients with acute migraine who have not responded to treatment with one or more NSAIDs.

Aspirin is unlikely to relieve acute migraine pain that has not responded to two NSAIDs and would be unnecessary for secondary stroke prevention in this patient.

The patient has not reported any clinical events suggestive of stroke or a demyelinating disease, and her normal neurologic examination findings and the absence of any larger or periventricular white matter lesions on MRI would be unusual in multiple sclerosis. Lumbar puncture is thus not warranted in this patient.

Magnetic resonance angiography is also unnecessary. Although migraine is a contributor to stroke risk in women, this patient has no features suggestive of cerebral ischemia and has no aura or other risk factors for cerebrovascular disease.

Timolol is a migraine prophylactic drug that is effective in reducing the frequency of migraine attacks. Pharmacologic prophylaxis of migraine is indicated for headache frequency greater than 2 days per week (or 8 days per month) or use of acute medications, successfully or unsuccessfully, more than 2 days per week. Migraine frequency in this patient is too low to warrant introduction of daily migraine preventive medication.

> **KEY POINT**
> - White matter signal abnormalities are typically seen on MRIs of patients with migraine, particularly in the posterior circulation and particularly in women; these lesions are benign and unrelated to neurologic examination abnormalities or cognitive anomalies

Bibliography

Palm-Meinders IH, Koppen H, Terwindt GM, et al. Structural brain changes in migraine. JAMA. 2012 Nov 14;308(18):1889-97. [PMID: 23150008]

Item 9   Answer: E

Educational Objective: Diagnose temporal lobe epilepsy.

This patient most likely has temporal lobe epilepsy. The rising epigastric sensation she describes is the most common epileptic aura that originates in the temporal lobe. Brief episodic anxiety with or without autonomic symptoms, such as dry mouth, also is characteristic of a temporal lobe seizure. These symptoms can occur independently or together (as in this patient) but are typically stereotyped in a given patient. The aura is a simple partial seizure, which can become a complex partial seizure and lead to altered sensorium and automatisms (such as "fidgety" behavior). The absence of focal findings on MRI and electroencephalography (EEG) does not rule-out a diagnosis of epilepsy and is in fact a common finding in temporal lobe epilepsy.

Frontal lobe epilepsy can present with different types of seizures, but a fearful and epigastric aura is not typical. Classically, frontal lobe seizures cause motor manifestations (focal jerking, bicycling movements) that awaken patients from sleep.

Juvenile absence epilepsy is a form of generalized epilepsy beginning at or after puberty that is characterized by absence seizures with or without convulsive seizures. An absence seizure is a brief loss of awareness, typically lasting 3 to 10 seconds. This type of seizure is not preceded by an aura.

Temporal lobe epilepsy is often misdiagnosed as panic disorder, which has some similar features. However, this patient's events are stereotyped and short in duration, characteristics that are more associated with temporal lobe seizures than panic attacks.

Although psychogenic nonepileptic seizures (PNES) can have numerous manifestations and should be part of the differential diagnosis, they are not the most likely cause of this patient's symptoms. PNES are less likely than epileptic seizures to be consistently stereotyped and brief in duration. The fact that episodes can be triggered by stress does not necessarily distinguish between epileptic and nonepileptic seizures. Given the characteristic and consistent features of this patient's events, she should be treated for presumed epilepsy. If the patient does not respond to treatment, inpatient video EEG monitoring should be considered to make a definitive diagnosis.

> **KEY POINT**
> - A rising epigastric sensation is the most common epileptic aura that originates in the temporal lobe; electroencephalographic and MRI findings are often normal.

Bibliography

Hurley RA, Fisher R, Taber KH. Sudden onset panic: epileptic aura or panic disorder? J Neuropsychiatry Clin Neurosci. 2006 Fall;18(4):436-43. [PMID: 17135371]

Item 10   Answer: B

Educational Objective: Obtain CT without contrast in a patient with acute stroke.

CT of the head without contrast is the most appropriate diagnostic test in this patient. She had sudden-onset severe headache followed by impaired consciousness, symptoms that are most concerning for hemorrhagic stroke caused by an aneurysmal subarachnoid hemorrhage or intracerebral hemorrhage. A neurologic examination by itself lacks sufficient predictive value to evaluate the source of impaired consciousness. Rapid imaging is required to initiate rapid treatment. CT of the head is readily available, can be performed quickly, and is the test of choice to rule out intracerebral hemorrhage, subarachnoid bleeding, and hydrocephalus, all of which may necessitate rapid neurosurgical intervention.

Catheter-based angiography is ultimately indicated in most patients with subarachnoid hemorrhage to determine the source of bleeding. However, CT of the head without contrast, which allows for more rapid imaging, should be performed first to evaluate for any condition (such as hydrocephalus from increased intracranial pressure) that can be rapidly reversed with emergency neurosurgical treatment.

Lumbar puncture should not be performed in a patient with stroke symptoms until the presence of a mass lesion has been excluded. If the patient has elevated intracranial pressure from mass effect, particularly in the cerebellum, lumbar puncture may worsen any cerebral herniation.

In the evaluation of a patient with symptoms of a stroke, MRI is time consuming, not readily available, and not cost-effective; this test also leaves the patient in a less monitored setting during the scanning than does CT. In the acute setting, stroke that requires rapid neurosurgical intervention should be diagnosed as quickly as possible.

> **KEY POINT**
> - CT of the head without contrast is the most appropriate diagnostic test in a patient with acute stroke.

Bibliography

Runchey S, McGee S. Does this patient have a hemorrhagic stroke? Clinical findings distinguishing hemorrhagic stroke from ischemic stroke. JAMA 2010 Jun 9; 303(22):2280-6. Epub 2010 Oct 21. [PMID: 20530782]

Item 11　　Answer:　E

Educational Objective: **Diagnose myotonic dystrophy.**

This patient most likely has myotonic dystrophy. Whereas muscle weakness and fatigue are present in a wide range of myopathies, neuromuscular junction disorders, and other conditions, the presence of myotonia—an impairment of muscle relaxation secondary to increased cellular membrane hyperexcitability—narrows the differential diagnosis. Myotonic dystrophy is the most common myotonic disorder, with accompanying symptoms of cataract, cardiomyopathy, cardiac conduction abnormalities, diabetes mellitus, and alopecia. This condition should be considered in all patients with weakness, fatigue, and a myopathic waddling gait who also have muscle stiffness and delayed grip relaxation. The diagnosis should be confirmed by electromyography; confirmatory genetic testing (for myotonic dystrophy type 1) is available commercially. Myotonic dystrophy type 1 is more common and preferentially involves distal limb and facial muscles, whereas the less common type 2 preferentially affects proximal muscles. An increased awareness of comorbidities of myotonic dystrophy and aggressive management of its cardiac complications, which can increase mortality, are recommended.

Becker muscular dystrophy typically starts in childhood, but its progression can be variable. Its pattern of weakness is predominantly proximal, and calf hypertrophy is present; myotonia is not.

Inclusion body myositis is a slowly progressive inflammatory myopathy that predominantly affects distal upper extremity flexors and quadriceps. Asymmetric involvement is common, but myotonia is not a feature.

Although fatigue and weakness can occur in Lambert-Eaton myasthenic syndrome and myasthenia gravis, neither of these conditions is associated with myotonia.

KEY POINT

- Myotonic dystrophy should be considered in all patients with weakness, fatigue, and a myopathic waddling gait who also have muscle stiffness and delayed grip relaxation.

Bibliography

Udd B, Krahe R. The myotonic dystrophies: molecular, clinical, and therapeutic challenges. Lancet Neurol. 2012 Oct;11(10):891-905. [PMID: 22995693]

Item 12　　Answer:　A

Educational Objective: **Diagnose a subarachnoid hemorrhage with lumbar puncture.**

This patient should undergo lumbar puncture. He reports sudden onset of a severe headache, most likely a thunderclap headache. Thunderclap headache is defined as a severe headache that reaches maximum intensity within 60 seconds of onset. Although classically associated with subarachnoid hemorrhage (SAH), thunderclap headache also may be caused by other conditions, ranging from benign to life-threatening ones. Because approximately 25% of thunderclap headache presentations result from an SAH, this type of headache should be approached as a neurologic emergency. Although other causes are possible, including dural sinus thrombosis, meningitis, and migraine, the presence of a dilated unreactive pupil suggests external compression of the left oculomotor nerve (cranial nerve III). In the presence of a normal mental status, cerebral herniation and increased intracranial pressure are unlikely, but an aneurysm of the left posterior communicating artery is possible that may not be visible on a noncontrast CT scan of the head. Patients with an aneurysmal SAH may first experience less extensive bleeding that also is not visible on a noncontrast head CT before more significant bleeding occurs. After this initial or "sentinel" bleeding, the patient is at high risk for a clinically significant SAH with associated high morbidity and mortality. Therefore, establishing the diagnosis is a priority.

When the suspicion of an SAH is high and the noncontrast CT scan of the head is normal, a lumbar puncture is required to evaluate the cerebrospinal fluid (CSF) for erythrocytes or xanthochromia. Xanthochromia describes a yellow discoloration of the CSF from breakdown of erythrocytes, which may not develop for at least 6 hours after the initial event.

Magnetic resonance angiography (MRA) is premature before SAH is excluded. Once SAH has been ruled out, MRA may be needed to exclude other arterial causes, such as cervicocephalic arterial dissection. Internal carotid artery dissection can cause pupillary abnormalities, but these are typically from a Horner syndrome, with a smaller pupillary diameter in the affected eye.

Similarly, magnetic resonance venography (MRV) of the brain should not be performed until SAH is excluded. MRV is used to diagnose deep venous thrombosis and cerebral venous sinus thrombosis. Although the latter disorder sometimes presents with thunderclap headache, it is unlikely to cause a dilated unreactive left pupil.

The usefulness of MRI for diagnosing SAH remains under investigation. MRI may ultimately be required if the CSF is normal to rule out other disorders.

KEY POINT

- When the suspicion of a subarachnoid hemorrhage is high and the noncontrast CT scan of the head is normal, a lumbar puncture is required to evaluate the cerebrospinal fluid for erythrocytes or xanthochromia.

Bibliography

Connolly ES Jr, Rabinstein AA, Carhuapoma JR, et al; American Heart Association Stroke Council; Council on Cardiovascular Radiology and Intervention; Council on Cardiovascular Nursing; Council on Cardiovascular Surgery and Anesthesia; Council on Clinical Cardiology. Guidelines for the management of aneurysmal subarachnoid hemorrhage: a guideline for healthcare professionals from the American Heart Association/American Stroke Association. Stroke. 2012 Jun;43(6):1711-37. [PMID: 22556195]

Item 13   Answer: C

Educational Objective: Treat primary progressive aphasia.

This patient should have speech and language therapy. His history is concerning for the initial stages of primary progressive aphasia, which is characterized by the progressive loss of language function with relative sparing of other cognitive domains early in the course of the disease. Primary progressive aphasia is most commonly associated with frontotemporal dementia but also may be a manifestation of Alzheimer disease. Different clinical subtypes of primary progressive aphasia exist that are based on the pattern of language impairment, but each progresses insidiously and eventually results in significant disturbance of communication. The disorder results in significant disability but can be very difficult to diagnose early in its course. Occupational therapy for speech and language can teach the patient and family compensatory strategies to improve communication. This treatment is most beneficial early in the disease when motivation, insight, and learning capabilities are greatest.

Determination of the patient's apolipoprotein E (*APOE ε4*) status could help define his risk for developing Alzheimer disease but would not confirm if he has this disorder. Additionally, the information obtained by assessing his genotype would not be informative if the underlying cause is frontotemporal dementia.

Observation with reevaluation in 3 to 6 months is not the most appropriate next step in management because it would delay intervention that could diminish early symptoms.

Donepezil, a cholinesterase inhibitor, is not FDA approved for the treatment of primary progressive aphasia or frontotemporal dementia. For primary progressive aphasia that is due to underlying Alzheimer disease, standard medications approved by the FDA for Alzheimer disease may be appropriate for symptomatic benefit. However, the first step in management should be occupational therapy for speech and language, especially before a diagnosis of Alzheimer disease is established.

KEY POINT

- In primary progressive aphasia, occupational therapy for speech and language can teach the patient and family compensatory strategies to improve communication.

Bibliography

Gorno-Tempini ML, Hillis AE, Weintraub S, et al. Classification of primary progressive aphasia and its variants. Neurology. 2011 Mar 15;76(11):1006-14. [PMID: 21325651]

Item 14   Answer: B

Educational Objective: Treat drug-induced tardive dyskinesia.

The most appropriate next step is to discontinue the dopamine receptor antagonist metoclopramide. This patient has prominent craniofacial features of chorea and dystonia that are characteristic of tardive dyskinesia. She most likely has medication-related dyskinesia, and discontinuation of the causative dopamine blocker agent is required. Physicians prescribing chronic dopamine blocker antinausea agents should warn their patients about the risk of tardive dyskinesia, a complication that can lead to long-lasting or permanent involuntary movements. Old age and female sex increase the risk of this complication.

Typical and most atypical antipsychotic agents can cause tardive dyskinesia. The main exceptions are quetiapine and clozapine. Because atypical antipsychotic agents also increase the risk of symptoms of tardive dyskinesia becoming permanent, risperidone should be avoided in this patient unless absolutely indicated.

Carbidopa-levodopa is appropriate treatment of Parkinson disease, and this patient's slow and narrow-based gait is typical of parkinsonism. However, carbidopa-levodopa can aggravate dyskinetic movements and thus should be avoided in this patient.

Tetrabenazine, a dopamine depleter, has been approved by the FDA for treatment of chorea in Huntington disease. Several studies also have shown its efficacy in reducing tardive dyskinesia, but this remains an off-label use. Because tardive dyskinesia often spontaneously resolves within several months of removal of the causative agent, the immediate use of tetrabenazine in this patient with a mood disorder is unjustified, especially in light of the drug's serious mood-related complications.

KEY POINT

- The most appropriate treatment of medication-related tardive dyskinesia is discontinuation of the causative dopamine blocker agent.

Bibliography

van Harten PN, Tenback DE. Tardive dyskinesia: clinical presentation and treatment. Int Rev Neurobiol. 2011;98:187-210. [PMID: 21907088]

Item 15   Answer: C

Educational Objective: Monitor patients for adverse effects of multiple sclerosis therapies.

This patient being treated with an interferon beta preparation should have her serum aminotransferase levels measured every 3 to 6 months. Interferon injections are associated with rare autoimmune hepatitis. Therefore, monitoring of liver status by periodic measurement of serum aminotransferase levels is appropriate in patients with multiple sclerosis (MS) who take an interferon beta preparation as a disease-modifying therapy. Although the optimal frequency of monitoring has not been established, most cases of severe hepatotoxicity appear to occur early in therapy. It is also recommended that concurrent use of potentially hepatotoxic agents, such as alcohol, be avoided while taking interferon therapy. Other more common adverse effects include injection site reactions, flu-like symptoms, and depression.

JC virus antibody screening is currently recommended as a risk mitigation strategy for patients with MS treated with natalizumab because elevated levels of JC virus antibody have been correlated with an increased risk of progressive multifocal leukoencephalopathy (PML) in patients taking this drug. However, no incidences of PML have been reported in patients (such as this one) treated with interferon beta injections. Therefore, monitoring for JC virus antibody is not indicated.

Frequent ophthalmologic examinations are recommended for patients taking fingolimod for MS because of the risk of macular edema. No specific ocular risks are associated with interferon injections.

Teriflunomide has been associated with pancreatitis, and monitoring of the serum amylase and lipase levels is indicated for patients with MS who take this medication. Interferon beta preparations have not been associated with this adverse effect.

KEY POINT

- In patients taking an interferon beta as a disease-modifying therapy for multiple sclerosis, serum aminotransferase levels should be measured every 3 to 6 months to monitor for autoimmune hepatitis.

Bibliography

Goodin DS, Frohman EM, Garmany GP Jr et al; Therapeutics and Technology Assessment Subcommittee of the American Academy of Neurology and the MS Council for Clinical Practice Guidelines. Disease modifying therapies in multiple sclerosis: report of the Therapeutics and Technology Assessment Subcommittee of the American Academy of Neurology and the MS Council for Clinical Practice Guidelines [erratum in Neurology. 2002 Aug 13;59(3):480]. Neurology. 2002 Jan 22;58(2):169-78. [PMID: 11805241]

Item 16   Answer: B

Educational Objective: Treat with antiplatelet agents for secondary stroke prevention.

Dipyridamole should be added to this patient's medication regimen. She had a small subcortical infarction despite taking daily aspirin before the stroke. The combination of aspirin and dipyridamole has been shown to be superior to aspirin alone in reducing the risk of recurrent stroke.

The combination of aspirin and clopidogrel versus aspirin alone in patients with small subcortical infarcts (lacunes) was associated with increased mortality without the benefit of reducing the risk of recurrent stroke in the Secondary Prevention of Small Subcortical Strokes (SPS3) trial. Similarly, in the Management of Atherothrombosis with Clopidogrel in High-Risk Patients with Recent Transient Ischemic Attacks or Ischemic Stroke (MATCH) trial, the combination of dual antiplatelet agents was associated with an increased risk of hemorrhagic complications that offset any potential clinical benefit. The combination of aspirin and clopidogrel thus has limited utility in the secondary prevention of stroke.

Ticlopidine is not first-line treatment for secondary stroke prevention. Although superior to aspirin in preventing a second stroke, ticlopidine is associated with the serious adverse effects of agranulocytosis and thrombotic thrombocytopenic purpura and thus is considered a second-line agent.

Warfarin should not be substituted for aspirin because no evidence of atrial fibrillation or other high-risk cardioembolic sources of stroke was detected in this patient.

KEY POINT

- The combination of aspirin and dipyridamole has been shown to be superior to aspirin alone in reducing the risk of recurrent stroke.

Bibliography

Furie KL, Kasner SE, Adams RJ, et al; American Heart Association Stroke Council, Council on Cardiovascular Nursing, Council on Clinical Cardiology, and Interdisciplinary Council on Quality of Car and Outcomes Research. Guidelines for the prevention of stroke in patients with stroke or transient ischemic attack: a guideline for healthcare professionals from the American Heart Association/American Stroke Association. Stroke. 2011 Jan;42(1):227-76. Epub 2010 Oct 21. [PMID: 20966421]

Item 17   Answer: C

Educational Objective: Treat epilepsy in a woman taking oral contraceptives.

This patient's epilepsy, which is strongly suggested by her MRI and electroencephalographic findings, should be treated with an antiepileptic drug (AED). Of the AEDs listed, levetiracetam is most appropriate for a woman who takes oral contraceptive pills for polycystic ovary syndrome (PCOS) and also relies on them for contraception because it has no significant interactions with synthetic hormones. Most AEDs, particularly older agents, induce hepatic enzymes that alter the metabolism of hormonal contraceptives. This alteration may lead to unpredictable levels of synthetic estrogens and progestin; additionally, when the contraceptives are used to prevent pregnancy, increased failure can occur in women taking AEDs.

Carbamazepine and oxcarbazepine induce cytochrome CYP3A4 and thus affect the metabolism of synthetic estrogens and progestins, which makes many forms of hormonal contraception ineffective. Neither drug is an appropriate treatment for this patient. An intrauterine device (IUD) is the preferred method of contraception for women taking enzyme-inducing AEDs, but an IUD would not address this patient's PCOS symptoms.

Lamotrigine has unique interactions with hormonal contraceptives. Synthetic estrogens induce the clearance of lamotrigine by as much as 50%, which means that higher dosages of lamotrigine have to be administered to patients taking an oral contraceptive and that AED levels will increase during the placebo week of contraceptive therapy. If needed, lamotrigine can be administered with extended-cycle oral contraceptives, but an IUD is the preferred method of contraception for patients taking lamotrigine. Lamotrigine also decreases levels of synthetic progestins by 20%, although the clinical significance of this decrease is unknown.

Topiramate also increases clearance of synthetic estrogens. Although the clinical significance of this effect with lower doses of topiramate is debated, the World Health Organization advises against combining oral contraceptives with any dose of topiramate and recommends an IUD for contraception in patients taking this drug. Furthermore, topiramate is considered a class D drug for pregnancy because of the increased risk of facial clefting in exposed children, Therefore, it should not be used as a first-line agent in women of childbearing age.

KEY POINT

- Levetiracetam has no major drug-to-drug interactions with hormonal contraceptives and thus is appropriate to use in women with epilepsy who take oral contraceptives.

Bibliography

Gaffield ME, Culwell KR, Lee CR. The use of hormonal contraception among women taking anticonvulsant therapy. Contraception. 2011 Jan;83(1): 16-29. [PMID: 21134499]

Item 18   Answer: D

Educational Objective: Treat stroke with admission to the stroke unit.

This patient has had an acute ischemic stroke and should be admitted to the inpatient stroke unit. Several studies have shown that admission of patients with stroke to an organized inpatient stroke unit compared with a general medical ward is associated with a reduction in mortality at 1 year, with benefits persisting up to several years after stroke. Stroke units are beneficial because of the multidisciplinary nature of care, with an emphasis on specialized nursing, early mobilization, removal of urinary bladder catheters, and adherence to stroke-specific protocols. An important component of the success of stroke units is early referral for rehabilitation services to promote stroke recovery.

Adding clopidogrel to this patient's medication regimen is inappropriate management because the combination of aspirin and clopidogrel has not been shown to be effective and may increase the risk of hemorrhage over the next 3 months. The combination of aspirin and clopidogrel recently was found to reduce the risk of recurrent stroke compared with aspirin alone when administered within 24 hours of transient ischemic attack or minor stroke (National Institutes of Health [NIH] Stroke Scale score less than 5). Because this patient is beyond the 24-hour mark and scored 8 on the NIH Stroke Scale, no evidence supports giving her combination therapy.

This patient's blood pressure is within the acceptable range for someone who has had an acute ischemic stroke. Immediate blood pressure lowering with labetalol or other antihypertensive agents in patients who do not receive intravenous thrombolysis is only recommended if the blood pressure is greater than 220/120 mm Hg or if a high risk or evidence of other end-organ damage exists; neither situation applies.

This patient is well beyond the acceptable timeframe for thrombolysis (3 hours).

KEY POINT

- In patients with newly diagnosed stroke, admission to an organized inpatient stroke unit compared with a general medical ward is associated with a reduction in mortality at 1 year, with benefits persisting up to several years after stroke.

Bibliography

Stroke Unit Trialists' Collaboration. Organised inpatient (stroke unit) care for stroke. Cochrane Database Syst Rev. 2013 Sep 11;9:CD000197. [PMID: 24026639]

Item 19   Answer: D

Educational Objective: Treat generalized epilepsy.

This patient should be treated with a broad-spectrum antiepileptic drug (AED), such as topiramate. Given his history of recurrent unprovoked seizures, he clearly has an epilepsy syndrome, but the seizure features and results of ancillary testing do not definitively identify what kind of epilepsy syndrome. When it is unclear if a patient has focal or generalized epilepsy, treatment should be a broad-spectrum AED that can be used to treat both generalized and partial epilepsy syndromes. Topiramate is a broad-spectrum agent appropriate for both focal and generalized epilepsy; other appropriate drugs are lamotrigine, levetiracetam, valproic acid, and zonisamide. Patients starting topiramate should be counseled about the risk of developing kidney stones and the need to stay hydrated. Topiramate may offer additional advantages to patients with comorbid headaches. It also is associated with weight loss and thus may be of added benefit in patients who are overweight. However, the drug may have cognitive adverse effects, such as word-finding difficulty, in some patients. The risk of rash and Stevens-Johnson syndrome should be discussed with all patients starting an AED.

Carbamazepine, gabapentin, and phenytoin are all narrow-spectrum AEDs used to treat partial-onset epilepsies. They have the potential to exacerbate generalized epilepsy and may provoke absence status epilepticus. They should be used when the seizure characteristics or MRI and electroencephalogram clearly support the diagnosis of a partial onset seizure. Typical features suggestive of partial onset include specific auras (déjà vu or a rising epigastric sensation) and unilateral clonic shaking before onset.

KEY POINT

- Topiramate is a broad-spectrum antiepileptic drug that is appropriate for treating both focal and generalized epilepsy, especially when the specific epilepsy syndrome is unknown.

Bibliography

Glauser T, Ben-Menachem E, Bourgeois B, et al; ILAE Subcommission on AED Guidelines. Updated ILAE evidence review of antiepileptic drug efficacy and effectiveness as initial monotherapy for epileptic seizures and syndromes. Epilepsia. 2013 Mar;54(3):551-63. [PMID: 23350722]

Item 20   Answer: B

Educational Objective: Diagnose normal pressure hydrocephalus.

Large-volume lumbar puncture is indicated in this patient with likely normal pressure hydrocephalus (NPH). NPH is the most likely diagnosis in the setting of the triad of gait abnormalities, cognitive impairment, and urinary disturbance, especially when neuroimaging studies show enlarged ventricles out of proportion to cortical atrophy. NPH is a potentially reversible cause of cognitive and motor decline. A large-volume lumbar puncture with measurement of intracranial pressure and removal of 30 to 50 mL of cerebrospinal fluid (CSF) should be performed before consideration of placement of a ventriculoperitoneal shunt. Cognitive, balance, and gait examinations before and after the lumbar puncture can be useful to evaluate for potential response to shunting. If a positive response to the initial lumbar puncture is not seen and the clinical suspicion remains high, serial lumbar punctures or continuous lumbar drainage can be considered.

Periventricular white matter changes can be seen on the brain MRI and may have an identical appearance to what is seen in small-vessel vascular disease. However, without additional clinical or neuroradiologic evidence of a previous infarction, extensive evaluation with neurovascular imaging to assess for a cause of these radiologic changes on brain MRI is not warranted. Periventricular hyperintensities are a frequent finding in normal pressure hydrocephalus and are thought to be related to transependymal resorption of CSF.

The cholinesterase inhibitor donepezil is sometimes effective in improving cognitive symptoms and function in patients with Alzheimer disease but has no benefit for the gait and cognitive disturbances typical of normal pressure hydrocephalus.

Although this patient has evidence of lower-body parkinsonism, he lacks other findings that suggest the presence of idiopathic Parkinson disease, such as a resting tremor, asymmetric onset of motor symptoms, and typical nonmotor symptoms. Therefore, levodopa is not likely to result in any symptomatic benefit.

KEY POINT

- Large-volume lumbar puncture should be performed before placement of a ventriculoperitoneal shunt in patients with normal pressure hydrocephalus.

Bibliography

Williams MA, Relkin NR. Diagnosis and management of idiopathic normal-pressure hydrocephalus. Neurol Clin Pract. 2013 Oct;3(5):375-85. [PMID: 24175154]

Item 21   Answer: A

Educational Objective: Diagnose carotid artery dissection.

The patient most likely has had a carotid artery dissection. Despite his migraine history, the report of a different type of headache should raise suspicion of a secondary headache. Cervicocephalic dissection is an uncommon but important cause of stroke, especially in persons younger than 50 years. The presence of ipsilateral neck pain and ischemic complications, such as transient monocular visual loss and Horner syndrome (miosis, ptosis, and anhidrosis), is characteristic of carotid artery dissection and may not be associated with preceding trauma. The cause of an associated stroke is primarily thrombus formation at the site of dissection with subsequent artery-to-artery embolism. The imaging modality of choice is an MRI of the soft tissues in the neck, which will demonstrate a crescent-shaped hematoma within the internal carotid artery wall on T1-weighted images. Aspirin is considered the treatment of choice to prevent ongoing ischemic complications or stroke.

Cluster headache is a primary headache disorder classified as a trigeminal autonomic cephalalgia. This type of headache presents with unilateral head pain, which is typically periorbital or temporal ("trigeminal") but sometimes may affect the face or neck. Cranial autonomic features, such as ptosis, miosis, tearing, and nasal congestion, are characteristic. Cluster headaches appear in a repetitive fashion, one to eight times daily, and are brief, with durations between 15 minutes and 3 hours. Related trigeminal autonomic cephalgias, such as chronic paroxysmal hemicrania or short-lasting unilateral neuralgiform headaches with conjunctival injection and tearing (SUNCT syndrome), occur with greater frequency and are of shorter duration, lasting minutes and seconds respectively. In this patient, the headache developed abruptly and has lasted an entire day, with no prior pattern indicative of these disorders.

The patient has a history of migraine, but his description of a "different" headache should raise concerns for secondary explanations. The duration of the attack is not outside the acceptable range for migraine (4 to 72 hours), and migraine can present with either unilateral or bilateral discomfort. Visual aura is described by 25% to 35% of those with established migraine, but monocular visual loss is much more uncommon than binocular hemifield impairment. Ptosis and miosis resulting from migraine are quite uncommon. Red flags in this patient's case include the "different" nature of the headache, the new symptoms of neck pain and monocular visual dysfunction, the abrupt onset of pain during physical exertion, and (most importantly) the abnormal physical examination findings. This combination renders migraine unlikely.

Vertebral artery dissection can present with acute head or neck pain associated with physical exertion or trauma but also can occur spontaneously. The most common symptom is headache, but neurologic symptoms or deficits also occur. As many as 25% of ischemic strokes in younger patients result from either carotid or vertebral artery dissection. Because the vertebrobasilar supply of the occipital cortex or cerebellum may be affected, symptoms of loss of vision or balance are common. Although ptosis and miosis may arise from infarction of the lateral medulla (Wallenberg syndrome) in vertebral dissection, they are always accompanied by other findings, such as vertigo, dysarthria, dysphagia, ataxia, and

CONT. loss of pain and temperature sensation ipsilaterally in the face and contralaterally in the body.

KEY POINT

- Carotid artery dissection should be suspected in a patient with acute headache and neck pain associated with Horner syndrome.

Bibliography

Kennedy F, Lanfranconi S, Hicks C, et al; CADISS Investigators. Antiplatelets vs anticoagulation for dissection: CADISS nonrandomized arm and meta-analysis. Neurology. 2012 Aug 14;79(7):686-9. [PMID: 22855862]

Item 22   Answer: C

Educational Objective: Diagnose oxcarbazepine-associated hyponatremia.

Oxcarbazepine is the drug most likely to be responsible for this patient's symptoms and abnormal laboratory findings, and its dosage should be reduced. The drug is associated with hyponatremia in 20% to 30% of the patients taking this medication. In most patients, symptoms associated with hyponatremia are generally mild and not clinically significant. However, severe hyponatremia occurs in 8% to 12% of these patients. Higher doses of oxcarbazepine and polytherapy with other drugs increase the risk of hyponatremia. Although a direct effect on the kidneys has been proposed, the exact mechanism of oxcarbazepine-induced hyponatremia is not well understood. Decreasing the dosage or discontinuing oxcarbazepine, if safe to do so, can help correct hyponatremia. Either of these steps should be taken in conjunction with standard evaluation and management of hyponatremia, including free water restriction. Hyponatremia also can occur with carbamazepine but is much more common and severe with oxcarbazepine use.

This patient's dizziness, end-gaze nystagmus, and ataxia also are likely adverse effects of oxcarbazepine use, although they could be related to the hyponatremia itself. These symptoms and findings can be seen with all antiepileptic drugs (AEDs), particularly in polytherapy, but are most common with AEDs that act on sodium channels, including oxcarbazepine, carbamazepine, lamotrigine, and phenytoin.

Clonazepam, levetiracetam, and topiramate are not associated with hyponatremia. Clonazepam can cause sedation, tolerance, and dependence. The most common adverse effect of levetiracetam is irritability and other adverse effects on mood. Topiramate can cause a mild, usually subclinical acidosis and a low serum bicarbonate level but does not affect the serum sodium level. It is also associated with kidney stones, weight loss, and acute angle-closure glaucoma.

KEY POINT

- Oxcarbazepine is associated with hyponatremia in 20% to 30% of the patients who take it; although symptoms are generally mild and not clinically significant, severe hyponatremia occurs in 8% to 12% of these patients.

Bibliography

Lin CH, Lu CH, Wang FJ, et al. Risk factors of oxcarbazepine-induced hyponatremia in patients with epilepsy. Clin Neuropharmacol. 2010 Nov-Dec;33(6):293-6. [PMID: 20881597]

Item 23   Answer: C

Educational Objective: Treat depression-related cognitive impairment.

The patient's symptoms are consistent with a major depressive episode, which should be treated with sertraline. More than half of patients with late-life major depression exhibit clinically significant cognitive impairment, most frequently affecting processing speed, executive function, and visuospatial ability. Her feelings of isolation and sadness, previous depressive episode, loss of interest in reading, loss of energy, poor concentration, indecisiveness, and significant weight loss are all suggestive of major depression. Depression-related cognitive impairment, historically known as pseudodementia, can be difficult to distinguish from early degenerative diseases. Cognitive testing may show objective impairment of working memory, attention, executive function, and processing speed. Psychomotor slowing, also known as psychomotor retardation, refers to reduced processing speed and motor activity, such as in speech and fine- and gross-motor skills. Psychomotor slowing is a common feature of severe depression. First-line treatment of major depression includes pharmacotherapy, with or without psychotherapy. Each patient should be clinically treated and then monitored for effectiveness of therapy, continued need for pharmacotherapy, and response of cognitive symptoms.

Carbidopa-levodopa is an effective medication for symptomatic treatment of Parkinson disease (PD). This patient exhibits psychomotor slowing but lacks the decremental response (decreased speed and amplitude) on repetitive movements typical of PD and also other defining features of PD. This medication is not effective in treating major depression.

Donepezil is a cholinesterase inhibitor that can be effective in improving cognitive symptoms and function in patients with Alzheimer disease. This patient's history and results of cognitive testing are not consistent with a diagnosis of dementia. Although depression can represent a prodrome to PD, Alzheimer disease, and other neurodegenerative conditions and often accompanies these conditions, cholinesterase inhibitors are not effective in treating major depression.

Depression is often unrecognized and undertreated in the elderly and is not a consequence of normal aging. Late-life depression has been associated with an increased risk of dementia and should be treated aggressively. Therefore, clinical observation is insufficient as management.

KEY POINT

- First-line treatment of major depression in patients with cognitive impairment is pharmacotherapy, with or without psychotherapy.

Answers and Critiques

Bibliography

Pellegrino LD, Peters ME, Lyketsos CG, Marano CM. Depression in cognitive impairment. Curr Psychiatry Rep. 2013 Sep;15(9):384. [PMID: 23933974]

Item 24   Answer: C

Educational Objective: Treat migraine with typical aura.

The patient should discontinue taking the combined oral contraceptive. She has a history of migraine with typical aura. Aura is considered typical if it involves any combination of visual, hemisensory, or language dysfunction, with sensory auras most typically affecting the face and upper extremities. Each neurologic feature of a typical aura typically lasts between 5 and 60 minutes before completely resolving and can occur before, during, or independent of a headache. Migraine with typical or other aura is a strong contributor to stroke risk in women. Data suggest that migraine with aura represents the second greatest risk factor for stroke in women (after hypertension), surpassing even diabetes mellitus. Estrogen-containing contraceptives, which further increase stroke risk, should be avoided by women with this diagnosis. Progesterone-only oral contraceptives, injections, implants, and intrauterine devices do not appear to increase the risk of stroke in these patients and are preferred means of contraception in this population.

Findings from physical examination and neuroimaging studies showed no evidence of a stroke in this patient. Therefore, aspirin therapy is unnecessary.

Topiramate is approved for use as migraine prophylaxis. Because this patient typically has a migraine only at onset of menses that is successfully treated with rizatriptan, she has no need for migraine preventive therapies.

Although basilar migraine and hemiplegic migraine are contraindications for triptan therapy, this patient has no symptoms indicating the presence of either subtype. Discontinuation of rizatriptan is thus unnecessary.

KEY POINT

- Because women with migraine with aura have an increased risk of stroke, estrogen-containing oral contraceptives, which further increase stroke risk, should be avoided.

Bibliography

MacGregor EA. Contraception and headache. Headache. 2013 Feb;53(2):247-76. [PMID: 23432442]

Item 25   Answer: D

Educational Objective: Treat essential tremor.

This patient should begin a trial of primidone for his worsening essential tremor. His long history of a bilateral action tremor, family history of tremor, and ethanol responsiveness are consistent with familial essential tremor. Although the severity of this type of tremor remains stable over a lifetime in most patients, a few experience tremor progression that can become disabling. Primidone and propranolol are FDA-approved first-line treatments of essential tremor. Because propranolol has already been administered without lasting relief, a trial of primidone is warranted.

Botulinum toxin injections can be effective in patients with essential tremor of the voice and head, but its benefit is more limited in the limbs because of the adverse effect of weakness. In this patient, primidone should be initiated first.

In patients with severe medication-refractory essential tremor, deep brain stimulation (DBS) of the thalamus is most likely to maximize tremor control. However, this option should be reserved for those who have not responded to medical therapy or have a marked disabling tremor. In this subset of patients, DBS has the potential to provide significant tremor control beyond that offered by the best medical therapy. DBS is premature for this patient who has not yet had a trial of primidone.

This patient does not have features of Parkinson disease, such as a tremor at rest. Therefore, levodopa therapy is not indicated.

Topiramate is a second-line treatment of essential tremor but is contraindicated in a patient with a history of kidney stones and glaucoma.

KEY POINT

- In patients with essential tremor, propranolol and primidone are FDA approved first-line therapies.

Bibliography

Zesiewicz TA, Elble RJ, Louis ED, et al. Evidence-based guideline update: treatment of essential tremor: report of the Quality Standards subcommittee of the American Academy of Neurology. Neurology. 2011 Nov 8;77(19):1752-5. [PMID: 22013182]

Item 26   Answer: C   H

Educational Objective: Treat compressive spinal cord lesions due to plasmacytoma.

This patient should undergo external beam radiation therapy for his epidural plasmacytoma in addition to continued high-dose glucocorticoid treatment. Skeletal lesions that occur as a result of plasmacytoma or myeloma are exquisitely radiosensitive; therefore, radiation therapy is the most appropriate specific and definitive treatment for this tumor type. Patients with compressive myelopathy due to very radiosensitive tumors who have a stable spine and minimal neurologic deficits may respond to this therapy, with recovery or improvement of their neurologic deficits.

Although radiation therapy is the preferred acute treatment for compressive myelopathy in patients with plasmacytomas because of their high level of radiosensitivity and rapid response to treatment, chemotherapy may be a reasonable second-line therapy for selected patients with compressive myelopathy due to myeloma.

High-dose intravenous glucocorticoids administered within the first 8 hours of traumatic spinal cord injury can be useful in the short term to reduce the effect of edema within the spinal cord caused by a compressive injury. However, these drugs will not treat the underlying neoplastic disease and thus are inappropriate as monotherapy in this patient.

Immediate surgical decompression is indicated with evidence of spinal instability or with severe neurologic deficits that require removal of the bulk of the tumor to prevent continued injury to the spinal cord. This intervention is usually followed by definitive radiation therapy for treatment of the local tumor.

KEY POINT

- Spinal cord compression by skeletal lesions resulting from plasmacytoma should be treated initially with radiation therapy in patients with no spinal instability and only minor neurologic deficits.

Bibliography
Tsutsumi S, Yasumoto Y, Ito M. Solitary spinal extradural plasmacytoma: a case report and literature review. Clin Neuroradiol. 2013 Mar;23(1):5-9. [PMID: 22706517]

Item 27 Answer: B

Educational Objective: Evaluate traumatic brain injury with CT of the head.

This patient should have CT of the head without contrast. The American College of Emergency Physicians and the Centers for Disease Control and Prevention have published guidelines for management of mild traumatic brain injury (TBI). Their recommendation is to consider a noncontrast head CT in patients with TBI who have had no loss of consciousness or posttraumatic amnesia but have a focal neurologic deficit, vomiting, severe headache, physical signs of a basilar skull fracture, Glasgow Coma Scale score less than 15, coagulopathy, or a dangerous mechanism of injury, such as ejection from a motor vehicle or a falling from a height of more than 3 feet. This patient sustained a TBI with a dangerous mechanism of injury several hours ago and has developed symptoms (worsening headache and vomiting) mentioned in the guideline. Therefore, noncontrast CT of the head is indicated. A finding of parenchymal, subdural, or epidural hemorrhage requires emergent neurosurgical evaluation and consideration of possible hematoma evacuation.

In the setting of acute head trauma, head CT without contrast is preferable to head CT with contrast and brain MRI because of its lower cost and wider availability. Contrast administration aids in the assessment of certain malignant and vascular lesions of the brain but adds nothing to the evaluation of acute head trauma. Head CT without contrast is also very sensitive for detecting skull fracture or acute hemorrhage, and a CT scan generally requires shorter examination times than a brain MRI requires, both important factors in the evaluation of a patient with acute head injury and symptoms of potential deterioration.

Hospital observation without first ruling out intracranial hemorrhage is inappropriate management of TBI.

Untreated intracranial hemorrhage can lead to an accumulation of blood and edema within the skull, which can cause compression or destruction of brain tissue, increased intracranial pressure, and even herniation and death.

KEY POINT

- Head CT without contrast is the appropriate imaging procedure for selected patients with acute traumatic brain injury.

Bibliography
Jagoda AS, Bazarian JJ, Bruns JJ Jr, et al; American College of Emergency Physicians; Centers for Disease Control and Prevention. Clinical policy: neuroimaging and decision making in adult mild traumatic brain injury in the acute setting. Ann Emerg Med. 2008 Dec;52(6):714-48. [PMID: 19027497]

Item 28 Answer: D

Educational Objective: Recognize adverse effects of cholinesterase inhibitors in a patient with Alzheimer disease.

This patient should stop taking rivastigmine. Given the results of her cognitive testing, she meets criteria for Alzheimer disease of mild severity. She began taking oral rivastigmine, a cholinesterase inhibitor, 12 weeks ago. All of the available cholinesterase inhibitors are approved for mild to moderate Alzheimer disease, except donepezil, which is also approved for the severe stage. Studies of cholinesterase inhibitors and memantine show consistent improvement on measures of cognition and global assessment of dementia, but the effect size is modest and evidence that they improve long-term outcome is lacking. In practice, individual response is variable. There is insufficient evidence to support one cholinesterase inhibitor over another, and choice of treatment in a patient should be based on cost, tolerability, and ease of using the specific formulation. There is also insufficient evidence of the optimal duration of treatment or when therapy should be discontinued. Medication decisions should be made on an individual basis. Cholinesterase inhibitors should be used with caution in patients with cardiac conduction abnormalities, active peptic ulcer disease (because of the risk of bleeding), and seizures. Gastrointestinal adverse effects are common to all cholinesterase inhibitors and include loss of appetite, weight loss, nausea, vomiting, and diarrhea. Insomnia also can occur. This patient has had a significant amount of weight loss, loss of appetite, and insomnia since starting rivastigmine. The most appropriate next step in management would be to discontinue the medication. A trial of a different type of cholinesterase inhibitor could be considered, but only after symptoms subside.

Donepezil, another cholinesterase inhibitor, might be considered as an alternative therapy for this patient. However, no indication supports prescribing multiple cholinesterase inhibitors concomitantly, and rivastigmine should be discontinued as the first step.

Memantine is a noncompetitive N-Methyl-D-aspartate receptor antagonist approved by the FDA for the treatment of moderate to severe Alzheimer disease. Although this drug could be added in the future, this patient's present symptoms should be addressed first.

Mirtazapine is a nonselective α_2-adrenoceptor antagonist effective in the treatment of depression. Stimulation of appetite, weight gain, and somnolence are frequently associated effects, and thus this medication may be the preferred treatment for depressed patients with Alzheimer disease who have insomnia or loss of appetite. This patient has apathy and loss of interest, which are common symptoms in Alzheimer disease, but lacks additional symptoms to suggest depression.

KEY POINT

- Gastrointestinal adverse effects can occur with cholinesterase inhibitor therapy.

Bibliography

Delrieu J, Piau A, Caillaud C, Voisin T, Vellas B. Managing cognitive dysfunction through the continuum of Alzheimer's disease: role of pharmacotherapy. CNS Drugs. 2011 Mar;25(3):213-26. [PMID: 21323393]

Item 29   Answer: A

Educational Objective: Treat blepharospasm with botulinum toxin in a patient with focal dystonia.

Botulinum toxin injection is the most effective treatment of focal forms of dystonia, including the blepharospasm experienced by this patient. Blepharospasm is characterized by involuntary and sustained contraction of the orbicularis oculi muscle. Similar to other forms of dystonia, this condition is a result of a dysregulation within a network that involves the basal ganglia, sensorimotor centers, and the cerebellum. Blepharospasm should be distinguished from hemifacial spasm, a form of focal myoclonus resulting from irritation of the facial nerve (cranial nerve VII). Hemifacial spasm is unilateral, involves other facial nerve–innervated muscles, is associated with blinking tics that are suppressible, and usually does not lead to sustained eyelid closure.

Clonidine is appropriate to treat tics but not blepharospasm. Tics are characterized by brief and typically suppressible movements that are distinct from the sustained and forceful contractions seen in dystonia.

Deep brain stimulation for dystonia should be considered only in the treatment of medication-refractory or severe generalized dystonia. Its utility in focal and segmental dystonias is less clear, and treatment with botulinum toxin, with or without other medications, should be attempted first.

Risperidone, an atypical antipsychotic agent, is not effective against dystonic movements and may aggravate them.

KEY POINT

- Botulinum toxin injection is the most effective treatment of focal forms of dystonia, including blepharospasm.

Bibliography

Tarsy D, Simon DK. Dystonia. New Engl J Med. 2006 Aug 24;355(8):818-29. [PMID: 16928997]

Item 30   Answer: A

Educational Objective: Diagnose small-fiber neuropathy associated with impaired glucose tolerance.

This patient should have a glucose tolerance test. He most likely has small-fiber neuropathy, a condition sometimes associated with impaired glucose tolerance. Although many classic neuropathies associated with diabetes mellitus occur later in the course of the disease, impaired glucose tolerance is being increasingly recognized as an underlying cause of distal peripheral neuropathies, especially those involving the small fibers, which are unmyelinated peripheral nerves that carry sharp pain, temperature, and autonomic nerve fibers. Pure small-fiber neuropathy can present with distal upper and lower extremity pain and paresthesia without sensory or motor deficit. Autonomic deficits also may be present. Clinical examination findings are typically normal, including normal results on sensory, motor, and reflex testing with the possible exception of a mild distal sensory deficit. Results of electromyography (EMG), which assesses the large nerve fibers, can be normal. The presence of glucose intolerance should be confirmed by a glucose tolerance test.

Given the normal results of the clinical examination and EMG, an MRI of the lumbosacral spine to assess for myelopathy and radiculopathy is not warranted.

Although vitamin D deficiency can cause myopathy and central nervous system–related symptoms, it usually does not cause small-fiber neuropathy. Although multiple other conditions may be associated with small-fiber neuropathy, impaired glucose metabolism is one of the most common causes, and evaluating for this possibility should be the initial investigation. Further evaluation of small-fiber neuropathy should consider the possibility of vitamin B_{12} deficiency, HIV infection, amyloidosis, Sjögren syndrome, paraproteinemia, celiac disease, and sarcoidosis.

Sural nerve biopsy has low sensitivity in detecting small-fiber disorders. The diagnosis is instead made on the basis of autonomic testing, including quantitative sudomotor axon reflex testing and skin biopsy, to assess intraepidermal nerve fiber density.

KEY POINT

- Impaired glucose tolerance is an underlying cause of distal peripheral neuropathies, especially those involving the small fibers that carry sharp pain, temperature, and autonomic nerve fibers

Bibliography

Lauria G, Merkies IS, Faber CG. Small fibre neuropathy. Curr Opin Neurol. 2012 Oct;25(5):542-9. [PMID: 22941266]

Item 31   Answer: D

Educational Objective: Diagnose nonepileptic seizures.

This patient should have continuous video electroencephalographic (EEG) monitoring for further evaluation of the seizures, which have become increasingly frequent and have not responded to two antiepileptic drugs (AEDs). Video EEG monitoring, performed in an epilepsy-monitoring unit, enables correlation of patient behavior with seizure activity on an electroencephalogram. This can lead to better characterization of seizure activity, such as the identification of specific localizing features, and allow assessment of potential non-seizure–related behaviors suggestive of nonepileptic seizures. This patient has several risk factors for psychogenic nonepileptic events. The long duration of the episodes is more typical of nonepileptic than epileptic seizures, as is the fact that his eyes remain closed during the event. The presence of incontinence does not exclude a nonepileptic episode. Although his previous closed head injury puts him at risk for epileptic seizures, it does not exclude the possibility of nonepileptic events. In fact, combat veterans, particularly those with posttraumatic stress disorder (PTSD), are at high risk for nonepileptic seizures. This diagnosis can be overlooked if a history of head trauma is present. Because epileptic and nonepileptic seizures can coexist in the same patient, a thorough description and characterization of the seizures are essential and best achieved by admission to an epilepsy monitoring unit.

Ambulatory EEG monitoring allows more prolonged evaluation of brain activity outside a clinical setting and may be helpful in identifying seizures or interictal epileptiform activity that may not have been seen on a routine interictal EEG study. However, inpatient video EEG monitoring allows analysis of both clinical and EEG characteristics of seizures to assist in diagnosis and management. The latter study is required for a diagnosis of nonepileptic seizures and presurgical evaluations in patients who have not responded to two or more AEDs. The inpatient setting also allows for withdrawal of AEDs in a monitored environment.

A definitive diagnosis is necessary before adding more AEDs, such as carbamazepine or levetiracetam. Furthermore, levetiracetam should be avoided in this patient with PTSD because it can exacerbate anxiety and irritability.

KEY POINT

- Video electroencephalography, performed in an epilepsy-monitoring unit, enables correlation of the patient's behavior with seizure activity on an electroencephalogram, which can lead to better characterization of seizure activity or allow assessment of potential non–seizure-related behaviors suggestive of nonepileptic seizures.

Bibliography

Salinsky M, Spencer D, Boudreau E, Ferguson F. Psychogenic nonepileptic seizures in US veterans. Neurology. 2011 Sep 6;77(10):945-50.[PMID: 21893668]

Item 32   Answer: C

Educational Objective: Treat urinary dysfunction in multiple sclerosis.

This patient should be treated with an anticholinergic medication, such as oxybutynin, for bladder spasticity due to myelopathy from multiple sclerosis (MS). Several different patterns of bladder dysfunction are associated with MS, with urge incontinence due to uninhibited detrusor function caused by denervation at the level of the spinal cord being the most common. This form of bladder dysfunction responds well to anticholinergic medications, which reduce the intensity and frequency of bladder spasms and reduce urgency, frequency, and incontinence. Other forms of dysfunction include bladder inactivity (leading to overflow incontinence), the loss of the sensation of bladder fullness, and other sensory deficits that also may impair bladder emptying. These conditions are more difficult to treat because anticholinergic agents can impair urinary retention and lead to predisposition to urinary tract infection. Patients with mixed bladder symptoms may require further diagnostic testing to better delineate the cause of incontinence.

Finasteride is a 5α-reductase inhibitor used to treat benign prostatic hyperplasia (BPH) and would have no effect on bladder spasticity. This patient is unlikely to have BPH given the normal findings on digital rectal examination and the absence of urinary hesitancy.

Intermittent urinary catheterization also has no role in isolated bladder spasticity. This patient had no symptoms or signs of urinary retention, which would be relieved by catheterization. It may, however, have a role in selected patients with complex bladder dysfunction due to MS who are not appropriate candidates for or do not respond to medical therapy.

Although patients with bladder dysfunction are at increased risk for urinary tract infection, assessing the type of bladder dysfunction present and providing appropriate treatment are indicated. Prophylactic antibiotics would not be indicated as management of this patient's urinary incontinence in the absence of evidence of infection or recurrent infections due to bladder dysfunction refractory to therapy.

KEY POINT

- In patients with multiple sclerosis, anticholinergic agents reduce the intensity and frequency of bladder spasms and thus may reduce symptoms of urgency, frequency, and incontinence.

Bibliography

de Sa JC, Airas L, Bartholome E, et al. Symptomatic therapy in multiple sclerosis: a review for a multimodal approach in clinical practice. Ther Adv Neurol Disord. 2011 May;4(3):139-68. [PMID: 21694816]

Item 33   Answer: D

Educational Objective: Diagnose cognitive impairment due to cerebrovascular disease.

This patient most likely has cognitive impairment due to cerebrovascular disease, otherwise known as vascular neurocognitive disorder (VND). VND comprises a group of pathophysiologically distinct processes and thus has heterogeneous clinical presentations. Because it encompasses a continuum of cognitive disorders, from mild cognitive

Answers and Critiques

impairment to dementia, that result from cerebrovascular disease, validated diagnostic criteria do not exist. Widely accepted clinical criteria require evidence of a cognitive disorder plus a previous clinical stroke or neuroimaging evidence that confirms the existence of cerebrovascular disease. A relationship between the cognitive decline and cerebrovascular disease should exist, as it does with this patient. The description of the "ministrokes" experienced by this patient is consistent with a history of previous lacunar strokes. Supportive features include gait disturbance, pseudobulbar affect (a neurologic disorder characterized by involuntary outbursts of laughing and/or crying that are out of proportion to the emotions being experienced), incontinence, depression, and focal neurologic signs. Cognitive impairment generally is characterized by executive dysfunction, slowed mental processing, and impaired attention, as is exhibited by this patient.

Coexisting Alzheimer disease is found at autopsy in a large number of patients with VND. However, the lack of prominent memory impairment, presence of focal neurologic symptoms and signs, and stepwise decline seen in this patient are more consistent with a clinical diagnosis of VND than Alzheimer disease.

Although this patient has some overlapping features typically associated with normal pressure hydrocephalus, such as urinary incontinence, magnetic gait, and cognitive decline, he lacks the neuroimaging findings of enlarged ventricles or hydrocephalus typically seen in this disorder.

This patient has some findings consistent with Parkinson disease, such as shuffling gait and executive dysfunction, but lacks other typical examination findings, such as asymmetric parkinsonism, resting tremor, stooped posture, and decline in fine motor movements. Underlying Parkinson disease is thus unlikely to be the cause of his symptoms.

KEY POINT

- Widely accepted clinical criteria for diagnosing vascular neurocognitive disorder require evidence of a cognitive disorder plus a previous clinical stroke or neuroimaging evidence that confirms the existence of cerebrovascular disease.

Bibliography

Gorelick PB, Scuteri A, Black SE, et al; American Heart Association Stroke Council, Council on Epidemiology and Prevention, Council on Cardiovascular Nursing, Council on Cardiovascular Radiology and Intervention, and Council on Cardiovascular Surgery and Anesthesia. Vascular contributions to cognitive impairment and dementia: a statement for healthcare professionals from the American Heart Association/American Stroke Association. Stroke. 2011 Sep;42(9):2672-2713. [PMID: 21778438]

Item 34   Answer: B

Educational Objective: **Treat an older patient with seizures.**

This patient should be treated with the antiepileptic drug (AED) lamotrigine. He has had several episodes consistent with complex partial seizures and is at high risk for recurrent seizures and associated morbidity, given his history of a previous stroke and age greater than 65 years. Older patients generally have difficulty tolerating the many adverse effects of AEDs. Lamotrigine, levetiracetam, and gabapentin are generally better tolerated in this population and thus are good first-line options. Because these medications have fewer adverse effects, older patients are more likely to continue taking them, which increases the likelihood of seizure freedom.

Carbamazepine, oxcarbazepine, and phenytoin are less well tolerated in older patients and have lower retention and seizure-freedom rates in this population. These drugs are thus inappropriate first-line treatments for this patient. Additionally, these drugs are enzyme-inducers and have drug-drug interactions with many other medications that are taken by older patients.

KEY POINT

- In older patients with seizures who are treated with an antiepileptic drug, lamotrigine, levetiracetam, and gabapentin are generally better tolerated and thus good first-line options.

Bibliography

Arif H, Buchsbaum R, Pierro J, et al. Comparative effectiveness of 10 antiepileptic drugs in older adults with epilepsy. Arch Neurol. 2010 Apr;67(4):408-15. [PMID: 20385905]

Item 35   Answer: C

Educational Objective: **Prophylactically treat asymptomatic extracranial carotid artery stenosis.**

This patient should be restarted on statin therapy for primary prevention of stroke and myocardial infarction. The patient has type 2 diabetes mellitus and coronary artery disease, and patients with these disorders benefit from high-intensity statin therapy to reduce the risk of atherosclerotic cardiovascular disease, including myocardial infarction and stroke. High-intensity statins also are recommended for patients with stroke or transient ischemic attack of a presumed atherosclerotic subtype (although this patient is not symptomatic). With improvements in medical therapy, particularly statins, the risk of stroke has been declining in patients with asymptomatic internal carotid artery (ICA) stenosis. In a recent study, the use of a statin in patients with this diagnosis was associated with a stroke risk of less than 2% per year. Although this patient developed apparent statin myopathy from rosuvastatin, switching to another statin less associated with statin myopathy is appropriate.

Although carotid endarterectomy may benefit some patients with greater than 60% asymptomatic ICA stenosis, its effectiveness is highly dependent on the patient's underlying risks and those associated with the procedure itself. The benefit of carotid surgery is modest in patients without symptoms, and this patient's multiple medical comorbidities make him a relatively poor surgical candidate. Some studies have suggested that additional clinical factors increase the risk of stroke further in patients with asymptomatic carotid stenosis, including rapidly progressive or greater than 80% stenosis, asymptomatic infarcts on brain imaging, or abnormal results of transcranial Doppler ultrasonography. However, the role that these factors should play in clinical decisions about treatment of asymptomatic carotid stenosis has not been established. Carotid revascularization with either endarterectomy or stenting can be considered in patients at low risk for perioperative cardiovascular morbidity.

Magnetic resonance angiography (MRA) of the neck is inappropriate in this patient because an additional diagnostic test is unlikely to change the medical management of his condition. The accuracy of MRA without contrast is likely similar to that of carotid ultrasonography.

No clear evidence supports the superiority of clopidogrel over aspirin for the primary prevention of stroke in the setting of asymptomatic ICA stenosis.

KEY POINT

- Using a statin to treat patients with asymptomatic internal carotid artery stenosis is associated with a stroke risk of less than 2% per year.

Bibliography

Marquardt L, Geraghty OC, Mehta Z, Rothwell PM. Low risk of ipsilateral stroke in patients with asymptomatic carotid stenosis on best medical treatment: a prospective, population-based study. Stroke. 2010 Jan; 41(1):e11-7. [PMID: 19926843]

Item 36   Answer: B

Educational Objective: Treat reversible cerebral vasoconstriction syndrome.

Normalization of blood pressure is recommended for this patient with reversible cerebral vasoconstriction syndrome (RCVS). This condition most commonly presents with thunderclap headaches that recur over several days or weeks. Thunderclap attacks may occur spontaneously or be triggered by bathing, exertion, or Valsalva maneuvers. The headaches may be complicated by focal neurologic deficits with corresponding areas of stroke, parenchymal hemorrhage, or edema visible on neuroimaging studies. The cerebrospinal fluid is typically normal or near normal. Cerebral angiographic studies reveal multifocal areas of vasospasm without evidence of aneurysm. RCVS can occur without an identifiable cause or may be associated with preeclampsia or eclampsia, exposure to certain medications (sympathomimetic agents, ergots, triptans) or blood products (transfused erythrocytes, immune globulin), or catecholamine-secreting tumors. Medications or illicit drugs are associated in up to 40% of affected patients, and women with the syndrome outnumber men at a ratio of 6:1. Migraine may be a predisposing factor. Transient neurologic deficits occur in 30% of patients with RCVS, and 10% may experience persistent deficits from parenchymal damage caused by ischemic or hemorrhagic infarctions.

No clinical trial data are available on which to base therapeutic recommendations. Conservative management, supported by expert consensus, includes headache control with analgesics, careful monitoring of blood pressure to maintain normotensive goals, and serial neurologic examinations.

Primary stabbing headache is a form of benign abrupt-onset headache that may respond to indomethacin. This type of headache typically lasts seconds, not 30 minutes as with this patient. Primary stabbing headache also occurs without visual blurring, focal numbness, or other neurologic symptoms. Although indomethacin is appropriate for treating several additional primary headache syndromes, such as chronic paroxysmal hemicrania, evidence does not support its effectiveness in RCVS.

Because reversible vasoconstriction and not thrombosis is the responsible mechanism for RCVS, tissue plasminogen activator is not indicated in this patient. The use of calcium channel antagonists, such as nimodipine or verapamil, is more appropriate.

No evidence suggests that anticoagulants, such as warfarin, or antiplatelet agents, such as aspirin, affect stroke risk or outcomes in RCVS. The mechanism of cerebral infarction, when present, is likely related to cerebral artery vasospasm and not thrombosis. Given this pathophysiology and the relatively high rate of hemorrhagic infarction in RCVS, antiplatelet or antithrombotic therapy has no role in disease management.

KEY POINT

- Normalization of blood pressure is recommended in patients with reversible cerebral vasoconstriction syndrome, which commonly presents with thunderclap headaches that recur over several days or weeks.

Bibliography

Yancy H, Lee-Iannotti JK, Schwedt TJ, Dodick DW. Reversible cerebral vasoconstriction syndrome. Headache. 2013 Mar;53(3):570-6. [PMID: 23489219]

Item 37   Answer: B

Educational Objective: Diagnose a primary central nervous system lymphoma.

This patient should undergo surgical biopsy of the brain lesion without resection. The MRI is suggestive of primary central nervous system lymphoma (PCNSL), a non-Hodgkin lymphoma that can affect any part of the central nervous system but commonly presents as a focal supratentorial lesion; visual symptoms are common because the tumor often involves the optic radiations. Cerebrospinal fluid (CSF) analysis can be diagnostic in up to 10% of patients, and ocular involvement may be found in 10% to 20%. However, in most patients, including this one with negative results on CSF analysis and slit lamp examination, pathologic analysis of a brain biopsy specimen is required to confirm the diagnosis. Treatment most commonly involves methotrexate-based chemotherapy and possible whole-brain radiation.

Bone marrow biopsy is not indicated in this patient. PCNSL is a whole-organ disease but is not typically systemic.

CONT.

Therefore, a bone marrow biopsy for diagnostic purposes would have low yield.

Because PCNSL tends to localize to a single organ system and may have multiple associated manifestations, such as diffuse brain and ocular involvement, resection of the presenting lesion is not helpful and can actually worsen patient outcomes.

Dexamethasone and similar glucocorticoids should be avoided if possible before brain biopsy in patients with suspected PCNSL because these agents can significantly decrease the yield of the biopsy. Furthermore, this patient does not have signs or symptoms of increased intracranial pressure that would necessitate urgent glucocorticoids.

Radiation is not indicated for PCNSL until after a tissue diagnosis is made and treatment with methotrexate-based chemotherapy has begun. Additionally, when patients with PCNSL receive radiation, it must be whole-brain radiation, not focal photon-beam radiation, which is more appropriate for gliomas and other primary brain tumors.

KEY POINT

- Pathologic analysis, usually of a brain biopsy specimen, to confirm primary central nervous system lymphoma is required before beginning treatment with methotrexate-based chemotherapy and possible whole-brain radiation.

Bibliography

Ricard D, Idbaih A, Ducray F, Lahutte M, Hoang-Xuan K, Delattre JY. Primary brain tumours in adults. Lancet. 2012 May 26;379(9830):1984-96. [PMID: 22510398]

Item 38   Answer: A

Educational Objective: Treat ischemic stroke in a patient with atrial fibrillation.

Aspirin should be added to this patient's medication regimen. She has had an acute ischemic stroke and has atrial fibrillation. No other obvious causes of stroke are present, and she is beyond the treatment window for recombinant tissue plasminogen activator therapy. According to two large clinical trials, aspirin administered within 48 hours of ischemic stroke onset modestly reduces the risk of recurrent ischemic stroke within the first 2 weeks without significantly increasing the risk of intracerebral hemorrhage. Administration of aspirin no later than the end of the second day after a stroke is an accepted quality-of-care core metric in primary and comprehensive stroke centers.

Anticoagulation with warfarin or a newer anticoagulant, such as dabigatran, is required to manage this patient's long-term risk of cardioembolic stroke. Some experts will initiate warfarin within 24 hours of stroke onset in medically stable patients with a small infarction, but withholding anticoagulation for 4 days to 2 weeks is typically recommended for patients with moderate to large infarctions. Until that time, patients are managed with aspirin.

In the acute ischemic stroke setting, intravenous heparin was ineffective compared with aspirin in patients with cardioembolic stroke in a randomized clinical trial. Furthermore, this patient's infarct is large enough to be associated with a risk of hemorrhaging into the bed of the infarct within the first 2 weeks of stroke.

KEY POINT

- In patients with acute ischemic stroke who are ineligible for recombinant tissue plasminogen activator therapy, aspirin should be administered within 48 hours of the stroke to reduce the risk of recurrent ischemic stroke.

Bibliography

Jauch, EC, Saver JL, Adams HP Jr, et al; American Heart Association Stroke Council, Council on Cardiovascular Nursing, Council on Peripheral Vascular Disease, Council on Clinical Cardiology. Guidelines for the early management of patients with acute ischemic stroke: a guideline for healthcare professionals from the American Heart Association/American Stroke Association. Stroke. 2013 Mar;44(3):870-947. [PMID: 23370205]

Item 39   Answer: C

Educational Objective: Treat a solitary metastatic brain tumor.

This patient should undergo surgical resection of the right frontal lesion. Her clinical history and imaging findings are most consistent with a solitary brain metastasis from the breast cancer. Standard-of-care treatment of a solitary brain metastasis in a patient with a good functional status and limited extracranial disease is complete resection of the lesion (when accessible) followed by radiation therapy. This treatment offers better symptom control, longer survival time, and longer periods of independent functional status compared with other therapies, including biopsy followed by radiation.

A PET scan of the brain is unlikely to be of additional diagnostic value in this patient whose MRI clearly reveals the lesion most likely responsible for her symptoms. MRI is more sensitive and specific than other imaging techniques in detecting the presence, location, and number of metastases.

Lumbar puncture is contraindicated in this patient with signs (papilledema) and symptoms (headache, nausea and vomiting) of increased intracranial pressure. Moreover, cerebrospinal fluid analysis is rarely diagnostic of metastatic disease. If an infectious process is also suspected, which often occurs in cancer patients, its presence can be determined by biopsy at the time of surgical resection.

Whole-brain radiation is an appropriate initial therapy for patients with multiple brain metastases but not for this patient whose single metastasis can be resected.

KEY POINT

- Complete resection followed by radiation therapy is standard-of-care treatment of an accessible solitary brain metastasis in patients with good functional status and limited extracranial disease.

Bibliography

Patel TR, Knisely JP, Chiang VL. Management of brain metastases: surgery, radiation, or both? Hematol Oncol Clin North Am. 2012 Aug;26(4):933-47. [PMID: 22794291]

Item 40   Answer: D

Educational Objective: Treat myasthenic crisis.

Treatment with plasmapheresis should be started immediately in this patient with myasthenic crisis. His several-month history of fluctuating proximal weakness with ocular and bulbar involvement is consistent with myasthenia gravis. His rapid decline most likely has been precipitated by recent exposure to ciprofloxacin. Fluoroquinolones can decrease transmission at the neuromuscular junction and exacerbate myasthenia gravis. Although Guillain-Barré syndrome (GBS) also can present with rapidly progressive respiratory failure, the slow clinical course and preserved reflexes in this patient are not consistent with GBS.

Patients with suspected myasthenic crisis (rapid respiratory failure) should be admitted to the ICU and have their respiratory parameters (vital capacity and negative inspiratory force) closely monitored. If myasthenic crisis is confirmed, treatment should be started emergently with either plasmapheresis or intravenous immune globulin (IVIG).

High-dose glucocorticoids can initially aggravate symptoms of myasthenia gravis. These agents can be started after therapy with plasmapheresis or IVIG has been initiated.

Magnesium deficiency usually presents as neuromuscular hyperexcitability, not muscular weakness. Furthermore, because magnesium administration can exacerbate myasthenia gravis by neuromuscular junction blockade, it is inappropriate for this patient. Other medications that need to be used with caution in this setting include fluoroquinolones, aminoglycosides, β-blockers, and calcium channel blockers.

Pyridostigmine can worsen respiratory secretions and should be avoided in the setting of acute respiratory failure with bulbar weakness.

KEY POINT

- Patients in myasthenic crisis should be treated emergently with either plasmapheresis or intravenous immunoglobulin.

Bibliography

Kumar V, Kaminski HJ. Treatment of myasthenia gravis. Curr Neurol Neurosci Rep. 2011 Feb;11(1):89-96. [PMID: 20927659]

Item 41   Answer: E

Educational Objective: Prevent cluster headache.

The patient should be treated with verapamil for episodic cluster headache. He experiences one or two daily attacks of severe, unilateral, periorbital pain lasting 2 to 3 hours if untreated that is accompanied by at least one ipsilateral cranial autonomic feature, such as ptosis, tearing, or rhinorrhea; he also exhibits motor restlessness during headache episodes. These features meet International Headache Society criteria for cluster headache. Cycles of cluster headache can last weeks to months, with attack frequency varying from 1 event every other day to 8 per day. Cluster headache typically affects young and middle-aged adults. Male sex and tobacco use are risk factors.

Oxygen therapy and subcutaneous sumatriptan are the most effective acute cluster headache treatments. Glucocorticoids can help reduce attack frequency and are effective as a bridge therapy to longer-term prophylactic agents. Verapamil is the drug of choice for cluster headache prevention. Because relatively high doses are sometimes required, regular electrocardiographic assessment for potential prolongation of the P-R interval or heart block is recommended.

Both amitriptyline and propranolol are effective agents for prevention of migraine but not cluster headache. The duration of the headaches described by this patient is too short to meet criteria for migraine.

Indomethacin is an effective treatment for chronic paroxysmal hemicrania (CPH) but not cluster headache. CPH also is characterized by repetitive episodes of unilateral pain with ipsilateral autonomic features but occurs at least 5 times daily with a typical duration between 3 and 20 minutes.

Anticonvulsants, such as topiramate, have limited effectiveness in cluster headache prevention and should be considered only after verapamil therapy proves ineffective or is poorly tolerated.

KEY POINT

- Oxygen therapy and subcutaneous sumatriptan are the most effective acute cluster headache treatments, and verapamil is the drug of choice for cluster headache prevention.

Bibliography

Ashkenazi A, Schwedt T. Cluster headache—acute and prophylactic therapy. Headache. 2011 Feb;51(2):272-86. [PMID: 21284609]

Item 42   Answer: B

Educational Objective: Treat cognitive dysfunction in multiple sclerosis.

This patient should be referred for counseling and cognitive therapy. Cognitive dysfunction is a common symptom in multiple sclerosis (MS), occurring in at least 50% of affected patients. The most common deficits involve short-term memory, processing speed, and executive function. This cognitive disability can have a significant effect on employment of patients with MS and can reduce their overall quality of life. Unfortunately no trials of pharmacologic therapy to reduce or prevent cognitive dysfunction in MS have as yet been successful. Formal neuropsychological testing, counseling, cognitive therapy, and accommodative strategies (such as creating checklists to overcome memory deficits) sometimes can be of benefit.

Amantadine is an appropriate treatment of the fatigue associated with MS but has not been shown to improve cognitive function in this disorder.

Donepezil has shown benefit for mild to moderate cognitive dysfunction due to Alzheimer disease. However, a randomized placebo-controlled trial of this medication in patients with MS who also had cognitive dysfunction showed no cognitive benefit.

The use of high-dose intravenous methylprednisolone is indicated only for acute exacerbations of MS, which the patient is not experiencing. The MRI also shows no evidence of breakthrough inflammatory activity.

Increasing the patient's fluoxetine dosage will not affect her cognition. Although depression is a common symptom in MS, and severe depression can be associated with a pseudodementia-like state, the patient did not report any worsening of depression and has a normal affect.

KEY POINT

- Formal neuropsychological testing, counseling, cognitive therapy, and accommodative strategies (such as creating checklists to overcome memory deficits) sometimes can be of benefit in patients with cognitive dysfunction related to multiple sclerosis.

Bibliography
Benedict RH, Zivadinov R. Risk factors for and management of cognitive dysfunction in multiple sclerosis. Nat Rev Neurol. 2011 May 10;7(6): 332-42. [PMID: 21556031]

Item 43   Answer: D

Educational Objective: Diagnose medication overuse headache.

This patient has developed medication overuse headache, which requires the presence of a headache-susceptible patient and excessive exposure to a causative medication. This patient has an underlying history of migraine treated with sumatriptan, and he has been exposed to hydrocodone for back pain. The use of opioid analgesics more than 10 days per month can contribute to the development of medication overuse headache. Daily analgesic exposure is not required. Patients with this condition may develop a worsening of their underlying headache disorder or a new milder, nonspecific headache.

Posttraumatic headaches have been reported to occur in as many as 70% of persons after mild traumatic brain injury (TBI). Posttraumatic headache types are classified similarly to nontraumatic headaches, with migraine and tension-type headaches being the most prevalent. Although this patient has a history of mild TBI, the timing of the TBI and the timing of the headache have no correlation. A true posttraumatic headache must develop within 7 days of the injury.

The headaches described by this patient have phenotypic features of chronic tension-type headache. However, this diagnosis requires the exclusion of secondary headache

disorders, such as medication overuse headache, and thus is premature at this time.

Given the absence of papilledema, the diagnosis of idiopathic intracranial hypertension is unlikely.

KEY POINT

- Medication overuse headache requires the presence of a headache-susceptible patient and excessive exposure to a causative medication, such as an opioid analgesic.

Bibliography
Johnson JL, Hutchinson MR, Williams DB, Rolan P. Medication-overuse headache and opioid-induced hyperalgesia: A review of mechanisms, a neuroimmune hypothesis and a novel approach to treatment. Cephalalgia. 2013 Jan;33(1):52-64. [PMID: 23144180]

Item 44   Answer: B

Educational Objective: Treat a multiple sclerosis relapse.

This patient should receive intravenous methylprednisolone. Her symptoms are consistent with a new multiple sclerosis (MS) relapse, most likely localizing to a new lesion in the pons and pontocerebellar pathways on the right. The standard of care for MS relapses is a high-dose glucocorticoid, usually intravenous methylprednisolone, 1 g/d for 3 to 5 days. Although this treatment has not been shown to reduce the amount of long-term disability sustained in a relapse, it substantially hastens the rate of recovery. Because of the unclear long-term benefit and the potential for adverse effects, acute high-dose glucocorticoid therapy is usually reserved for attacks resulting in sustained impairment in functional status that interferes substantially with activities of daily living.

In addition to treatment of individual relapses, most patients with relapsing-remitting MS receive chronic maintenance therapy with immunomodulatory or immunosuppressive medications, such as the interferon beta-1a that this patient takes. These disease-modifying therapies have been shown to reduce the relapse rate, slow disability progression, and reduce the accumulation of new demyelinating lesions on MRI. Glatiramer acetate is another disease-modifying drug that has been shown to reduce the relapse rate by approximately one third compared with placebo and appears equivalent to the interferon beta preparations in head-to-head studies. Combining glatiramer acetate with an interferon beta provides no added benefit compared with what either drug achieves alone. Additionally, disease-modifying medications are not effective in hastening recovery in a patient with a functionally significant acute exacerbation of MS.

Although an increasing number of studies suggest the equivalency of oral treatment with prednisone and intravenous treatment with another glucocorticoid for MS, the reported equivalent dose of prednisone is 1250 mg/d, which is a very high dose. In the original Optic Neuritis Treatment Study, which compared treatment of optic neuritis with oral prednisone (1 mg/kg), intravenous methylprednisolone (1 g/d), or placebo, the oral prednisone group had worse outcomes after treatment than even the placebo group. Thus, oral prednisone in the range of 1 mg/kg may actually be detrimental in treating acute demyelination.

Relapses that are refractory to glucocorticoid treatment may respond to rescue therapy with plasmapheresis. Since this patient has not received a trial of intravenous methylprednisone, treatment with plasmapheresis is premature.

KEY POINT

- The standard of care for multiple sclerosis relapses is a high-dose glucocorticoid, usually intravenous methylprednisolone.

Bibliography

Rubin SM. Management of multiple sclerosis: an overview. Dis Mon. 2013 Jul;59(7):253-60. [PMID:23786659]

Item 45   Answer: D

Educational Objective: Manage hypertension in a patient with acute ischemic stroke.

This patient should receive no pharmacologic treatment. He has an ischemic stroke in the pons, which is commonly caused by hypertensive changes in penetrator vessels originating from the basilar artery. He is not a candidate for intravenous thrombolysis because 18 hours have passed since he was known to be well. He has an elevated blood pressure but no evidence of end-organ damage. Treatment guidelines advise treatment of hypertension in the setting of acute ischemic stroke only if blood pressure is greater than 220/120 mm Hg or evidence of other end-organ damage exists. The rationale for these guidelines is to prevent neurologic worsening from expansion of the cerebral infarct; in recent clinical trials, acute lowering of blood pressure with candesartan within 36 hours of stroke was associated with neurologic worsening. When appropriate, antihypertensive medications are commonly started close to the day of discharge home or to a rehabilitation facility.

Neither oral captopril nor oral metoprolol is appropriate for this patient, who does not require immediate treatment of hypertension. Additionally, he should not be given any oral medication until a dysphagia evaluation documents the ability to swallow.

Sublingual nitroglycerin is also inappropriate because the patient does not require therapy to lower blood pressure at this time.

KEY POINT

- Treatment guidelines advise treatment of hypertension in patients with acute ischemic stroke only if blood pressure is greater than 220/120 mm Hg or evidence of end-organ damage exists.

Bibliography

Jauch EC, Saver JL, Adams HP Jr, et al; American Heart Association Stroke Council, Council on Cardiovascular Nursing, Council on Peripheral Vascular Disease, Council on Clinical Cardiology. Guidelines for the early management of patients with acute ischemic stroke: a guideline for healthcare professionals from the American Heart Association/American Stroke Association. Stroke. 2013 Mar;44(3):870-947. [PMID: 23370205]

Item 46   Answer: C

Educational Objective: Evaluate facial nerve palsy with incomplete recovery after 3 months.

An MRI of the brain should be obtained in this patient who has limited recovery despite appropriate treatment 3 months after onset of complete facial nerve (cranial nerve VII) palsy to rule out an underlying structural abnormality. He has acute weakness involving both upper and lower facial muscles, which favors a peripheral rather than central weakness. The initial presence of hyperacusis and the impaired taste noted on examination are also consistent with facial nerve involvement. In patients with typical isolated facial nerve paralysis, immediate brain imaging is unnecessary. Most of these patients have idiopathic Bell palsy, and 70% to 90% achieve complete recovery within 3 months. Severe residual weakness occurs in a minority of patients with Bell palsy, but the persistence of significant deficits at 3 months should prompt further investigation, including evaluation for alternative causes of facial nerve paralysis (such as diabetes mellitus, Lyme disease, vasculitis, HIV infection, sarcoidosis, paraproteinemia, and Sjögren syndrome) and an MRI of the brain to rule out structural causes. If results of this evaluation do not reveal a cause of the persistent symptoms, the diagnosis is incomplete recovery after Bell palsy, and clinical monitoring is then recommended.

Acute monotherapy with antiviral medications, such as acyclovir, does not improve prognosis. Early adjunctive use of antiviral therapy in addition to prednisone is favored by some experts, but the evidence supporting this treatment is inconsistent.

Evidence supporting the benefit of physical therapy for rehabilitation after facial nerve palsy is insufficient. In this patient, a structural cause of the deficits should first be excluded.

KEY POINT

- MRI of the brain is an appropriate next step in management for patients with incomplete recovery 3 months after onset of facial nerve palsy despite appropriate initial treatment.

Bibliography

Baugh RF, Basura GJ, Ishii LE, et al. Clinical practice guideline: Bell's palsy. Otolaryngol. Head Neck Surg. 2013 Nov;149(3 Suppl):S1-27. [PMID: 24189771]

Item 47   Answer: B

Educational Objective: Evaluate a first seizure in a patient at high risk of recurrent seizure.

This patient should receive an antiepileptic drug (AED), such as carbamazepine. His seizure was unprovoked. The 2-year risk of recurrence after a single unprovoked seizure is approximately 40%. On the basis on this estimate, most experts do not recommend starting an AED for a first seizure unless the patient has risk factors that increase the likelihood for future

H
CONT.

events. This patient, however, has several risk factors for future seizures, including previous head trauma with loss of consciousness, a focal brain lesion on MRI, and postictal Todd paralysis of the right arm (focal weakness after a seizure). His risk of future seizures is high, and he should be treated with an AED. In this patient, the brain injury involving the contra-lateral parietal lobe is likely the source of the seizure, with the abnormal sensation experienced at seizure onset representing a sensory aura. He most likely had a simple partial seizure starting in the parietal lobe that spread to the motor cortex, which led to the dystonic posture of his hand and subsequent tonic-clonic seizure.

Ambulatory electroencephalography (EEG) is an out-patient test that can be useful to exclude the presence of unrecognized seizures and provide a more sensitive evalua-tion of interictal discharges than a 30-minute EEG. This test, however, is not performed in the emergency department and does not have to be completed before starting treatment in this patient, who had a witnessed seizure and has a high risk of recurrent seizure.

Clinical observation is appropriate management of a single unprovoked seizure only in patients with no risk fac-tors for future seizures.

A lumbar puncture is indicated in some patients with a first seizure if they have symptoms or signs of infection or have altered mental status. In this patient with a clear reason for a partial seizure, a normal mental status, and no signs of infection, a lumbar puncture is unnecessary.

KEY POINT

- In a patient with a first seizure and risk factors for future seizures, treatment with an antiepileptic drug is appropriate.

Bibliography

Berg AT. Risk of recurrence after a first unprovoked seizure. Epilepsia. 2008;49 Suppl 1:13-8. [PMID: 18184149]

Item 48   Answer: E

Educational Objective: Treat migraine with aura.

The patient has migraine with aura and should be given sumatriptan. The pattern of his headaches has been stable for more than a decade and meets diagnostic criteria for migraine, namely, that migraine attacks should last between 4 and 72 hours if untreated, and the pain must possess two of the following four features: unilateral location, throbbing nature, moderate or severe intensity, and aggravation with physical activity. The quality and duration of the episodic visual distortion are compatible with migraine aura. Aura occurs in 25% to 35% of those with migraine and, most commonly, is visual. By definition, migraine aura should last between 5 and 60 minutes with complete resolution. Symptoms often precede headache but may accompany or even occur separately from the pain of an attack. Episodes of hemisensory symptoms or language disturbance of a similar duration are also described as "typical" aura and warrant no

specific restrictions or acute migraine therapy. Because of their lower cost, NSAIDs are considered first-line options in acute migraine management. Because this patient has not responded to NSAIDs, acute treatment with a triptan is now appropriate.

CT of the head and MRI of the brain may be appropri-ate in the setting of potential secondary headache, but this patient has no "red flags" raising concern for this type of headache and instead exhibits classic signs and symptoms of migraine with aura. The headache pattern is stable, the visual loss is periodic and always reversible over the course of many years, and both headache and visual loss meet diagnostic criteria for migraine with aura. Neuroimaging is inappropriate in the evaluation of uncomplicated headache.

Similarly, electroencephalography has no role in the assessment of headache disorders, according to the Amer-ican Academy of Neurology's five "Choosing Wisely" initia-tives. Compared with standard clinical evaluation, it offers no diagnostic advantage, does not improve outcomes, and adds to medical costs.

Measurement of the erythrocyte sedimentation rate would be reasonable in the setting of suspected temporal arteritis. However, the young age of this patient and stable migraine pattern—episodic headaches with occasional tran-sient visual impairment over 18 years—are incompatible with this diagnosis. Visual loss that occurs with temporal arteritis is typically monocular and more compatible with ischemic events, such as amaurosis fugax. Although the visual loss in typical migraine aura is benign and fully reversible, that noted with temporal arteritis is concerning and may become permanent following retinal artery occlusion.

KEY POINT

- Neuroimaging is inappropriate in the evaluation of uncomplicated headache.

Bibliography

Langer-Gould AM, Anderson WE, Armstrong MJ, et al. The American Academy of Neurology's top five choosing wisely recommendations. Neurology. 2013 Sep 10;81(11):1004-11. [PMID: 23430685]

Item 49   Answer: D

Educational Objective: Diagnose medical complications after stroke.

This patient should be referred for polysomnography. His chief symptom of fatigue is highly prevalent among patients in the poststroke period. Common reversible causes of fatigue after stroke include depression, sleep apnea of the central or obstructive type, and heart failure. This patient has had no recent depression and has normal findings on cardiac examination. He has an elevated BMI and hyper-tension, both of which are associated with sleep apnea. The diagnosis of sleep apnea is typically confirmed by polysom-nography. Appropriate treatment of the sleep apnea can lead to lessening of fatigue symptoms and improved control of hypertension.

Cardiovascular stress testing is inappropriate in this patient who reports no exercise-induced fatigue and has normal findings on a recent electrocardiogram and echocardiogram. Myocardial ischemia is thus unlikely as an explanation of his symptoms. Patients with ischemic stroke are nonetheless at high risk for myocardial infarction, and a previous ischemic stroke is a coronary risk equivalent for the purposes of cardiovascular disease risk factor management strategies.

Depression is highly prevalent after stroke and is associated with poorer recovery and nonadherence to medical therapy. Use of antidepressant medications or cognitive behavioral psychotherapy (or both) is standard treatment of patients with stroke who experience depression. Although this patient has a remote history of depression, and fatigue can be a symptom of depression, he does not exhibit depressed mood or anhedonia, which are both elements of the two-question depression screening instrument. Treatment with citalopram or another antidepressant medication is therefore not necessary, although he should continue to be screened for this complication on routine visits.

Stimulants, including amphetamines, have shown no clinical benefits in stroke recovery and may exacerbate patients' hypertension. Dextroamphetamine is thus not appropriate in the management of this patient's poststroke fatigue.

KEY POINT

- Common reversible causes of fatigue after stroke include depression, sleep apnea of the central or obstructive type, and heart failure.

Bibliography
Kumar S, Selim MH, Caplan LR. Medical complications after stroke. Lancet Neurol. 2010 Jan;9(1):105–18. [PMID: 20083041]

Item 50   Answer: C

Educational Objective: Diagnose multiple sclerosis in a patient with optic neuritis.

This patient should have an MRI of the brain. She has symptoms and signs consistent with optic neuritis, including pain with eye movement, central scotoma, and an afferent pupillary defect. Although idiopathic optic neuritis can occur, the most common cause is multiple sclerosis (MS). An MRI of the brain should be obtained to evaluate for brain lesions consistent with MS. If they are present, a diagnosis of MS is likely on the basis of the official diagnostic criteria. These criteria require clinical and radiologic dissemination of lesions in space and time. In this patient, the occurrence of two disparate clinical events happening at separate times satisfies criteria for dissemination in time, and the presence of an optic nerve (cranial nerve II) lesion (detected on clinical examination) and additional brain lesions (if shown by MRI) would satisfy criteria for dissemination in space.

Determination of the erythrocyte sedimentation rate (ESR) has no role in the evaluation of MS. ESR elevation can

occur in giant cell arteritis, a potential cause of visual loss, but this is typically a condition of older patients. In addition, this patient has not had the symptom of a headache.

Although a lumbar puncture is often performed when evaluating a patient for MS, the presence or absence of oligoclonal bands in the cerebrospinal fluid (CSF) is not part of any MS diagnostic criteria. Approximately 10% to 15% of patients with MS do not have these bands in their CSF, and their presence, by itself, is a nonspecific finding. If an MRI confirms the diagnosis of MS, CSF examination is unnecessary.

A rapid plasma reagin test is a screening test for syphilis. The classic pupillary abnormality of neurosyphilis is the Argyll-Robertson pupil, in which pupils are unreactive to light but constrict to accommodation. This patient instead manifested an afferent pupillary defect, which is a sign of reduced optic nerve (cranial nerve II) conductance. Although optic nerve inflammation can be a complication of meningovascular neurosyphilis, this scenario is quite rare, and this patient shows no other concerning signs or symptoms for this condition.

KEY POINT

- In patients with optic neuritis, an MRI of the brain should be obtained to evaluate for brain lesions consistent with multiple sclerosis, which is the most common cause.

Bibliography
Polman CH, Reingold SC, Banwell B, et al. Diagnostic criteria for multiple sclerosis: 2010 revisions to the McDonald criteria. Ann Neurol. 2011 Feb;69(2):292–302. [PMID: 21387374]

Item 51   Answer: C

Educational Objective: Prevent worsening of traumatic brain injury.

Contact sports should be prohibited for this patient with symptoms after sustaining a mild traumatic brain injury, which occurred when head trauma resulted in a transient alteration of neurologic function. The patient exhibited the typical physical symptoms of this type of injury, including headache, dizziness, and nausea. Although the symptoms have largely resolved, he still requires acetaminophen to control headache pain. Prohibiting contact sports is recommended for a patient who is still symptomatic. This restriction should remain in place even when the patient is in an asymptomatic state after taking medication. Not until the patient is asymptomatic without taking any medication should a return to contact sports be considered.

In the presence of normal findings on physical examination, a head CT scan or MRI of the brain is unlikely to provide any useful information and thus has no role. A noncontrast head CT scan is recommended in the setting of acute head injury when skull fracture or intracranial hemorrhage is suspected. Risk factors for these findings include prolonged loss of consciousness, posttraumatic amnesia, focal neurologic deficit(s), vomiting, severe headache, physical evidence of a basilar skull fracture, a Glasgow Coma Scale score less than 15, coagulopathy, or a dangerous mechanism of injury. MRI of the brain may be more sensitive in the detection of small areas of parenchymal damage or hemorrhage in the patient who is seen days or weeks after an injury, but suspicion of such damage would be low in this patient who has shown significant improvement 1 week after the trauma.

Gradual reintroduction of cognitive and normal physical activities is recommended for patients with concussion. Those with significant cognitive symptoms or neuropsychological examination deficits should have restrictions placed on cognitive activity. Immediate resumption of normal levels of cognitive activity (such as full days of classroom work) may delay recovery in some patients. Typically, cognitive rest is recommended for 3 to 7 days, followed by gradual reintroduction of cognitive activity periods. These periods initially should be limited to the threshold of concussion symptom aggravation but, over time, should be lengthened. Given the wide variability of recovery timeframes, management must be individualized. In this patient without any cognitive or significant physical symptoms 1 week after the injury, returning to school is appropriate, and restriction of classroom participation is not required.

KEY POINT

- Contact sports should be prohibited in patients who are symptomatic after sustaining a mild traumatic brain injury.

Bibliography

Giza CC, Kutcher JB, Ashwal S, et al. Summary of evidence-based guideline update: evaluation and management of concussion in sports: report of the Guideline Development Subcommittee of the American Academy of Neurology. Neurology 2013 Jun 11;80(24):2250-7. [PMID: 23508730]

Item 52   Answer: B

Educational Objective: Treat generalized epilepsy in a woman of childbearing age.

This patient should begin taking levetiracetam and be weaned off valproic acid. She has juvenile myoclonic epilepsy, which responds particularly well to valproic acid. However, valproic acid should be avoided whenever possible in women of childbearing age because this antiepileptic drug (AED) is associated with a significantly elevated risk (6%-16%) of major congenital malformations, which is much higher than that of other AEDs. In utero exposure to valproic acid also is associated with a 7- to 10-point decrease in intelligence quotient (IQ) on average and an increased risk for autism and autism spectrum disorders in the offspring. Therefore, whenever possible, a trial of another suitable AED should be attempted before pregnancy. This patient should be advised to switch to levetiracetam, which has shown a relatively low risk of birth defects when used in pregnancy. Lamotrigine is another reasonable option, but starting lamotrigine while a patient is still taking valproic acid carries an increased risk of

Stevens-Johnson syndrome. If she does not respond to levetiracetam or the drug has adverse effects, lamotrigine, with or without levetiracetam, would be another reasonable choice. If a woman does not respond to treatment with other suitable medications and needs to remain on valproic acid, the dose should be adjusted during pregnancy to the minimum therapeutic dose required. Women should be counseled to use contraception during any period of drug transition from valproic acid because of the drug's significantly increased teratogenic risk.

Carbamazepine is not a good choice for this patient because it is a narrow-spectrum drug used to treat focal epilepsies. Carbamazepine potentially can exacerbate generalized epilepsies, such as juvenile myoclonic epilepsy, and should be avoided in this patient.

Topiramate can be used to treat juvenile myoclonic epilepsy. However, early data suggest that this drug is associated with a moderately increased risk of major congenital abnormalities, particularly cleft lip/cleft palate and small-for-gestational-age infants.

Stopping all AEDs can be considered in some women who have been seizure free for 2 or more years. However, it is rarely an option for patients with juvenile myoclonic epilepsy. These patients typically need life-long AED treatment, and the risk of seizures during pregnancy typically outweighs the potential complications of AED therapy, when selected carefully. The fact that this patient had a seizure after stopping her AED strongly suggests that she should stay on her medication during pregnancy.

KEY POINT

- Valproic acid should not be used by women with epilepsy who are or wish to become pregnant because of its association with a significantly elevated risk of major congenital malformations and other abnormalities in the fetus.

Bibliography

Christensen J, Grønborg TK, Sørensen MJ, et al. Prenatal valproate exposure and risk of autism spectrum disorders and childhood autism. JAMA. 2013 Apr 24;309(16):1696-703. [PMID: 23613074]

Item 53   Answer: A

Educational Objective: Diagnose a Parkinson-plus syndrome.

The combination of parkinsonism, cerebellar ataxia, and early postural instability and falls in this patient is most consistent with multiple system atrophy (MSA), a Parkinson-plus syndrome. MSA (Shy-Drager subtype) also can be associated with prominent autonomic deficits, such as orthostatic hypotension and urinary symptoms. Her history of acting out of dreams during sleep (rapid eye movement sleep behavior disorder [RBD]) is another clue suggestive of a synucleinopathy (such as Parkinson disease or MSA). Patients with MSA are at higher risk for falls, dysautonomia, and sleep-related complications, including nocturnal stridor.

Many of this patient's symptoms also can occur in idiopathic Parkinson disease, but her early prominent imbalance, recurrent falls, and cerebellar features are atypical for this disorder.

Progressive supranuclear palsy is the main differential diagnosis, given the patient's early prominent postural instability. She does not, however, have the characteristic impairment in vertical extraocular movements. Additionally, her cerebellar features, asymmetric tremor, hyposmia, and RBD are more typical of multiple system atrophy than progressive supranuclear palsy.

Patients with vascular parkinsonism have sudden or step-wise onset of symptoms and exhibit disproportionate involvement of the lower extremities. The involvement of the upper body, gradual course, and nonmotor symptoms in this patient make this diagnosis unlikely.

KEY POINT

- The combination of parkinsonism, cerebellar ataxia, and early postural instability and falls is most consistent with a diagnosis of multiple system atrophy.

Bibliography

Aerts MB, Esselink RA, Post B, van de Warrenburg BP, Bloem BR. Improving the diagnostic accuracy in parkinsonism: a three-pronged approach. Pract Neurol. 2012 Apr;12(2):77-87. [PMID: 22450452]

Item 54   Answer: A

Educational Objective: Treat carpal tunnel syndrome.

Decompression surgery is the most appropriate treatment for this patient with carpal tunnel syndrome. Patients with this disorder who have active denervation on nerve conduction studies and have muscle weakness and atrophy on clinical examination should undergo decompression surgery to prevent irreversible motor weakness. Uncontrolled pain and sensory symptoms can be another indication for surgery, but in the absence of motor weakness and active denervation, conservative measures to treat pain and control paresthesia should be attempted first.

Symptomatic treatment, such as NSAIDs, gabapentin, and glucocorticoid injections, and conservative treatment, such as nocturnal neutral position wrist splinting and occupational therapy, may be appropriate therapy for patients with mild to moderate carpal tunnel syndrome, but only if they have no evidence of weakness, atrophy, or active motor denervation on nerve conduction studies. Weight reduction also can be helpful in patients with obesity.

Diabetes mellitus can cause (or predispose one to) compressive mononeuropathies, including median neuropathy at the wrist and ulnar neuropathy at the elbow. However, patients with diabetes who experience hand numbness also should be assessed for carpal tunnel syndrome. The criteria for using surgical decompression to treat carpal tunnel syndrome and the expected response to surgery are similar in patients with and without diabetes.

KEY POINT

- Patients with carpal tunnel syndrome who have active denervation on nerve conduction studies and have muscle weakness and atrophy on clinical examination should undergo decompression surgery to prevent irreversible motor weakness.

Bibliography

Alfonso C, Jann S, Massa R, Torreggiani A. Diagnosis, treatment and follow-up of the carpal tunnel syndrome: a review. Neurol. Sci. 2010 Jun;31(3):243-52. [PMID: 20145967]

Item 55   Answer: A

Educational Objective: Treat hypertension after an intracerebral hemorrhage.

This patient should receive labetalol intravenously. He most likely has an intracerebral hemorrhage induced by hypertension. In patients with this type of hemorrhage and a systolic blood pressure greater than 180 mm Hg, acute blood pressure lowering is indicated. Hematoma expansion is a significant source of morbidity and mortality in intracerebral hemorrhage, particularly with extension into the ventricles, and commonly occurs within the first 3 hours after hemorrhage onset. Uncontrolled hypertension is a strong risk factor for hematoma expansion. In this patient, the blood pressure should be lowered to less than 160/90 mm Hg, according to American Heart Association guidelines. A recent clinical trial even reported that lowering blood pressure to less than 140/80 mm Hg was safe and led to a trend in improvement in neurologic outcomes. Labetalol is a fast-acting agent that can be titrated easily.

Intravenous nitroprusside can increase intracranial pressure and thus should be avoided in this patient with a likely intracerebral hemorrhage. The mechanism of action is thought to be related to an increase in cerebral blood volume from either a direct increase in venous volume or impaired venous drainage.

No evidence supports the use of platelet transfusion to improve outcomes in intracerebral hemorrhage or prevent hematoma expansion in patients taking antiplatelet agents. Associated risks of platelet transfusion include transfusion syndrome and volume overload.

Recombinant factor VIIa is inappropriate treatment for this patient. Studies have not shown a beneficial role of hemostatic agents in intracerebral hemorrhage without coagulopathy. In fact, a phase 3 trial that compared recombinant factor VIIa with placebo showed no improvement in neurologic outcomes but a significant increase in the rate of thrombotic complications.

KEY POINT

- In patients with intracranial hemorrhage and a systolic blood pressure greater than 180 mm Hg, blood pressure should be lowered to less than 160/90 mm Hg.

Answers and Critiques

Bibliography

Morgenstern LB, Hemphill JC 3rd, Anderson C, et al; American Heart Association Stroke Council and Council on Cardiovascular Nursing. Guidelines for the management of spontaneous intracerebral hemorrhage: a guideline for healthcare professionals from the American Heart Association/American Stroke Association. Stroke. 2010 Sep;41(9): 2108-29. [PMID: 20651276]

Item 56   Answer: D

Educational Objective: Treat convulsive status epilepticus.

This patient should be treated with intravenous (IV) lorazepam followed by IV phenytoin. She is exhibiting convulsive status epilepticus (CSE), which is defined as convulsive seizures lasting longer than 5 minutes without a return to baseline mental status. CSE is a medical emergency requiring immediate treatment. First-line therapy for CSE is IV lorazepam followed by IV phenytoin or fosphenytoin. This combination has been shown to be superior to a benzodiazepine or phenytoin alone for stopping and providing ongoing control of CSE. When available, fosphenytoin, a prodrug of phenytoin, is preferred over phenytoin because it can be administered faster and does not cause the skin necrosis sometimes seen with phenytoin. Valproic acid also can be used after lorazepam to treat CSE, with several studies showing a similar efficacy to phenytoin. In some patients with known generalized epilepsy syndromes, valproic acid may be a better choice because phenytoin has the potential to provoke absence seizures or absence status epilepticus in these patients.

IV diazepam is less effective that IV lorazepam in treating CSE and thus should not be used if IV lorazepam is available. Rectal diazepam can be used if IV access cannot be obtained. Intramuscular midazolam recently also has been shown to be a good alternative to lorazepam for out-of-hospital CSE or patients without IV access. IV access has been established in this patient.

Levetiracetam has not shown efficacy in the treatment of CSE or been approved by the FDA for use in this clinical scenario. No antiepileptic drugs besides fosphenytoin, phenytoin, and valproic acid are recommended as first-line treatment of CSE.

KEY POINT

- First-line therapy for convulsive status epilepticus is intravenous (IV) lorazepam followed by IV phenytoin or fosphenytoin.

Bibliography

Brophy GM, Bell R, Claassen J, et al; Neurocritical Care Society Status Epilepticus Guideline Writing Committee. Guidelines for the evaluation and management of status epilepticus. Neurocrit Care. 2012 Aug;17(1): 3-23. [PMID: 22528274]

Item 57   Answer: B

Educational Objective: Diagnose chronic inflammatory demyelinating polyradiculoneuropathy.

This patient most likely has chronic inflammatory demyelinating polyradiculoneuropathy (CIDP). His rapidly progressive symmetric distal and proximal weakness that plateaued 3 months after onset is consistent with this diagnosis. The diffuse areflexia and sensory and motor neuropathy noted on physical examination and the demyelinating pattern (conduction blocks and slowing of conduction velocities) detected on nerve conduction studies all support the diagnosis of CIDP. CIDP can be idiopathic or associated with a range of systemic conditions, including diabetes mellitus, paraproteinemia, and HIV infection. Recognition of CIDP is essential because the disorder is responsive to glucocorticoids and other forms of immunomodulatory therapy.

Patients with Charcot-Marie-Tooth disease type 1 also have uniform demyelination on nerve conduction studies. However, the clinical course is much slower than in this patient, and symptoms are more prominent in the distal extremities.

Diabetic amyotrophy, also known as proximal lumbosacral radiculoneuropathy, presents with subacute pain and weakness in the proximal lower extremities. The simultaneous involvement of the upper extremities, diffuse areflexia, and diffuse motor nerve abnormalities on nerve conduction studies in this patient are inconsistent with this diagnosis.

The clinical features of CIDP are very similar to those of Guillain-Barré syndrome, but the latter condition has a faster progression and reaches its nadir within 4 weeks, whereas CIDP progression continues beyond 8 weeks from onset.

KEY POINT

- Progressive weakness, areflexia, and sensorimotor neuropathy with a progression extending beyond 8 weeks since onset of symptoms are characteristic of chronic inflammatory demyelinating polyradiculoneuropathy.

Bibliography

Peltier AC, Donofrio PD. Chronic inflammatory demyelinating polyradiculoneuropathy: from bench to bedside. Semin Neurol. 2012 Jul;32(3): 187-95. [PMID: 23117943]

Item 58   Answer: A

Educational Objective: Treat idiopathic intracranial hypertension.

The patient should be treated with acetazolamide. Although the headache described has many features of a tension-type headache, the findings of papilledema, partial left palsy of the abducens nerve (cranial nerve VI), and a cerebrospinal fluid (CSF) opening pressure of 350 mm H_2O suggests the presence of a secondary headache syndrome. Documentation of an elevated CSF opening pressure without evidence of a space-occupying lesion on neuroimaging confirms the diagnosis of idiopathic intracranial hypertension (IIH). This condition is most frequently seen in young women with an elevated BMI. The use of a combined oral contraceptive is an additional risk factor. Headache is the most common symptom, and papilledema is the most common physical examination finding. Carbonic anhydrase inhibitors, such as acetazolamide, are the only reliably effective medications for IIH. These inhibitors have been shown to reduce headache and improve visual impairment in patients with IIH.

Amitriptyline is an effective preventive medication for migraine or tension-type headache but would not address this patient's elevated intracranial pressure and thus is inappropriate.

An epidural blood patch is used in the treatment of intracranial hypotension arising spontaneously or occurring after lumbar puncture. This patient has intracranial hypertension.

Optic nerve sheath fenestration involves an incision in the meninges surrounding the optic nerve (cranial nerve II) to relieve elevated intracranial pressure. Optic nerve sheath fenestration can be used in the treatment of IIH but only after the failure of medical management. If acetazolamide does not relieve this patient's symptoms, then optic nerve fenestration may be appropriate.

Spironolactone is a recognized therapy for polycystic ovary syndrome but has no reported effect on headaches or intracranial pressure.

KEY POINT

- Carbonic anhydrase inhibitors, such as acetazolamide, are the only reliably effective medications for idiopathic intracranial hypertension.

Bibliography
Hoffmann J, Goadsby PJ. Update on intracranial hypertension and hypotension. Curr Opin Neurol. 2013 Jun;26(3):240-7. [PMID: 23594732]

Item 59   Answer: C

Educational Objective: Monitor for atrial fibrillation in cryptogenic ischemic stroke.

The most appropriate next step is cardiac rhythm monitoring. The patient has an acute infarction in the anterior cerebral artery territory, which is typically the result of artery-to-artery embolic sources or cardiac embolism. This diagnosis is supported by the abrupt termination of the artery seen on magnetic resonance angiography. Until final stroke classification can be confirmed, the patient has a cryptogenic stroke. The patient's vascular imaging did not show extracranial or intracranial internal carotid artery stenosis, which makes cardiac embolism more likely. In several reports, as many as 25% of patients with cryptogenic ischemic stroke have paroxysmal atrial fibrillation on prolonged cardiac monitoring of up to 30 days; patients who have premature atrial contractions and other findings of ectopy on short-term telemetry may be more likely to have this finding. Continued cardiac rhythm monitoring to detect atrial fibrillation is thus advisable in this patient.

Clopidogrel should not be added to this patient's medication regimen because the combination of aspirin and clopidogrel was associated with an increased risk of major

hemorrhage without any associated clinical benefit in several clinical trials in the subacute setting.

Dabigatran and other novel anticoagulants have only been approved for stroke prevention in the setting of atrial fibrillation, which has not yet been diagnosed in this patient.

Patent foramen ovale (PFO) closure did not reduce the risk of ischemic stroke more than best medical therapy in patients with cryptogenic stroke in the recently completed CLOSURE I trial. The risk of recurrent stroke in patients with an otherwise isolated PFO, with or without an atrial septal aneurysm, is low in most clinical trials. In older patients, a PFO frequently is an incidental finding and unlikely to be causally related to the infarct.

KEY POINT

- Patients with cryptogenic ischemic stroke require prolonged cardiac monitoring to detect atrial fibrillation, which is found in as many as 25% of these patients.

Bibliography
Tayal AH, Tian M, Kelly KM, et al. Atrial fibrillation detected by mobile cardiac outpatient telemetry in cryptogenic TIA or stroke. Neurology. 2008 Nov 18;71(21):1696-701. Epub 2008 Sep 24. [PMID: 18815386]

Item 60   Answer: A

Educational Objective: Treat advanced Parkinson disease with motor complications.

Deep brain stimulation is the appropriate treatment of this patient with advanced Parkinson disease who continues to benefit from dopaminergic medications but experiences medication-related complications. His initial marked benefit from carbidopa-levodopa wears off before he takes the next dosage. Appropriate initial steps to alleviate this problem included increasing the frequency of carbidopa-levodopa dosing and adding entacapone to prolong the effect of the carbidopa-levodopa after it is taken. However, he developed prominent medication-induced dyskinesia and visual hallucinations, which both limit further medical management. Deep brain stimulation of the subthalamic nucleus is likely to provide more sustained control of his medication-responsive motor deficits and allow a reduction in his medications; this, in turn, should resolve any medication-induced hallucinations or dyskinesia.

Discontinuing entacapone is likely to diminish the patient's dyskinesia but at the same time would remove the beneficial effect of prolonging the action of the carbidopa-levodopa and thus lead to earlier wearing off of its benefit.

Although amantadine can be effective against dyskinesia, increasing the dosage further may worsen the hallucinations.

Adding a dopamine agonist, such as ropinirole, may boost the dopaminergic effect of the carbidopa-levodopa, but this medication also is likely to worsen the patient's hallucinations and dyskinesia and should be avoided.

Answers and Critiques

Adding a monoamine oxidase B inhibitor, such as selegiline, also is likely to worsen his dyskinesia and thus is inappropriate.

KEY POINT

- Deep brain stimulation is the appropriate treatment of patients with advanced Parkinson disease who continue to benefit from dopaminergic medications but experience medication-related complications.

Bibliography

Okun MS. Deep-brain stimulation for Parkinson's disease. New Engl J Med 2012 Oct 18;367(16):1529-38. [PMID: 23075179]

Item 61   Answer: C

Educational Objective: Identify the cause of delirium in a patient with dementia.

This patient should undergo testing for concurrent illnesses. She has had an acute change in cognitive symptoms accompanied by fluctuating symptoms, inattention, and a depressed level of consciousness. This presentation is consistent with delirium, which should be recognized early and treated by correction of the underlying cause. Underlying cognitive impairment or dementia is a significant risk factor for delirium. The acute change in mental status experienced by this patient is unlikely to be due to worsening dementia, given that the disease course has been slowly progressive to this point. Features of inattention and a depressed level of arousal are not common in Alzheimer disease until late in the disease course. The initial evaluation should focus on ruling out the most common metabolic and infectious causes of delirium in older patients by obtaining a complete blood count, serum electrolyte and plasma glucose levels, liver chemistry and kidney function tests, urinalysis, and a chest radiograph. Additional tests should be tailored to the clinical presentation.

Initiation of quetiapine is premature in this patient. Immediate therapy should focus on identifying and treating the underlying cause of delirium. For agitation, nonpharmacologic interventions should be tried first, such as frequent reorientation, avoiding immobilization and catheterization, restoring normal sleep patterns, and minimizing disruptions in the environment. Only if these steps prove inadequate should treatment with dopamine antagonists be considered.

Although cholinesterase inhibitors, such as donepezil, may be associated with cholinergic adverse effects in some patients, these effects tend to occur shortly after starting the medication or increasing the dose. This patient has tolerated a stable dose of donepezil for at least 1 year, and so it would not be appropriate to attribute her acute delirium to this medication. Evaluation for another cause should be pursued.

Neuroimaging is not indicated in the immediate evaluation of this patient because the findings on neurologic examination were nonfocal. If the initial testing for concurrent illnesses is unrevealing, additional evaluation would include neuroimaging to rule out hemorrhage, territorial infarction, or mass lesion.

KEY POINT

- Underlying cognitive impairment or dementia is a significant risk factor for delirium; identification of any concurrent illness(es) causing the delirium should be the first step in management.

Bibliography

Young J, Murthy L, Westby M, Akunne A, O'Mahony R; Guideline Development Group. Diagnosis, prevention, and management of delirium: summary of NICE guidance. BMJ. 2010 Jul 28;341:c3704. [PMID: 20667955]

Item 62   Answer: C

Educational Objective: Treat multiple sclerosis–related spasticity.

This patient should be treated with a skeletal muscle relaxant, such as oral baclofen. He is experiencing muscle spasms and cramps as a long-term consequence of corticospinal tract injury from multiple sclerosis. Damage to upper motoneuron pathways has resulted in reduced inhibition of reflex arcs in the spinal cord, which allows for tonic activation of the lower motoneuron and resultant spasms and cramps. These symptoms can be reduced with the use of skeletal muscle relaxant medications, including baclofen, tizanidine, and cyclobenzaprine. Some patients may require intrathecal baclofen pumps or botulinum toxin injections for refractory symptoms.

Electroencephalography would be an appropriate test if a high suspicion of seizure was present. This patient's history and clinical evaluation do not suggest seizure, and his symptoms are highly consistent with upper motoneuron spasticity.

Because the physical examination findings are clearly consistent with an upper motoneuron injury, electromyography (EMG) (nerve conduction studies and needle electrode examination) is inappropriate. EMG is most appropriate for disorders of the lower motoneuron, neuromuscular junction, or muscle. The lack of fasciculations makes lower motoneuron injury even less likely, and the normal serum creatine kinase level and lack of pain on muscle palpation make an inflammatory myopathy very unlikely.

Pramipexole would be an appropriate treatment for restless legs syndrome (RLS), but this patient is not experiencing RLS symptoms. RLS does not result in upper motoneuron signs on examination or daytime muscle cramps. Also, patients with RLS experience feelings of discomfort in the legs or periodic limb movements while sleeping, not tonic leg spasms and cramps as with this patient.

KEY POINT

- Baclofen is appropriate for treatment of muscle spasms and cramps due to corticospinal tract injury from multiple sclerosis.

Answers and Critiques

Bibliography

Kheder A, Nair KP. Spasticity: pathophysiology, evaluation and management. Pract Neurol. 2012 Oct;12(5):289-98. [PMID: 22976059]

Item 63   Answer: C

Educational Objective: **Treat refractory temporal lobe epilepsy.**

Right temporal lobectomy is the intervention most likely to make this patient seizure free and thus improve her quality of life. She has refractory epilepsy, defined as the persistence of disabling seizures for longer than 1 year despite treatment with adequate doses of two or more antiepileptic drugs (AEDs). Surgery is the most likely intervention to stop the seizures, and seizure freedom is closely tied to quality of life in a patient with refractory epilepsy. Given her history of febrile seizures in infancy and the presence of mesial temporal sclerosis on the MRI, her chances of seizure freedom 2 years after surgery are at least 70%.

Patients who do not respond to either their first or their second AED (in sequence or conjunction) have a less than 10% chance of experiencing seizure remission with pharmacotherapy. Therefore, adding a third agent, such as carbamazepine, to her medication regimen is unlikely to stop the seizures or improve her quality of life. Although carbamazepine could be offered in an attempt to temporize the situation while she awaits a surgical evaluation, it would not be the most effective management.

The ketogenic diet and vagal nerve stimulation are palliative treatments that can lessen the seizure burden in patients who are not candidates for epilepsy surgery. Both options rarely lead to seizure freedom.

KEY POINT

- In patients with refractory temporal lobe epilepsy, surgery is the most likely intervention to stop seizures and thus improve quality of life.

Bibliography

Jette N, Quan H, Tellez-Zenteno JF, et al; CASES Expert Panelists. Development of an online tool to determine appropriateness for an epilepsy surgery evaluation. Neurology. 2012 Sep 11;79(11):1084-93. Epub 2012 Aug 15. [PMID: 22895589]

Item 64   Answer: D

Educational Objective: **Treat parkinsonian-hyperpyrexia syndrome secondary to dopaminergic medication withdrawal.**

Levodopa should be restarted in this patient. Sudden withdrawal from dopaminergic medications, as may occur during hospitalization in patients with Parkinson disease, can lead to an acute dopamine agonist withdrawal syndrome, termed parkinsonian-hyperpyrexia syndrome, which resembles neuroleptic malignant syndrome (NMS). Patients who abruptly stop taking dopaminergic medications can develop acute altered mental status, hyperthermia, rhabdomyolysis, and extrapyramidal symptoms, including severe rigidity and dystonia. A high index of suspicion for parkinsonian-hyperpyrexia syndrome is required in these patients because mortality rates of up to 4% have been reported and may be prevented by early recognition and treatment. The differential diagnosis also includes central nervous system infection and status epilepticus. Aggressive supportive care, which may include intensive care and respiratory support, is appropriate. The primary medical therapy is restoration of dopaminergic medication.

Administration of the skeletal muscle relaxant baclofen may be helpful in patients with severe spasticity or progressive encephalomyelitis with rigidity and myoclonus, but not in those with Parkinson disease or disorders due to withdrawal from dopaminergic medications.

Dantrolene is a skeletal muscle relaxant that has proven efficacy in treating malignant hyperthermia and NMS. However, its effectiveness in parkinsonian-hyperpyrexia syndrome has not been established.

The clinical manifestations of serotonin syndrome may overlap with those of parkinsonian-hyperpyrexia syndrome and NMS, although serotonin syndrome is more often associated with hyperreflexia and myoclonus and not extrapyramidal symptoms. It typically occurs in patients taking high doses of serotoninergic agents (such as citalopram) and would not be expected in this patient in whom this medication has been withheld. Restarting the citalopram would not address the underlying disease process in this patient.

KEY POINT

- In hospitalized patients with Parkinson disease, sudden withdrawal of dopaminergic medications can lead to parkinsonian-hyperpyrexia syndrome, an acute syndrome resembling neuroleptic malignant syndrome; restarting the medications is the mainstay of therapy.

Bibliography

Newman EJ, Grosset DG, Kennedy PG . The parkinsonism-hyperpyrexia syndrome. Neurocrit Care. 2009;10(1):136-40. [PMID: 18712508]

Item 65   Answer: C

Educational Objective: **Treat status migrainosus.**

The patient has status migrainosus and should receive repetitive intravenous infusions of dihydroergotamine. Status migrainosus is defined as a migraine attack extending beyond 72 hours and is the most common complication of acute migraine. The condition is characterized by persistent severe pain that often is accompanied by protracted nausea with vomiting and profound sensory sensitivities. Hormonal factors are extremely common as inciting events. Life stressors, mood or anxiety disorders, and acute medication overuse may be other contributing factors. Triptans are often unsuccessful in resolving a migraine of this duration, but parenteral hydration and antiemetic medications sometimes provide some relief. Because this patient has not responded to either of

CONT. these treatments or to the ketorolac administered in the emergency department, the next step is repetitive administration of intravenous dihydroergotamine. This drug is administered in conjunction with either prochlorperazine or metoclopramide over the course of 1 to 3 days. Outpatient treatment options include a several-day course of oral glucocorticoids.

The patient has normal findings on neurologic examination. An MRI of the brain is unlikely to provide any additional useful information.

Combined oral contraceptives should be avoided in patients with migraine with aura because they further increase stroke risk, which is already elevated in this patient.

Opioids, such as hydromorphone, may provide analgesia but often contribute to worsening migraine frequency or intensity. They should be avoided in patients with acute migraine when other options are available.

Sertraline may help control anxiety but contributes nothing to the acute or preventive treatment of migraine and thus is inappropriate for this patient.

KEY POINT

- Repetitive administration of intravenous dihydroergotamine is the most appropriate in-patient treatment of status migrainosus.

Bibliography

Nagy AJ, Gandhi S, Bhola R, Goadsby PJ. Intravenous dihydroergotamine for inpatient management of refractory primary headaches. Neurology. 2011 Nov 15;77(20):1827-32. [PMID: 22049203]

Item 66   Answer: B

Educational Objective: Modify pharmacologic therapy for multiple sclerosis in the setting of pregnancy.

In addition to discontinuing the oral contraceptive in preparation for attempting conception, fingolimod should be stopped. An oral disease-modifying therapy for multiple sclerosis (MS), fingolimod is a sphingosine-1-phosphate receptor modulator that restricts activated lymphocytes to lymph nodes and may also have direct neuroprotective effects. Fingolimod significantly reduces the relapse rate, risk of disability progression, and accumulation of new lesions on MRI. This drug has been associated with rare but potentially harmful side effects, including increased rates of serious herpesvirus infection, hypertension, bradycardia, lymphopenia, liver function abnormalities, and macular edema. Fingolimod is classified as a pregnancy category C drug, and thus its safety in human pregnancy is not clearly established. Although category C medications are indicated in some patients if the benefits outweigh the risks, the hormonal state of pregnancy itself is protective against MS activity, and thus discontinuing a disease-modifying drug during pregnancy is considered relatively safe.

Advising this patient against pregnancy is clearly inappropriate. The adverse effect of pregnancy on MS progression is a commonly held misconception. In fact, observational studies have found reduced risks for conversion to clinically

definite MS from clinically isolated syndromes and reduced risks for conversion from relapsing MS to secondary progressive MS in women with multiple pregnancies.

Mitoxantrone is an anthracenedione chemotherapeutic agent that reduces lymphocyte proliferation and decreases the relapse rate and disability progression in MS. Despite mitoxantrone's efficacy, cardiac toxicity and the risk of secondary leukemia have significantly limited its use. Mitoxantrone is classified as a pregnancy category X drug and is contraindicated during pregnancy.

The MS drug teriflunomide is the active metabolite of leflunomide, which inhibits pyrimidine biosynthesis and interferes with the interaction between T lymphocytes and antigen-presenting cells. Substituting teriflunomide for fingolimod is inappropriate because teriflunomide is classified as pregnancy category X drug and is contraindicated during pregnancy.

KEY POINT

- Fingolimod is classified as a pregnancy category C drug (safety in human pregnancy not clearly established) and thus should not be used by women who are pregnant or planning to become pregnant.

Bibliography

D'hooghe MB, Nagels G, Uitdehaag BM. Long-term effects of childbirth in MS. J Neurol Neurosurg Psychiatry. 2010 Jan;81(1):38-41. [PMID: 19939856]

Item 67   Answer: C

Educational Objective: Prevent neurologic complications with nimodipine after subarachnoid hemorrhage.

This patient should receive oral nimodipine. Nimodipine is an L-type calcium channel blocker that has reduced the incidence of vasospasm in clinical trials involving patients with subarachnoid hemorrhage; morbidity and mortality also were reduced, even among patients who did not have cerebral vasospasm. Nimodipine may improve outcomes by preventing vasospasm and by a neuroprotective mechanism, particularly because calcium influx into neurons is a common pathway of cell injury in ischemia. Administration of oral nimodipine for 21 days after the hemorrhage is indicated in all patients with aneurysmal subarachnoid hemorrhage. This patient had an aneurysmal subarachnoid hemorrhage that was appropriately treated. In the first 48 hours after subarachnoid hemorrhage, rebleeding and hydrocephalus can cause neurologic worsening that is associated with significant morbidity and mortality.

Because the patient has no evidence of cerebral artery vasospasm, such as deterioration in level of consciousness or new focal neurologic deficits, treatment with intravenous dopamine is inappropriate. Vasospasm with subsequent cerebral ischemia is a significant contributor to neurologic worsening and poor long-term outcomes in patients with aneurysmal hemorrhage. Patients with a thick clot in the base of the brain are at higher risk of vasospasm, which can be detected before symptom onset on a transcranial Doppler ultrasound. This patient, however, has no clinical, objective, or imaging signs of vasospasm that would warrant prophylactic treatment with a vasopressor.

Intravenous insulin should not be given to this patient. Her blood glucose levels are mildly elevated, but acute management of mild hyperglycemia has not shown benefit in patients with all stroke subtypes. Because of the risk of hypoglycemia, the American College of Physicians (ACP) and other organizations recommend not using intensive insulin therapy to normalize blood glucose levels in critically ill patients with or without diabetes mellitus. If insulin therapy is required, the ACP recommends target blood glucose levels of 140 mg/dL to 200 mg/dL (7.8-11.1 mmol/L).

The efficacy of statins for secondary stroke prevention or as a neuroprotective agent in subarachnoid hemorrhage has not been established. Statins are indicated for secondary stroke prevention in patients with ischemic stroke or transient ischemic attack of a presumed atherosclerotic subtype.

KEY POINT

* Oral nimodipine is indicated in all patients with aneurysmal subarachnoid hemorrhage.

Bibliography

Connolly ES Jr, Rabinstein AA, Carhuapoma JR, et al; American Heart Association Stroke Council; Council on Cardiovascular Radiology and Intervention; Council on Cardiovascular Nursing; Council on Cardiovascular Surgery and Anesthesia; Council on Clinical Cardiology. Guidelines for the management of aneurysmal subarachnoid hemorrhage: a guideline for healthcare professionals from the American Heart Association/American Stroke Association. Stroke. 2012 Jun;43(6):1711-37. [PMID: 22556195]

Item 68   Answer: B

Educational Objective: Provide preventive therapy in multiple sclerosis.

This patient should have a yearly influenza vaccination. She takes the disease-modifying drug glatiramer acetate, a pregnancy category B drug, for her multiple sclerosis (MS). The patient already exercises at least 3 hours weekly, takes a daily calcium–vitamin D supplement, and does not smoke, all recommended preventive measures against osteoporosis or conversion to secondary progression in patients with MS. According to a position statement by the American Academy of Neurology, there is no evidence of adverse outcomes of routine vaccinations in patients with MS beyond what is expected in the general population. In fact, these vaccinations are recommended to prevent infections leading to a heightened immune state and potential MS relapse.

Moderate alcohol usage has not been shown to adversely affect MS outcomes and has no effect on the metabolism of glatiramer acetate. Therefore, alcohol cessation is not necessary.

Although urinary tract infections (UTIs) are more common among patients with MS because of neurogenic bladder dysfunction, screening urinalysis is not indicated as a preventive medicine strategy in this patient population, barring UTI symptoms.

Despite the commonly held belief that pregnancy results in adverse events in MS, all evidence points instead toward to the protective effect of the hormonal state of pregnancy. Multiparous women with MS have equivalent, or perhaps better, outcomes than women with MS who have never been pregnant. Initiating an oral contraceptive is indicated only if the patient wishes to avoid pregnancy, but not as a preventive strategy for worsening of MS.

KEY POINT

* Routine vaccinations, such as an annual influenza vaccination, are recommended for patients with multiple sclerosis (MS) to prevent infections leading to a heightened immune state and potential MS relapse.

Bibliography

Rutschmann OT, McCrory DC, Matchar DB; Immunization Panel of the Multiple Sclerosis Council for Clinical Practice Guidelines. Immunization and MS: a summary of published evidence and recommendations. Neurology. 2002 Dec 24;59(12):1837-43. [PMID: 12499473]

Item 69   Answer: C

Educational Objective: Treat migraine without aura with an NSAID.

The patient should receive naproxen to treat his headaches, which meet criteria for migraine without aura. Episodes of migraine without aura typically last between 4 and 72 hours if untreated. Two of four pain features are necessary for the diagnosis to be made: unilateral location, throbbing quality, moderate to severe intensity, and worsening with physical activity. Either nausea or a combination of photophobia and phonophobia also is required. Patients with this diagnosis commonly report sinus pressure or drainage with these episodes, which often leads to the incorrect diagnosis of sinus headache. Common triggers include stress, hormonal or weather changes, alterations in sleep or meal patterns, or strong light, noise, or odor stimuli. Neurologic examination findings are normal. Evidence-based guidelines suggest that NSAIDs (such as naproxen), triptans, and dihydroergotamine are effective therapy for this type of acute migraine but that NSAIDs are preferred as initial treatment because of their greater cost-effectiveness.

In the context of a stable pattern of headaches that meets the criteria for migraine, CT of the head in unnecessary. Similarly, the headache pattern described by this patient—weekly headache episodes lasting 6 to 8 hours—is incompatible with an acute or chronic sinus pathology, which makes CT of the sinuses also unlikely to add any useful information.

Pseudoephedrine is effective in alleviating sinus congestion but has no role in the treatment of migraine. Headache is a relatively late-appearing and minor symptom of acute sinusitis; major symptoms include facial pain, purulent discharge, fever, and hyposmia, none of which this patient reports.

KEY POINT

- Evidence-based guidelines suggest that NSAIDs, triptans, and dihydroergotamine are effective treatments for acute migraine without aura and that NSAIDs are preferred as initial treatment because of their greater cost-effectiveness.

Bibliography

Taylor FR, Kaniecki RG. Symptomatic treatment of migraine: when to use NSAIDs, triptans, or opiates. Curr Treat Options Neurol. 2011 Feb;13(1): 15-27. [PMID: 21125432]

Item 70   Answer: D

Educational Objective: Treat amyotrophic lateral sclerosis with riluzole.

This patient should receive riluzole. Clinical and electromyographic evidence of simultaneous upper and lower motoneuron signs in multiple body regions is most consistent with a diagnosis of amyotrophic lateral sclerosis (ALS). Onset in a single limb, rapid progression, bulbar involvement, and MRI evidence of a corticospinal tract abnormality further support the diagnosis, which was confirmed by results of the needle electrode examination. The absence of an alternative likely cause of his symptoms, such as Lyme disease, hyperparathyroidism, vitamin B_{12} or copper deficiency, lead intoxication, or combined cervical myelopathy and neuropathy, also suggests the diagnosis.

Riluzole is the only FDA-approved medication for ALS and can increase the survival of affected patients by a modest average of 3 months. It should be offered to all patients with a new diagnosis of ALS who wish to maximize their survival.

Bilevel positive airway pressure and other similarly noninvasive respiratory support methods can increase survival in ALS and should be started in the presence of respiratory symptoms and hypercarbia, which are absent in this patient.

Although intravenous immune globulin (IVIG) can be used in the management of chronic inflammatory demyelinating polyradiculoneuropathy (CIDP), this patient's clinical history and findings on needle electrode examination, especially the prominent upper motoneuron signs and absence of sensory deficits, are inconsistent with CIDP. IVIG is not indicated for the management of ALS.

Percutaneous endoscopic gastrostomy should be considered in patients with ALS and dysphagia before they reach the advanced stages of the disease to improve nutrition and increase survival. This intervention would be premature in this patient, however, who has no signs of dysphagia.

KEY POINT

- Riluzole, the only FDA-approved medication for amyotrophic lateral sclerosis, can increase the survival of affected patients by an average of 3 months

Bibliography

Kiernan MC, Vucic S, Cheah BC, et al. Amyotrophic lateral sclerosis. Lancet. 2011 Mar 12;377(9769):942-55. Epub 2011 Feb 4.[PMID: 21296405]

Item 71   Answer: A

Educational Objective: Diagnose a secondary headache.

The patient should undergo brain MRI. Although she has a long-standing history of migraine with aura, the recent escalation in headache frequency and intensity is concerning. The pattern of her headaches has fundamentally changed, and she exhibits several other red flags, such as the development of a new headache condition after age 50 years and neurologic symptoms lasting more than 1 hour, that are compatible with the presence of a secondary headache. Diplopia, when present in migraine aura, should be accompanied by other features seen in migraine with brainstem aura (basilar migraine), such as vertigo, ataxia, dysarthria, diplopia, tinnitus, hyperacusis, or alteration in consciousness; this patient has none of these features. Additionally, the maximum duration of aura in basilar migraine is 60 minutes or less, not the 2 hours she experienced. MRI is the preferred study to confirm the diagnosis of a secondary headache.

Discontinuation of ibuprofen would be helpful in the setting of medication overuse headache. Excessive analgesic intake can result in worsening of the underlying headache or the appearance of a milder, nonspecific headache. However, this medication would not cause new neurologic symptoms, such as diplopia.

In this patient with a probable secondary headache, neuroimaging is necessary before consideration of lumbar puncture to exclude any space-occupying lesion that could affect intracranial pressure.

Switching from naratriptan to sumatriptan may have been a consideration if the diagnosis were only worsening migraine. However, this patient most likely has a secondary headache disorder, so changing triptans in unlikely to be helpful.

Substituting topiramate for amitriptyline may be an appropriate treatment in patients with escalating migraine frequency, but not in those suspected to have a secondary headache disorder.

KEY POINT

- Recent escalation of headache frequency in patients with migraine suggests a secondary headache disorder and should be evaluated with brain MRI.

Bibliography

Detsky ME, McDonald DR, Baerlocher MO, Tomlinson GA, McCrory DC, Booth CM. Does this patient with headache have a migraine or need neuroimaging? JAMA. 2006 Sep 13;296(10):1274-83. [PMID: 16968852]

Item 72   Answer: C

Educational Objective: Counsel a patient with an unruptured cerebral aneurysm about smoking cessation.

This patient should be counseled about smoking cessation and provided with smoking cessation aids as appropriate, including nicotine replacement or pharmacologic treatment. She has an unruptured intracranial aneurysm of the left middle cerebral artery. A subarachnoid hemorrhage (SAH) has been ruled out by neuroimaging and lumbar puncture findings. She has no history of a previous SAH, and the aneurysm measures less than 7 mm, both of which indicate a low risk of rupture. The major risk factors for cerebral aneurysms and their rupture are hypertension and tobacco use. Her hypertension is well controlled by the amlodipine. Smoking cessation is indicated to prevent further aneurysmal expansion and rupture.

Neither aneurysmal clipping nor endovascular coiling is necessary because the aneurysm is less than 12 mm and located in the anterior circulation, which suggests a low risk of rupture (0.05% annually). The surgical morbidity associated with either technique is too great given the low risk of rupture. Repeat neuroimaging on an annual basis can be considered to track any change in the aneurysm's size.

The calcium channel blocker nimodipine has been shown to improve outcomes in SAH and is the standard of care for all patients with aneurysmal SAH. SAH has been ruled out in this patient, whose blood pressure is well controlled by amlodipine. No evidence suggests that switching to nimodipine from amlodipine will prevent aneurysmal expansion or rupture.

KEY POINT

- Patients with unruptured intracranial aneurysms should be counseled to stop smoking because of the increased risk of aneurysmal rupture.

Bibliography
Wiebers DO, Whisnant JP, Huston H 3rd, et al; International Study of Unruptured Intracranial Aneurysms Investigators. Unruptured intracranial aneurysms: natural history, clinical outcome, and risks of surgical and endovascular treatment. Lancet. 2003 Jul 12;362(9378):103-10. [PMID: 12867109]

Item 73   Answer: D

Educational Objective: Diagnose early Parkinson disease.

This patient most likely has early Parkinson disease (PD) on the basis of his clinical examination findings and does not require additional diagnostic testing. This diagnosis requires the presence of bradykinesia (in this patient, the decrements in speed and amplitude of repetitive movements) and at least one other cardinal feature (resting tremor, rigidity, or postural instability, with only postural instability absent in this patient). In addition, the absence of atypical features, such as early dementia, early falls, vertical gaze palsy, or prominent dysautonomia, is consistent with the diagnosis of PD. Reemergence of a resting tremor with posturing and ambulation also is seen in PD. The presence of bilateral kinetic tremor, although more typical of essential tremor, is still consistent with this diagnosis. Further diagnostic testing is not necessary in this patient before a diagnosis can be made.

A dopamine transporter scan can confirm degeneration of nigrostriatal dopaminergic terminals in Parkinson disease and differentiate between Parkinson disease and essential tremor in patients in whom the diagnosis cannot be made on clinical grounds (which is not the case in this patient). The sensitivity of this expensive test, however, is not superior to that of expert clinical assessment.

An MRI of the brain can be used to assess for vascular parkinsonism and hydrocephalus but should not be obtained before a clinical diagnosis is made. This patient does not have symptoms of vascular parkinsonism (predominant lower extremity involvement, gait impairment, and a step-wise course) or normal pressure hydrocephalus (the triad of gait impairment, urinary incontinence, and cognitive impairment), which makes these diagnoses unlikely.

Needle electrode electromyography can be helpful in studies of nerve and muscle disease but has no role in the diagnosis of Parkinson disease.

KEY POINT

- The diagnosis of Parkinson disease can be made on the basis of clinical findings and requires the presence of bradykinesia and at least one of the other cardinal features of resting tremor, rigidity, or postural instability.

Bibliography
Stoessl AJ, Martin WW, McKeown MJ, Sossi V. Advances in imaging in Parkinson's disease. Lancet Neurol. 2011 Nov;10(11): 987-1001. [PMID: 22014434]

Item 74   Answer: D

Educational Objective: Treat a pseudorelapse of multiple sclerosis, differentiating it from an actual relapse.

This patient should be treated with supportive care and clinical observation. His clinical picture is consistent with a likely viral upper respiratory tract infection, which is causing a pseudorelapse of his multiple sclerosis (MS). MS pseudorelapses involve a worsening of baseline neurologic symptoms (or recurrence of previous symptoms) that occurs in the setting of physiologic stressors. In this patient, the viral syndrome and associated systemic inflammatory response are the underlying cause of the pseudorelapse. Supportive treatment of these symptoms and observation to ensure that the patient returns to baseline status is the most appropriate management to avoid unnecessary treatments or changes in medication. Because actual inflammatory relapses can sometimes be triggered by pseudorelapses (and similar causes), treatment with glucocorticoids can be considered if improvement does not occur within days of resolution of the causative condition.

The patient most likely has a viral upper respiratory tract infection, with no evidence of a urinary tract infection. Without evidence of bacterial infection, antibiotic therapy, such as administration of amoxicillin-clavulanate, is not indicated.

The increased postvoid residual urine volume suggests that this patient has moderate urinary retention. An increase in the oxybutynin dosage would cause relaxation of the

Answers and Critiques

muscles of the bladder wall and would likely worsen the patient's retention.

Although glucocorticoid therapy might be appropriate therapy for a true MS relapse, treatment with methylprednisolone in this patient with a likely pseudorelapse is inappropriate.

KEY POINT

- A pseudorelapse of multiple sclerosis is a worsening of baseline neurologic symptoms or recurrence of previous symptoms that occurs in the setting of physiologic stressors, such as a superimposed infection.

Bibliography

Thrower BW. Relapse management in multiple sclerosis. Neurologist. 2009 Jan;15(1):1-5. [PMID: 19131851]

Item 75   Answer: A

Educational Objective: Select the appropriate diagnostic test to evaluate for complications after subarachnoid hemorrhage.

This patient should undergo CT angiography of the brain to assess for cerebral vasospasm. He is now at day 7 after a subarachnoid hemorrhage due to a left middle cerebral artery aneurysm. In the first 48 hours after a subarachnoid hemorrhage, rebleeding from an unsecured aneurysm and hydrocephalus are the principal causes of neurologic deterioration. This patient's aneurysm has been successfully clipped, and hydrocephalus is being managed with the use of an external ventricular drain. Potential neurologic complications after the first 48 hours include seizures, hydrocephalus, infection, and symptomatic cerebral vasospasm; the incidence of cerebral vasospasm peaks on days 5 to 10 after a hemorrhage. Cerebral vasospasm can manifest as a decline in neurologic function in patients who are awake enough for a neurologic examination. Although transcranial Doppler ultrasonography may reveal a vasospasm, CT angiography is more sensitive at detecting vasospasm that can be treated with the initiation of vasopressors to augment the blood pressure or with endovascular treatment in more refractory cases. CT angiography has the additional benefit of imaging the brain parenchyma for evidence of cerebral edema or infarction and the ventricles for evidence of hydrocephalus that may be amenable to shunting.

Electroencephalography (EEG) is inappropriate as the next diagnostic step in this patient with an aneurysmal subarachnoid hemorrhage. Convulsive and nonconvulsive status epilepticus is common and underdiagnosed after hemorrhagic stroke and is associated with poor neurologic outcome. If imaging does not identify a clear cause of the patient's decline that can be treated with medical or surgical therapy before irreversible damage occurs, then continuous EEG monitoring may help in diagnosing seizures.

Lumbar puncture may be useful for measuring intracranial pressure in this patient with an external ventricular drain. However, repeat imaging would first be required, independent of the presence of the drain, to rule out mass effect that could precipitate cerebral herniation after a lumbar puncture.

MRI requires too long a time to complete in the setting of a neurologic emergency and may not adequately detect arterial narrowing. Vasospasm is more readily detected with CT angiography.

KEY POINT

- Cerebral vasospasm is a potential complication of subarachnoid hemorrhage that most often occurs 5 to 10 days after the hemorrhage and is best detected by CT angiography of the brain.

Bibliography

van Gijn J, Kerr RS, Rinkel GJ. Subarachnoid hemorrhage. Lancet. 2007 Jan 27;369(9558): 306-18. [PMID: 17258671]

Item 76   Answer: C

Educational Objective: Treat restless legs syndrome.

This patient has restless legs syndrome (RLS) and should be treated with ropinirole. Dopamine agonists, such as ropinirole, pramipexole, or rotigotine, are first-line treatments for RLS. This syndrome is characterized by the clinical features of abnormal sensations in the lower extremities, an urge to move the extremities in response to these sensations (with movement resulting in a transient relief of symptoms), emergence of symptoms at rest, and a circadian pattern (with symptoms more prominent at night). Diagnosis is clinical and based on history. Additional treatment options include gabapentin, gabapentin enacarbil, levodopa, and opioids.

Patients with RLS should be screened for iron deficiency. Iron supplementation can improve or resolve the symptoms of RLS in patients with iron deficiency and those with low-normal (15-45 ng/mL [15-45 µg/L]) serum ferritin levels. This patient's serum ferritin level is well above this range, and no evidence suggests that iron supplementation in this setting is beneficial.

Pentoxifylline is a peripheral vasodilator used in the treatment of peripheral arterial disease. Arterial insufficiency is not associated with RLS, and nothing suggests its presence in this patient. Therefore, this treatment is not indicated.

Zolpidem may help with insomnia but does not treat the underlying problem of RLS.

KEY POINT

- Dopamine agonists, such as ropinirole, pramipexole, or rotigotine, are first-line treatment for restless legs syndrome.

Bibliography

Garcia-Borreguero D, Kohnen R, Silber MH, et al. The long-term treatment of restless legs syndrome/Willis-Ekbom disease: evidence-based guidelines and clinical consensus best practice guidance: a report from the International Restless Legs Syndrome Study Group. Sleep Med. 2013 Jul;14(7): 675-84. [PMID: 23859128]

Item 77　　Answer:　B

Educational Objective: Evaluate mild cognitive impairment.

This patient should have an MRI of the brain. He most likely has mild cognitive impairment (MCI), as evidenced by cognitive difficulties that are greater than those typical of normal aging but do not impair activities of daily living and have minimal effect on instrumental activities of daily living. MCI is a clinical diagnosis made exclusively on the basis of history and the results of cognitive testing. Although neuroimaging cannot be used to detect whether or not a cognitive disorder is present, structural neuroimaging studies, specifically head CT and brain MRI, can play a key role in the routine diagnostic evaluation of patients with established cognitive impairment to exclude structural lesions of the brain, such as strokes, hematomas, brain tumors, or other mass lesions.

Amyloid PET imaging allows for in vivo detection of amyloid plaques, which are a core pathologic feature of Alzheimer disease. However, positive results are not synonymous with the presence of Alzheimer disease because cognitively normal persons can have abnormal scans. Amyloid PET imaging may provide prognostic information in patients with MCI by identifying those whose cognitive impairment may be related to underlying Alzheimer disease pathology, but much more research is still required before the routine use of this technology in clinical practice.

Screening for carotid stenosis with ultrasonography or any imaging modality has no role in the routine evaluation of cognitive impairment in an asymptomatic patient. An asymptomatic patient in this context is one without previous hemispheric neurologic symptoms—such as transient ischemic attack, stroke, or amaurosis fugax—or the presence of a carotid bruit on examination.

The apolipoprotein E gene (*APOE ε4*) located on chromosome 19 has been identified as a genetic risk factor for late-onset Alzheimer disease. *APOE ε4* genotyping has marginal additive value over clinical diagnoses but is neither necessary nor sufficient to predict who will develop Alzheimer disease and thus is not recommended for broad clinical use.

A fluorodeoxyglucose-PET scan of the brain or any other metabolic scan of the brain cannot determine if a patient's cognitive symptoms indicate cognitive impairment. Abnormal results of fluorodeoxyglucose-PET scanning also occur in persons who are cognitively normal. Although these abnormal results may indicate a future risk of cognitive impairment, this relationship has not been established.

KEY POINT

- Structural neuroimaging studies, specifically head CT and brain MRI, can play a key role in the routine diagnostic evaluation of patients with established cognitive impairment to exclude structural lesions of the brain, such as strokes, hematomas, brain tumors, or other mass lesions.

Bibliography

Petersen RC. Clinical practice. Mild cognitive impairment. N Engl J Med. 2011 Jun 9;364(23):2227-34. [PMID: 21651394]

Item 78　　Answer:　D

Educational Objective: Diagnose an acute complication of thrombolytic therapy.

This patient should undergo repeat noncontrast CT of the head. She had an ischemic stroke that was likely due to subtherapeutic anticoagulation. Findings from physical examination, notably an elevated National Institutes of Health Stroke Scale (NIHSS) score, and the initial CT scan of the head suggest a large cerebral infarction in the entire territory of the left middle cerebral artery. She was appropriately given intravenous recombinant tissue plasminogen activator within the recommended treatment window because of the high risk of a poor neurologic outcome. At the time of treatment, she did not meet any exclusion criterion for thrombolysis, such as an elevated blood pressure or an INR greater than 1.7. The patient has several risk factors for intracerebral hemorrhage after thrombolysis, including a high NIHSS score and a cardioembolic cause of the stroke. Any change in the neurologic examination, particularly in patients treated with thrombolysis, should prompt consideration of hemorrhage, which is associated with a high mortality rate. Hemorrhage after thrombolysis can be detected on a noncontrast CT scan of the head.

Intra-arterial thrombectomy is inappropriate in this patient. The new right-leg paralysis noted in the second neurologic examination is most concerning for intracerebral hemorrhage after thrombolysis. However, the benefit of intra-arterial treatment modalities, after or instead of intravenous thrombolysis, has not been established in randomized clinical trials.

This patient also should not be given intravenous labetalol. Administering treatment to lower her blood pressure is inappropriate because her blood pressure is already less than the recommended target of 180/105 mm Hg after thrombolysis.

Aspirin is appropriate stroke therapy in patients not eligible for thrombolysis and can be administered rectally in patients who are unable to swallow. However, in patients who have received thrombolysis, early administration of antiplatelet agents can increase the risk of hemorrhage. In addition, although aspirin is associated with a reduction in recurrent stroke risk when administered within 48 hours of ischemic stroke onset, aspirin has not been shown to prevent or reverse neurologic worsening.

KEY POINT

- Hemorrhage after thrombolysis for ischemic stroke can be detected on a noncontrast CT scan of the head.

Bibliography

Jauch, EC, Saver JL, Adams HP Jr, et al; American Heart Association Stroke Council; Council on Cardiovascular Nursing; Council on Peripheral

Answers and Critiques

Vascular Disease; Council on Clinical Cardiology. Guidelines for the early management of patients with acute ischemic stroke: a guideline for healthcare professionals from the American Heart Association/American Stroke Association. Stroke. 2013 Mar;44(3):870-947. [PMID: 23370205]

Item 79   Answer: E
Educational Objective: Treat acute refractory migraine.

The patient should be treated with subcutaneous sumatriptan for migraine without aura. She no longer responds to NSAIDs and oral triptans. The headaches are associated with emesis, and she is awakening with attacks. Migraine episodes have been so severe that she has visited an urgent care facility recently for parenteral treatment of refractory migraine. Self-administered injectable migraine medications would be of value for this patient. Although nasal spray options exist for several acute medications, they are less potent than their injectable counterparts. According to guidelines, no first-line agent for acute migraine treatment is available in suppository form.

Neither butalbital compounds nor opioids (such as hydrocodone) are recommended as first-line treatments of recurrent headache disorders. Little evidence of benefit in acute migraine exists for either class of drugs, and both contribute to an increased future risk of transformation into chronic migraine, compared with first-line agents.

Evidence supports the use of naproxen in the management of acute migraine, and the drug is listed by evidence-based guidelines as first-line therapy. In the setting of migraine that occurs upon awakening or with vomiting, however, it is unlikely to be beneficial, especially in a patient who has not responded to another NSAID or oral triptan.

The orally dissolvable versions of rizatriptan and zolmitriptan require gastrointestinal absorption and thus should not be used in the setting of migraine with vomiting.

KEY POINT

- Self-administered subcutaneous sumatriptan is appropriate as therapy for migraine without aura in patients not responding to NSAIDs or oral triptans, especially those with vomiting.

Bibliography
Kelley NE, Tepper DE. Rescue therapy for acute migraine, part 1: triptans, dihydroergotamine, and magnesium. Headache. 2012 Jan;52(1):114-28. [PMID: 22211870]

Item 80   Answer: A
Educational Objective: Diagnose a posttraumatic epidural hematoma.

This patient most likely has an epidural hematoma. Traumatic epidural hematoma classically presents with precipitous neurologic decline after head trauma. Most patients with this diagnosis have a skull fracture with associated rupture of an underlying artery, typically the middle meningeal artery. Blood under arterial pressure accumulates between the inner table of the skull and the dural membranes. The most common symptoms are severe headache and vomiting. Impairment of consciousness may develop immediately or after a lucid interval. Uncal or subfalcine brain herniation can occur and is characterized by ipsilateral occulomotor nerve (cranial nerve III) palsy, contralateral paresis, and stupor or coma. Hypertension with bradycardia (the Cushing response) can be another sign of increased intracranial pressure. A CT scan of the head confirms the diagnosis, and immediate surgical evacuation is required. Mortality rates are commonly reported to be 10% to 20%.

Dissection of the left internal carotid artery typically results in ipsilateral Horner syndrome with ptosis, miosis, and anhidrosis but not oculomotor nerve (cranial nerve III) palsy. Contralateral hemiparesis could result if a secondary stroke were to occur in the left frontal lobe after the dissection, but rapidly declining consciousness would be unexpected.

Postconcussion syndrome is defined by a constellation of neurologic, psychological, and constitutional symptoms without significant abnormalities on physical examination. Minor neurologic findings noted on the examination of a patient with mild traumatic brain injury may include ocular convergence insufficiency or mild ataxia, but typically examination findings are normal. This patient's clinical findings do not fit this pattern.

Seizures occur in approximately 5% of persons hospitalized for acute head trauma. They may be classified as "immediate" if occurring within the first 24 hours, "early" if noted within the first week, or "late" if occurring more than 1 week after the injury. Half of the seizures occurring within the first week will occur in the first 24 hours, and the risk decreases with time. Some correlation between the severity of injury and the risk of posttraumatic seizures exists. This patient shows no signs of involuntary motor activity, so convulsive status epilepticus is not present. Nonconvulsive status epilepticus might manifest as stupor, but the presence of focal cranial nerve and motor deficits in this patient is more indicative of a progressive structural lesion.

KEY POINT

- Traumatic epidural hematoma classically presents with precipitous neurologic decline after head trauma; common symptoms are severe headache and vomiting, with possible impairment of consciousness developing immediately or after a lucid interval.

Bibliography
Zammit C, Knight WA. Severe traumatic brain injury in adults. Emerg Med Pract. 2013 Mar;15(3):1-28. [PMID: 23452439]

Item 81   Answer: D
Educational Objective: Diagnose a tic disorder.

This patient's clinical presentation is most consistent with a tic disorder. Tics are repetitive, stereotyped, suppressible movements typically preceded by an abnormal sensation (premonitory urge). She previously has experienced simple motor tics and has a positive family history of facial twitching. The presence of vocal (repetitive throat clearance) and complex motor (shoulder elevation followed by neck rolling) tics, the persistence of symptoms for 1 year, and the comorbid obsessive-compulsive disorder are all consistent with Tourette syndrome. Tics can wax and wane, and old tics can be replaced by new ones over time, but at any given time, a limited number of stereotyped movements are present during clinical examination.

Chorea involves typically random, diffuse, and nonsuppressible involuntary abnormal movements. The focal distribution, suppressibility, and stereotyped character of this patient's movements make chorea unlikely.

Dystonia consists of patterned and directional movements limited to certain parts of the body. However, dystonia is typically sustained and nonsuppressible. The presence of vocal tic, the premonitory urge, and the long history of waxing and waning of various types of movements in this patient also make dystonia unlikely.

Myoclonus consists of a single, rapid, shocklike muscle jerk. Complex stereotyped movements (such as shoulder elevation followed by neck rolling) and suppressibility are inconsistent with myoclonus.

KEY POINT

- Tics are repetitive, stereotyped, suppressible movements typically preceded by an abnormal sensation (premonitory urge).

Bibliography

Jankovic J. Treatment of hyperkinetic movement disorders. Lancet Neurol. 2009 Sep;8(9):844-56. [PMID: 19679276]

Item 82   Answer: C

Educational Objective: Treat seizures in a patient with a brain tumor.

This patient should be treated with valproic acid. In patients with brain tumors and one or more seizures, antiepileptic drug (AED) regimens that do not induce hepatic enzymes and thus have limited interaction with commonly used chemotherapy regimens are favored. Valproic acid is a non–enzyme-inducing AED that is appropriate to treat this patient. Other AEDs that would be reasonable to use include lacosamide, lamotrigine, and levetiracetam.

Carbamazepine and phenytoin are enzyme-inducing AEDs that can diminish the efficacy of the chemotherapy and other drugs this patient may receive. Additionally, because they are metabolized by the same enzyme pathways, chemotherapeutic agents also may alter AED levels unpredictably, which makes them potentially less effective in controlling seizures.

Deferring AED therapy in this patient is not appropriate. He had a clear focal seizure, and the presence of a known brain lesion puts him at risk for subsequent seizures. However, AED treatment is not appropriate as prophylaxis in patients with brain tumors who have not had any clinical seizures.

KEY POINT

- In patients with metastatic brain tumors and one or more seizures, antiepileptic drug regimens that do not induce hepatic enzymes and thus have limited interaction with commonly used chemotherapy regimens are favored.

Bibliography

Maschio M, Dinapoli L. Patients with brain tumor-related epilepsy. J Neurooncol. 2012 Aug;109(1):1-6. Epub 2012 Apr 22.[PMID: 22528794]

Item 83   Answer: C

Educational Objective: Diagnose dementia with Lewy bodies.

This patient most likely has dementia with Lewy bodies, the second most common cause of degenerative dementia. Core features of dementia with Lewy bodies are fluctuating attention and alertness; recurrent, well-formed visual hallucinations; and spontaneous parkinsonism. Sensitivity to neuroleptic medications also is commonly seen. Suggestive features include rapid eye movement sleep behavior disorder and low dopamine transporter uptake in the basal ganglia on single-photon emission CT or PET scans. The patient's features of cognitive fluctuations (episodic disorganized speech and functional disability, daytime sleepiness), parkinsonism, visual hallucinations, and severe sensitivity to haloperidol all support a diagnosis of dementia with Lewy bodies.

Although visual hallucinations and parkinsonism can occur in Alzheimer disease, these features generally present relatively late in the disease course. Severe sensitivity to neuroleptic medications also is less common in Alzheimer disease than dementia with Lewy bodies. Alzheimer disease is predominantly characterized by a decline in memory that can be accompanied by deficits in other cognitive domains. Typical behavioral changes in the earlier stages of Alzheimer disease include irritability, anxiety, and depression.

Delirium is characterized by disturbances of attention, cognition, and perception, with fluctuations in symptoms during the day. These disturbances typically develop over the course of hours to days, rather than over 1 year as occurred in this patient. A careful history obtained from a reliable informant often easily distinguishes delirium from dementia with Lewy bodies.

Major depression with psychotic features is characterized by hallucinations, more often auditory than visual, and delusions that are typically mood congruent, such as guilt, nihilism, or deserved punishment. Although the patient is being treated for depression, no evidence that supports a diagnosis of major depression, such as suicidal ideation, hopelessness, or guilt, has been reported.

KEY POINT

- Core features of dementia with Lewy bodies are fluctuating attention and alertness; recurrent, well-formed visual hallucinations; or spontaneous parkinsonism.

Bibliography

McKeith IG, Dickson DW, Lowe J, et al; Consortium on DLB. Diagnosis and management of dementia with Lewy bodies: third report of the DLB Consortium [erratum in Neurology. 2005 Dec 27;65(12):1992]. Neurology. 2005 Dec 27;65(12):1863–72. [PMID: 16237129]

Item 84   Answer: D

Educational Objective: Diagnose trigeminal neuralgia.

This patient has developed trigeminal neuralgia. Although more common among older patients, trigeminal neuralgia can be seen in young adults, particularly those with multiple sclerosis. Affected patients describe brief episodes of lancinating pain affecting either the second or third distribution of the trigeminal nerve (cranial nerve V_2 or V_3). The pain may occur spontaneously or be triggered by sensory stimulation of the face or mouth. The diagnosis is made clinically. Brain MRI may be indicated in patients with atypical presentations, including those developing symptoms in young adulthood. As many as 15% of patients with trigeminal neuralgia may have a structural explanation for their disease, such as cerebellopontine angle tumors in older patients or demyelinating disease in younger patients. Brain MRI is also indicated in the course of surgical evaluation, if appropriate. Glucocorticoids are typically ineffective. Carbamazepine is the drug of choice for initial management, with a greater than 50% response rate. Oxcarbazepine, a structural derivative of carbamazepine, is also effective and has fewer adverse effects and drug interactions but is a more expensive medication.

Chronic paroxysmal hemicrania is typically expressed along the first branch of the trigeminal nerve (cranial nerve V_1). Pain attacks are brief but generally last a mean of 15 minutes rather than seconds and may recur between 8 to 40 times daily. The diagnosis also requires concomitant ipsilateral autonomic findings, such as tearing, nasal congestion, or rhinorrhea, none of which this patient has.

The eruption of herpes zoster is preceded by a prodrome of constant pain or burning, commonly for up to several days. The patient's intermittent sharp facial pain is most consistent with trigeminal neuralgia.

Primary stabbing headaches are brief paroxysms of pain lasting seconds, without associated autonomic features. The face is typically spared. This patient's pain does not fit this description.

KEY POINT

- Trigeminal neuralgia typically results in brief episodes of lancinating pain affecting either the second or third distribution of the trigeminal nerve (cranial nerve V_2 or V_3); the pain can occur spontaneously or be triggered by sensory stimulation of the face or mouth.

Bibliography

Bigal ME. Diagnostic evaluation and treatment of trigeminal neuralgia. Curr Pain Headache Rep. 2009 Aug;13(4):256–7. [PMID: 19586587]

Item 85   Answer: C

Educational Objective: Adjust medication dosage in glucocorticoid-induced myopathy.

Tapering the prednisone dosage while monitoring the patient's response is the most appropriate method to distinguish between weakness caused by a flare of inflammatory myopathy and glucocorticoid-induced toxic myopathy. The latter diagnosis is more likely in this patient with a normal serum creatine kinase level. In contrast, a flare of inflammatory myopathy, which can present the same way clinically, is associated with a marked increase in the serum creatine kinase level and evidence of irritable myopathy on electromyography (such as abnormal spontaneous necrosis or active muscle membrane damage from inflammation). If weakness improves after prednisone tapering, the patient should be given a glucocorticoid-free holiday or, if needed, switched to another agent. In contrast, if weakness worsens with tapering, an inflammatory flare should be suspected, and increasing the glucocorticoid dosage or adding another immunosuppressive therapy should be considered.

Intravenous immunoglobulin (IVIG) is a second-line therapy for severe inflammatory myopathies that are refractory to treatment with a glucocorticoid and at least one other immunosuppressive agent. Because glucocorticoid-induced myopathy is suspected in this patient, IVIG treatment is not warranted.

Increasing the prednisone dosage without evidence of active inflammation would be inappropriate and could worsen the patient's weakness, which is likely associated with glucocorticoid therapy.

A repeat muscle biopsy might show type 2 muscle fiber atrophy due to glucocorticoid myopathy, but these changes also are seen in disuse atrophy and other conditions and thus are nonspecific. Biopsy is also likely to show inflammatory changes but is unlikely to provide a definitive differentiation between a flare of inflammatory myopathy and glucocorticoid-induced myopathy.

KEY POINT

- Glucocorticoid tapering is the most appropriate method to distinguish between a flare of inflammatory myopathy and glucocorticoid-induced toxic myopathy in a patient with persistent myopathy.

Bibliography

Hanaoka BY, Peterson CA, Horbinski C, Crofford LJ. Implications of glucocorticoid therapy in idiopathic inflammatory myopathies. Nat Rev Rheumatol. 2012 Aug;8(8):448–57. [PMID: 22688888]

Item 86   Answer: A

Educational Objective: Treat elevated blood pressure after recombinant tissue plasminogen activator therapy for stroke.

The patient should receive intravenous nicardipine in an attempt to lower her blood pressure to the target range. She

CONT. met no exclusion criteria and was correctly treated with intravenous recombinant tissue plasminogen activator (rtPA) for an acute ischemic stroke within the optimal 3-hour window from onset of symptoms. Her blood pressure before treatment was less than 185/110 mm Hg, as recommended by guidelines. The most serious complication of thrombolysis with intravenous rtPA is intracerebral hemorrhage, which occurs in as many as 6% of patients. The main risk factors for hemorrhage after thrombolysis are a large-volume cerebral infarction, a high National Institutes of Health Stroke Scale score, a cardioembolic origin of the stroke, and protocol violations. The postthrombolysis protocol includes avoiding antiplatelet and anticoagulant agents for 24 hours until a repeat head CT scan shows no hemorrhage, frequent neurologic and vital sign evaluation, and maintenance of the blood pressure at less than 180/105 mm Hg. When the blood pressure exceeds this limit, as in this patient, intravenous labetalol or nicardipine is the best option to reduce the blood pressure and thereby avoid intracerebral hemorrhage.

Oral aspirin and subcutaneous heparin are inappropriate treatments for this patient at this point because antithrombotic medications should not be administered until follow-up CT of the head is obtained 24 hours after rtPA infusion is completed. If the repeat CT scan shows no hemorrhage, and no systemic bleeding complications have occurred, then aspirin should be initiated for secondary stroke prevention and deep venous thrombosis prophylaxis should be started with low-molecular-weight or unfractionated subcutaneous heparin.

Although sublingual nitroglycerin can lower blood pressure, the inability to rapidly titrate the dose to maintain a blood pressure of less than 180/105 mm Hg makes non-intravenous medications a poor choice. Nitrates also have a relative contraindication in the treatment of blood pressure in acute stroke, particularly hemorrhagic stroke, because of the possibility of raising intracranial pressure.

KEY POINT

- After patients with acute ischemic stroke are treated with intravenous recombinant tissue plasminogen activator, their blood pressure should be maintained at less than 180/105 mm Hg to avoid intracerebral hemorrhage.

Bibliography

Jauch, EC, Saver JL, Adams HP Jr, et al; American Heart Association Stroke Council; Council on Cardiovascular Nursing; Council on Peripheral Vascular Disease; Council on Clinical Cardiology. Guidelines for the early management of patients with acute ischemic stroke: a guideline for healthcare professionals from the American Heart Association/American Stroke Association. Stroke. 2013 Mar;44(3):870-947. [PMID: 23370205]

Item 87   Answer: D

Educational Objective: Treat chronic migraine.

The patient should be treated with topiramate for chronic migraine, which is headache occurring on 15 or more days per month for more than 3 months. Chronic migraine is characterized by increasingly frequent attacks of migraine that are eventually accompanied by an interval milder headache. By definition, on at least 8 days of the month, the headache of chronic migraine must be severe, possess migraine features, or respond to migraine-specific therapy. The interval headache may have no migraine features and appear to be a tension-type or sinus headache. A medication overuse element is often present and may interfere with the efficacy of preventive and acute migraine treatments. Headache frequency and acute medication use of greater than 10 days per month are significant risk factors for transformation to chronic migraine. Because the development of secondary brain pathology also occasionally may contribute to the transformation to chronic migraine, MRI of the brain is indicated.

Topiramate has level A evidence of effectiveness in treating episodic migraine. Topiramate and onabotulinumtoxinA are the only agents that have shown efficacy in studies of chronic migraine. Topiramate is less expensive than onabotulinumtoxinA.

Carbamazepine is the drug of choice for treating trigeminal neuralgia but has shown no effect on migraine prevention.

Although the serotonin-norepinephrine reuptake inhibitor venlafaxine has demonstrated benefit in migraine prevention studies, no such data are available for duloxetine, which is in the same drug class and is used to treat major depressive disorder and generalized anxiety disorder.

Propranolol has level A evidence of effectiveness in the prevention of episodic migraine but has the potential to worsen both depression and asthma. No evidence supports it use for chronic migraine.

Verapamil is the treatment of choice in cluster headache prevention. The drug, however, has neither level A (effective) nor level B (probably effective) evidence supporting its use in migraine prevention.

KEY POINT

- Topiramate and onabotulinumtoxinA are the only agents that have shown efficacy in studies of chronic migraine.

Bibliography

Silberstein SD, Holland S, Freitag F, Dodick DW, Argoff C, Ashman E; Quality Standards Subcommittee of the American Academy of Neurology and the American Headache Society. Evidence-based guideline update: pharmacologic treatment for episodic migraine prevention in adults: report of the Quality Standards Subcommittee of the American Academy of Neurology and the American Headache Society. Neurology. 2012 Apr 24;78(17):1337-45. [PMID: 22529202]

Item 88   Answer: D

Educational Objective: Diagnose paraneoplastic limbic encephalitis.

This patient has limbic encephalitis, or inflammation of the emotional and memory structures of the brain. The subacute progression of this patient's symptoms of personality change,

Answers and Critiques

H
CONT.

psychosis, and seizures is most consistent with a paraneoplastic antibody syndrome, which is usually mediated by autoantibodies. Paraneoplastic limbic encephalitis is most commonly associated with lung tumors (usually small cell lung cancer), breast cancer, thymoma, germ cell tumors, and Hodgkin lymphoma. Patients frequently have the neurologic symptoms before discovery of the causative tumor. In this patient, the possible presence of the concomitant syndrome of inappropriate antidiuretic hormone secretion (SIADH), as suggested by the low serum sodium level, makes the particular diagnosis of anti-LG1 (formerly anti–voltage-gated potassium channel) antibody syndrome most likely because it is associated with both limbic encephalitis and SIADH. A definitive diagnosis is usually made after laboratory testing of serum and/or cerebrospinal fluid (CSF) for paraneoplastic antibodies in the appropriate clinical context. Treatment involves immunotherapy and treatment of the underlying tumor, if available. Although these syndromes traditionally have been characterized as "paraneoplastic" because they often are associated with an underlying cancer, many, including most anti-LG1 syndromes, are primarily autoimmune.

Although paranoia and seizures can be seen in Alzheimer disease, they typically occur late in the disease course. Alzheimer disease also is not generally associated with mesial temporal MRI changes.

Reactivation of human herpesvirus 1 also can cause an encephalitis with cognitive problems, psychiatric disturbance, and bitemporal seizures. However, the progression of this type of encephalitis is acute, occurring over days, not weeks. If not treated emergently, herpes encephalitis is lethal. Patients suspected of having human herpesvirus 6 encephalitis will need a lumbar puncture to rule out other viral causes of limbic encephalitis, such as human herpesvirus 3 (varicella-zoster virus), human herpesvirus 8, and cytomegalovirus.

The course of Lewy body dementia is typically longer than that described in this patient. Also, the seizures and imaging findings would be atypical.

KEY POINT

- The subacute progression of the symptoms of personality change, psychosis, and seizures is most consistent with an antibody-mediated cause, such as a paraneoplastic antibody syndrome.

Bibliography

Tüzün E, Dalmau J. Limbic encephalitis and variants: classification, diagnosis and treatment. Neurologist. 2007 Sep;13(5):261-71. [PMID: 17848866]

H **Item 89**   **Answer: A**

Educational Objective: Diagnose delirium.

This patient most likely has delirium. Tests such as spelling a word backwards or reciting the days of the week in reverse are rapid ways to measure attention at the bedside. Frequent redirection during the course of an interview is another indicator of inattention. A tangential thought process is often

misinterpreted as part of normal aging, but it actually is an indicator of disorganized thinking. Acute onset of cognitive dysfunction over hours to days, impairment of attention, disorganized thinking, and fluctuating mental status are core features of delirium. Increased or decreased psychomotor activity, disorientation, and perceptual disturbances are other supportive features. The use of a screening instrument (such as the Confusion Assessment Method) allows for improved recognition and diagnosis of delirium.

Delirium is an underrecognized disorder in older patients who are hospitalized and may result from various causes, including organ failure (such as the worsening kidney function in this patient), metabolic disturbances, medications, or infection. A key to the likely cause of delirium in this patient is myoclonus seen on physical examination. Myoclonus is a sudden involuntary muscle contraction (positive myoclonus) or sudden brief loss of muscle activity (negative myoclonus, or asterixis); this patient's examination shows asterixis, a common finding in metabolic disturbances (uremia, liver failure, or hypoglycemia) and toxic encephalopathy (due to antibiotics, pain medications, and immunosuppressants).

Although the presence of delirium significantly increases the risk of developing dementia and, conversely, dementia is a significant risk factor for developing delirium, this patient was previously functioning independently. The onset of dementia is typically insidious. The diagnosis of dementia requires 6 months of progressive cognitive decline.

Nonconvulsive status epilepticus (NCSE), or alteration in mental status without overt convulsive activity as a result of continuous or near continuous epileptiform discharges, is often unrecognized in older patients with mental status changes and should be considered as part of the differential diagnosis of acute confusional state if the cause remains unknown. However, the cause of delirium is often identifiable by a careful history, physical examination, and review of medical conditions or interventions that may be contributing to a change in mental status. Additionally, the negative myoclonus seen in this patient would be unlikely in a patient with NCSE without a history of preexisting epilepsy.

Although stroke presents with an abrupt onset, and this patient is at higher risk for stroke because of his recent myocardial infarction, this patient does not have any focal neurologic signs, such as dysarthria, facial droop, hemiparesis, or dysmetria, to suggest that a stroke has occurred.

KEY POINT

- Acute onset of cognitive dysfunction over hours to days, impairment of attention, disorganized thinking, and fluctuating mental status are core features of delirium, an underrecognized disorder in older patients who are hospitalized.

Bibliography

Young J, Murthy L, Westby M, Akunne A, O'Mahony R; Guideline Development Group. Diagnosis, prevention, and management of delirium: summary of NICE guidance. BMJ. 2010 Jul 28;341:c3704. [PMID: 20667955]

Item 90   Answer: C

Educational Objective: **Treat fatigue in multiple sclerosis.**

This patient should be treated with modafinil. She is experiencing fatigue related to her multiple sclerosis (MS). Fatigue is a very common symptom of MS but is often underevaluated and undertreated. Given this patient's decreased work performance and need for daytime sleep, pharmacologic treatment is indicated. The stimulant medications modafinil and armodafinil are frequently used in patients with MS. Amantadine also is an effective therapy for fatigue. For fatigue refractory to these medications, methylphenidate or other amphetamines may be considered.

Iron supplementation is an appropriate treatment for iron deficiency anemia, which can sometimes result in fatigue and always should be excluded as a cause in patients with MS. However, this patient's normal hemoglobin level and normal mean corpuscular volume argue against her being iron deficient.

Although hypothyroidism also can result in fatigue, this patient is clinically euthyroid, and her thyroid-stimulating hormone level is normal. Thyroid hormone supplementation in the absence of hypothyroidism is not appropriate treatment for the fatigue associated with MS.

Nocturnal continuous positive airway pressure (CPAP) can be an appropriate treatment of obstructive sleep apnea (OSA) and other causes of daytime sleepiness, such as primary sleep disorder. OSA should be considered in patients with MS and severe fatigue. However, this patient has no clinical history consistent with OSA, and thus prescribing CPAP without diagnostic polysomnography would not be appropriate.

This patient's history, physical examination, and imaging findings give no indication that her disease-modifying drug is resulting in treatment failure. Therefore, the teriflunomide does not have to be replaced with dimethyl fumarate or any other drug. In addition, fatigue is not a known adverse effect of teriflunomide, and this patient's fatigue is not a sign of medication intolerance.

KEY POINT

- Modafinil is often a successful treatment of fatigue in multiple sclerosis.

Bibliography

Amato MP, Portaccio E. Management options in multiple sclerosis-associated fatigue. Expert Opin Pharmacother. 2012 Feb;13(2):207-16. [PMID: 22220738]

Item 91   Answer: C

Educational Objective: **Treat statin-related toxic myopathy with a hydrophilic statin.**

Rosuvastatin is the most appropriate treatment for this patient with hyperlipidemia. Hydrophilic statins, especially rosuvastatin but also pravastatin and fluvastatin, are less likely than lipophilic statins (such as atorvastatin, simva-

statin, and lovastatin) to cause statin-induced myopathy and can be used at low doses in patients with previous statin-related myalgia, myopathy, or mild rhabdomyolysis. Hydrophilic statins also are much less likely than lipophilic statins to cause muscle weakness and elevated serum creatine kinase levels. Lipophilic statins should be avoided in patients with previous statin-related myopathy or rhabdomyolysis. Recently, an immune-mediated necrotizing form of statin myopathy that is associated with anti-HMGCR autoantibodies has been identified in some statin-exposed patients; this form continues to progress even after removal of the statin and may require immunosuppression as treatment. This patient, whose symptoms have resolved after discontinuation of the simvastatin, has no evidence of this type of statin myopathy.

Gemfibrozil is a fibric acid derivative that is typically used for the treatment of hypertriglyceridemia. If added to statin therapy, gemfibrozil raises the serum concentration of statins by twofold, which increases the risk of rhabdomyolysis. Cytochrome P3A4 inhibitors, such as antifungal agents, macrolides, immunophilin ligands, and tricyclic antidepressants, also can increase risk of statin-induced myopathy.

Although selenium supplementation does not treat hyperlipidemia, it has been suggested as a potential method of preventing statin-induced myopathy. Available evidence, however, does not allow a definitive conclusion to be drawn.

KEY POINT

- Hydrophilic statins, such as rosuvastatin, are less likely than lipophilic statins to cause statin-induced myopathy.

Bibliography

Mohassel P, Mammen AL. Statin-associated autoimmune myopathy and anti-HMGCR autoantibodies. Muscle Nerve. 2013 Oct;48(4): 477-83. [PMID: 23519993]

Item 92   Answer: D

Educational Objective: **Diagnose behavioral variant frontotemporal dementia.**

This patient likely has the behavioral variant type of frontotemporal dementia (FTD). This form of FTD is a clinical syndrome characterized by the insidious onset of changes in behavior, personality, and executive function. This patient demonstrates the typical features of hyperorality (as evidenced by excessive alcohol intake), loss of insight, loss of empathy, compulsive behaviors, and impaired social conduct. An early age of onset is typical for the disease. Behavioral variant FTD is the second most common cause of early-onset dementia, second only to Alzheimer disease. A family history of a related neuropsychiatric disorder is evident in approximately 40% of patients with FTD; this patient's family history of a father being institutionalized in his 50s is thus concerning. Patients with behavioral variant FTD typically do well on the Mini–Mental State Examination because executive function is not well assessed by this screening test, and this cognitive domain is most likely to be impaired in patients with FTD.

Although Alzheimer disease is the most common cause of early-onset dementia, the disease presentation in this patient is not typical for this diagnosis. On cognitive testing, patients with Alzheimer disease typically exhibit impairment on tests of learning, memory, and visuospatial function. This patient showed none of these impairments.

This patient's decline in functioning can be attributed to behavioral dysfunction rather than cognitive impairment, which is the cause of impaired functioning in patients with dementia with Lewy bodies. In addition, he lacks other supportive features of dementia with Lewy bodies, such as parkinsonism, formed visual hallucinations, fluctuating cognition, rapid eye movement sleep behavior disorder, or autonomic dysfunction.

Patients with behavioral variant FTD are frequently misdiagnosed with a psychiatric illness, such as depression, bipolar disorder, or another mood or personality disturbance, especially early in the disease course. Although this patient has a few symptoms of depression, such as apathy and loss of interest, the prominent changes in behavior and lack of additional depressive symptoms make behavioral variant FTD the more likely diagnosis.

KEY POINT

- Behavioral variant frontotemporal dementia is characterized by the typical features of hyperorality, loss of insight, loss of empathy, compulsive behaviors, impaired social conduct, and an early age of onset.

Bibliography

Rascovsky K, Hodges JR, Knopman D, et al. Sensitivity of revised diagnostic criteria for the behavioural variant of frontotemporal dementia. Brain. 2011 Sep;134(Pt 9):2456-77. [PMID: 21810890]

Item 93   Answer: B

Educational Objective: Diagnose Creutzfeldt-Jakob disease.

This patient most likely has Creutzfeldt-Jakob disease (CJD), a dementing illness that occurs subacutely over weeks to months and is classified as a rapidly progressive dementia. This patient has the hallmark neuroradiologic finding of sporadic CJD, namely, hyperintensities on diffusion-weighted imaging (DWI), in this instance involving the basal ganglia and insular and left parietal cortices. DWI hyperintensities also can occur in the cerebral cortex (as cortical ribboning) and thalamus in CJD. DWI is highly sensitive and specific for the diagnosis of sporadic CJD.

Alzheimer disease can present as a rapidly progressive dementia, but not commonly. The MRI findings seen in this patient are not consistent with Alzheimer disease, in which the MRI is typically normal or shows focal atrophy involving the temporal and/or parietal lobes.

Rapidly progressive dementias are relatively uncommon and are more likely to be due to treatable, reversible causes than are the more typical dementing conditions that develop over years. Herpes simplex virus 1 (HSV-1) encephalitis typically results in an acute neurologic decline occurring over days to 1 week rather than months as with this patient. Fever, focal neurologic findings, and focal seizures are common. T2 hyperintensities (and occasionally DWI hyperintensities), with a predilection for the temporal lobes, are strongly suggestive of HSV-1 encephalitis, rather than the DWI abnormalities seen in this patient.

Vascular neurocognitive disorder is characterized by cognitive impairment occurring after a clinical stroke or in the presence of neuroimaging findings of cerebrovascular disease. The prevalence of poststroke dementia is approximately 30%. This patient has neither the history nor focal neurologic signs (such as hemiparesis, facial droop, or dysarthria) to suggest that a clinical stroke has occurred. Although DWI is very sensitive in the detection of early ischemic infarction, the DWI abnormalities seen in this patient do not follow vascular territories and are instead classic for sporadic CJD.

KEY POINT

- Creutzfeldt-Jakob disease can be diagnosed by the presence of hyperintensities in the cerebral cortex (cortical ribboning), basal ganglia, or thalamus on diffusion-weighted imaging, which is highly sensitive and specific for the diagnosis.

Bibliography

Paterson RW, Takada LT, Geschwind MD. Diagnosis and treatment of rapidly progressive dementias. Neurol Clin Pract. 2012 Sep;2(3):187-200. [PMID: 23634367]

Item 94   Answer: D

Educational Objective: Treat acute ischemic stroke with thrombolysis.

This patient should receive intravenous recombinant tissue plasminogen activator (rtPA). He is within the 3-hour window for treatment of patients who do not meet any of the exclusion criteria for thrombolysis. In the National Institute of Neurological Diseases and Stroke (NINDS) rtPA trial, patients who received intravenous rtPA within 3 hours of stroke onset had a greater likelihood of clinical improvement at 3 months compared with those who received placebo. The trial included patients with atrial fibrillation and all ischemic stroke subtypes and showed no significant safety difference between stroke subtypes. Because he has no contraindications to thrombolysis, it is the treatment of choice in this patient.

High-dose (325-mg) aspirin would be an appropriate initial treatment if the patient met any of the exclusion criteria for thrombolysis, which he does not. As long as a follow-up CT scan of the head shows no hemorrhage, aspirin should be initiated 24 hours after administration of rtPA.

Hyperglycemia is common in patients with acute ischemic stroke and, if persistent in the first 24 hours after stroke onset, is associated with poor functional outcomes. To date, no definitive clinical trials have outlined the best approach to treatment or the most appropriate targets. Acute ischemic stroke guidelines are thus in keeping with general recommendations for all critically ill hospitalized patients who have mild hypertension, with or without diabetes mellitus, which are not to use intensive insulin therapy to normalize plasma glucose levels. If insulin therapy is required, the American College of Physicians recommends target plasma glucose levels of 140 mg/dL to 200 mg/dL (7.8-11.1 mmol/L) while monitoring carefully for hypoglycemia. Insulin therapy is thus not indicated in this patient whose plasma glucose level falls in the target range.

Intravenous heparin does not reduce the 14-day risk of recurrent stroke or mortality in patients with atrial fibrillation who have a new stroke and is therefore not indicated.

KEY POINT

- In patients with focal neurologic symptoms suggestive of an acute ischemic stroke, recombinant tissue plasminogen activator should be administered within 3 hours of symptom onset to patients who do not meet any of the exclusion criteria.

Bibliography

Jauch, EC, Saver JL, Adams HP Jr, et al; American Heart Association Stroke Council; Council on Cardiovascular Nursing; Council on Peripheral Vascular Disease; Council on Clinical Cardiology. Guidelines for the early management of patients with acute ischemic stroke: a guideline for healthcare professionals from the American Heart Association/American Stroke Association. Stroke. 2013 Mar;44(3):870-947. [PMID: 23370205]

Item 95   Answer: A

Educational Objective: Diagnose nonconvulsive status epilepticus with continuous electroencephalographic monitoring.

This patient should have continuous monitoring with electroencephalography (EEG) because his presentation is concerning for nonconvulsive status epilepticus (NCSE). Approximately 48% of patients treated for convulsive status epilepticus (CSE) will continue to have subtle or subclinical seizures on EEG. Persistently altered mental status, particularly with waxing and waning features and focal neurologic deficits (such as aphasia), is a characteristic feature of NCSE. Patients with intracranial structural abnormalities who are comatose also are at high risk for this disorder. Intracerebral hemorrhage is an additional risk factor for nonconvulsive seizures and status epilepticus.

Continuous EEG monitoring is twice as sensitive as a routine 30-minute EEG for detecting seizures, especially the intermittent seizures that are common in patients already treated for CSE. All patients with altered mental status after CSE should have continuous EEG monitoring for at least 24 hours to detect nonconvulsive seizures or a changed status. Comatose patients should be evaluated for 24 to 48 hours. Continuous EEG monitoring is indicated

in patients with acute structural intracranial lesions and altered mental status, even if clinically evident seizures have not occurred.

Flumazenil should not be administered to any patient with seizures or at risk for seizures because the drug can precipitate status epilepticus. Because the patient is not showing any signs of respiratory depression or other adverse effects of medication, there is no urgent need to reverse the benzodiazepine he received as part of appropriate CSE treatment.

Cavernous malformations usually have self-limited bleeding, and this patient does not have any mass effect or other urgent need for surgery. Although he ultimately may be a surgical candidate, given that refractory seizures are associated with cavernous malformations, surgical resection is not the most appropriate next step. He first should be evaluated and treated for NCSE.

Maintenance antiepileptic drugs (AEDs) should not be withheld in a patient with CSE at presentation unless the drugs are clearly causing severe adverse effects. In this patient, NCSE is a more likely explanation of the patient's mental state than is an adverse effect of the AED.

KEY POINT

- All patients with altered mental status after convulsive status epilepticus should have continuous electroencephalographic monitoring for at least 24 hours to detect nonconvulsive seizures.

Bibliography

Kennedy JD, Gerard EE. Continuous EEG monitoring in the intensive care unit. Curr Neurol Neurosci Rep. 2012 Aug;12(4):419-28. [PMID: 22653639]

Item 96   Answer: B

Educational Objective: Anticipate the potential adverse effects of medications used for symptomatic treatment of patients with multiple sclerosis.

This patient's dalfampridine (4-aminopyridine) should be discontinued. Dalfampridine is a voltage-gated potassium channel antagonist that can potentiate action potentials along demyelinated axons and is used in patients with multiple sclerosis (MS) for potassium channel blockade. This medication can improve lower extremity function and walking speed and endurance. Because of its mechanism of action, seizures have been reported as a rare, dose-dependent adverse effect of this medication. Dalfampridine is excreted through the kidneys and thus is contraindicated in patients with kidney disease because its resultant decreased clearance would significantly increase the seizure risk. For this reason, this medication should be discontinued in this patient.

Baclofen can alleviate the spasticity often associated with MS. There is no reason to discontinue the drug in this patient with acute kidney injury because no specific adverse effects of this drug due to kidney toxicity or related to kidney

CONT.

clearance have been reported. Dosing may have to be modified in patients with severe kidney failure, however.

Glatiramer acetate is a disease-modifying medication used in the treatment of MS to impede disease activity and prevent relapses. This drug has no known adverse effects on the kidneys due to poor clearance or direct toxicity.

Vitamin D supplementation is now suggested for all patients with MS to reduce the accumulation of new lesions on MRI. No adverse effects on kidney function or kidney clearance have been reported.

KEY POINT

- Dalfampridine is renally excreted and thus is contraindicated in patients with kidney disease.

Bibliography

Egeberg MD, Oh CY, Bainbridge JL. Clinical overview of dalfampridine: an agent with a novel mechanism of action to help with gait disturbances [erratum in Clin Ther. 2013 Jun;35(6):900]. Clin Ther. 2012 Nov;34(11): 2185-94. [PMID: 23123001]

Index

A **NAME AND ADDRESS (Please complete.)**

_____
Last Name   First Name   Middle Initial

_____
Address

_____
Address cont.

_____
City   State   ZIP Code

_____
Country

_____
Email address

B **Order Number**

(Use the Order Number on your MKSAP materials packing slip.)

[ ][ ][ ][ ][ ][ ][ ][ ][ ][ ][ ][ ][ ][ ][ ][ ][ ]

C **ACP ID Number**

(Refer to packing slip in your MKSAP materials
for your ACP ID Number.)

[ ][ ][ ][ ][ ][ ][ ][ ][ ][ ][ ][ ][ ][ ][ ][ ][ ]

ACP®
American College of Physicians
Leading Internal Medicine, Improving Lives

Medical Knowledge Self-Assessment Program® 17

TO EARN _AMA PRA CATEGORY 1 CREDITS™_ YOU MUST:

1. Answer all questions.
2. Score a minimum of 50% correct.

TO EARN _FREE_ INSTANTANEOUS _AMA PRA CATEGORY 1 CREDITS™_ ONLINE:

1. Answer all of your questions.
2. Go to **mksap.acponline.org** and enter your ACP Online username and password to access an online answer sheet.
3. Enter your answers.
4. You can also enter your answers directly at **mksap.acponline.org** without first using this answer sheet.

To Submit Your Answer Sheet by Mail or FAX for a $15 Administrative Fee per Answer Sheet:

1. Answer all of your questions and calculate your score.
2. Complete boxes A–F.
3. Complete payment information.
4. Send the answer sheet and payment information to ACP, using the FAX number/address listed below.

COMPLETE FORM BELOW ONLY IF YOU SUBMIT BY MAIL OR FAX

Last Name   First Name   MI

[ ]

Payment Information. Must remit in US funds, drawn on a US bank.

The processing fee for each paper answer sheet is $15.

☐ Check, made payable to ACP, enclosed

Charge to ☐ **VISA**   ☐ **MasterCard**   ☐ **AMERICAN EXPRESS**   ☐ **DISCOVER**

Card Number _____

Expiration Date _____/_____   Security code (3 or 4 digit #s) _____
                    MM   YY

Signature _____

Fax to: 215-351-2799

Mail to:
Member and Customer Service
American College of Physicians
190 N. Independence Mall West
Philadelphia, PA 19106-1572

D

TEST TYPE

	Maximum Number of CME Credits
◯ Cardiovascular Medicine	21
◯ Dermatology	12
◯ Gastroenterology and Hepatology	16
◯ Hematology and Oncology	22
◯ Neurology	16
◯ Rheumatology	16
◯ Endocrinology and Metabolism	14
◯ General Internal Medicine	26
◯ Infectious Disease	19
◯ Nephrology	19
◯ Pulmonary and Critical Care Medicine	19

E

CREDITS CLAIMED ON SECTION
(1 hour = 1 credit)

Enter the number of credits earned on the test to the nearest quarter hour. Physicians should claim only the credit commensurate with the extent of their participation in the activity.

F

Enter your score here.

Instructions for calculating your own score are found in front of the self-assessment test in each book.

You must receive a minimum score of 50% correct.

_____ %

Credit Submission Date: _____

1 Ⓐ Ⓑ Ⓒ Ⓓ Ⓔ   46 Ⓐ Ⓑ Ⓒ Ⓓ Ⓔ   91 Ⓐ Ⓑ Ⓒ Ⓓ Ⓔ   136 Ⓐ Ⓑ Ⓒ Ⓓ Ⓔ
2 Ⓐ Ⓑ Ⓒ Ⓓ Ⓔ   47 Ⓐ Ⓑ Ⓒ Ⓓ Ⓔ   92 Ⓐ Ⓑ Ⓒ Ⓓ Ⓔ   137 Ⓐ Ⓑ Ⓒ Ⓓ Ⓔ
3 Ⓐ Ⓑ Ⓒ Ⓓ Ⓔ   48 Ⓐ Ⓑ Ⓒ Ⓓ Ⓔ   93 Ⓐ Ⓑ Ⓒ Ⓓ Ⓔ   138 Ⓐ Ⓑ Ⓒ Ⓓ Ⓔ
4 Ⓐ Ⓑ Ⓒ Ⓓ Ⓔ   49 Ⓐ Ⓑ Ⓒ Ⓓ Ⓔ   94 Ⓐ Ⓑ Ⓒ Ⓓ Ⓔ   139 Ⓐ Ⓑ Ⓒ Ⓓ Ⓔ
5 Ⓐ Ⓑ Ⓒ Ⓓ Ⓔ   50 Ⓐ Ⓑ Ⓒ Ⓓ Ⓔ   95 Ⓐ Ⓑ Ⓒ Ⓓ Ⓔ   140 Ⓐ Ⓑ Ⓒ Ⓓ Ⓔ

6 Ⓐ Ⓑ Ⓒ Ⓓ Ⓔ   51 Ⓐ Ⓑ Ⓒ Ⓓ Ⓔ   96 Ⓐ Ⓑ Ⓒ Ⓓ Ⓔ   141 Ⓐ Ⓑ Ⓒ Ⓓ Ⓔ
7 Ⓐ Ⓑ Ⓒ Ⓓ Ⓔ   52 Ⓐ Ⓑ Ⓒ Ⓓ Ⓔ   97 Ⓐ Ⓑ Ⓒ Ⓓ Ⓔ   142 Ⓐ Ⓑ Ⓒ Ⓓ Ⓔ
8 Ⓐ Ⓑ Ⓒ Ⓓ Ⓔ   53 Ⓐ Ⓑ Ⓒ Ⓓ Ⓔ   98 Ⓐ Ⓑ Ⓒ Ⓓ Ⓔ   143 Ⓐ Ⓑ Ⓒ Ⓓ Ⓔ
9 Ⓐ Ⓑ Ⓒ Ⓓ Ⓔ   54 Ⓐ Ⓑ Ⓒ Ⓓ Ⓔ   99 Ⓐ Ⓑ Ⓒ Ⓓ Ⓔ   144 Ⓐ Ⓑ Ⓒ Ⓓ Ⓔ
10 Ⓐ Ⓑ Ⓒ Ⓓ Ⓔ   55 Ⓐ Ⓑ Ⓒ Ⓓ Ⓔ   100 Ⓐ Ⓑ Ⓒ Ⓓ Ⓔ   145 Ⓐ Ⓑ Ⓒ Ⓓ Ⓔ

11 Ⓐ Ⓑ Ⓒ Ⓓ Ⓔ   56 Ⓐ Ⓑ Ⓒ Ⓓ Ⓔ   101 Ⓐ Ⓑ Ⓒ Ⓓ Ⓔ   146 Ⓐ Ⓑ Ⓒ Ⓓ Ⓔ
12 Ⓐ Ⓑ Ⓒ Ⓓ Ⓔ   57 Ⓐ Ⓑ Ⓒ Ⓓ Ⓔ   102 Ⓐ Ⓑ Ⓒ Ⓓ Ⓔ   147 Ⓐ Ⓑ Ⓒ Ⓓ Ⓔ
13 Ⓐ Ⓑ Ⓒ Ⓓ Ⓔ   58 Ⓐ Ⓑ Ⓒ Ⓓ Ⓔ   103 Ⓐ Ⓑ Ⓒ Ⓓ Ⓔ   148 Ⓐ Ⓑ Ⓒ Ⓓ Ⓔ
14 Ⓐ Ⓑ Ⓒ Ⓓ Ⓔ   59 Ⓐ Ⓑ Ⓒ Ⓓ Ⓔ   104 Ⓐ Ⓑ Ⓒ Ⓓ Ⓔ   149 Ⓐ Ⓑ Ⓒ Ⓓ Ⓔ
15 Ⓐ Ⓑ Ⓒ Ⓓ Ⓔ   60 Ⓐ Ⓑ Ⓒ Ⓓ Ⓔ   105 Ⓐ Ⓑ Ⓒ Ⓓ Ⓔ   150 Ⓐ Ⓑ Ⓒ Ⓓ Ⓔ

16 Ⓐ Ⓑ Ⓒ Ⓓ Ⓔ   61 Ⓐ Ⓑ Ⓒ Ⓓ Ⓔ   106 Ⓐ Ⓑ Ⓒ Ⓓ Ⓔ   151 Ⓐ Ⓑ Ⓒ Ⓓ Ⓔ
17 Ⓐ Ⓑ Ⓒ Ⓓ Ⓔ   62 Ⓐ Ⓑ Ⓒ Ⓓ Ⓔ   107 Ⓐ Ⓑ Ⓒ Ⓓ Ⓔ   152 Ⓐ Ⓑ Ⓒ Ⓓ Ⓔ
18 Ⓐ Ⓑ Ⓒ Ⓓ Ⓔ   63 Ⓐ Ⓑ Ⓒ Ⓓ Ⓔ   108 Ⓐ Ⓑ Ⓒ Ⓓ Ⓔ   153 Ⓐ Ⓑ Ⓒ Ⓓ Ⓔ
19 Ⓐ Ⓑ Ⓒ Ⓓ Ⓔ   64 Ⓐ Ⓑ Ⓒ Ⓓ Ⓔ   109 Ⓐ Ⓑ Ⓒ Ⓓ Ⓔ   154 Ⓐ Ⓑ Ⓒ Ⓓ Ⓔ
20 Ⓐ Ⓑ Ⓒ Ⓓ Ⓔ   65 Ⓐ Ⓑ Ⓒ Ⓓ Ⓔ   110 Ⓐ Ⓑ Ⓒ Ⓓ Ⓔ   155 Ⓐ Ⓑ Ⓒ Ⓓ Ⓔ

21 Ⓐ Ⓑ Ⓒ Ⓓ Ⓔ   66 Ⓐ Ⓑ Ⓒ Ⓓ Ⓔ   111 Ⓐ Ⓑ Ⓒ Ⓓ Ⓔ   156 Ⓐ Ⓑ Ⓒ Ⓓ Ⓔ
22 Ⓐ Ⓑ Ⓒ Ⓓ Ⓔ   67 Ⓐ Ⓑ Ⓒ Ⓓ Ⓔ   112 Ⓐ Ⓑ Ⓒ Ⓓ Ⓔ   157 Ⓐ Ⓑ Ⓒ Ⓓ Ⓔ
23 Ⓐ Ⓑ Ⓒ Ⓓ Ⓔ   68 Ⓐ Ⓑ Ⓒ Ⓓ Ⓔ   113 Ⓐ Ⓑ Ⓒ Ⓓ Ⓔ   158 Ⓐ Ⓑ Ⓒ Ⓓ Ⓔ
24 Ⓐ Ⓑ Ⓒ Ⓓ Ⓔ   69 Ⓐ Ⓑ Ⓒ Ⓓ Ⓔ   114 Ⓐ Ⓑ Ⓒ Ⓓ Ⓔ   159 Ⓐ Ⓑ Ⓒ Ⓓ Ⓔ
25 Ⓐ Ⓑ Ⓒ Ⓓ Ⓔ   70 Ⓐ Ⓑ Ⓒ Ⓓ Ⓔ   115 Ⓐ Ⓑ Ⓒ Ⓓ Ⓔ   160 Ⓐ Ⓑ Ⓒ Ⓓ Ⓔ

26 Ⓐ Ⓑ Ⓒ Ⓓ Ⓔ   71 Ⓐ Ⓑ Ⓒ Ⓓ Ⓔ   116 Ⓐ Ⓑ Ⓒ Ⓓ Ⓔ   161 Ⓐ Ⓑ Ⓒ Ⓓ Ⓔ
27 Ⓐ Ⓑ Ⓒ Ⓓ Ⓔ   72 Ⓐ Ⓑ Ⓒ Ⓓ Ⓔ   117 Ⓐ Ⓑ Ⓒ Ⓓ Ⓔ   162 Ⓐ Ⓑ Ⓒ Ⓓ Ⓔ
28 Ⓐ Ⓑ Ⓒ Ⓓ Ⓔ   73 Ⓐ Ⓑ Ⓒ Ⓓ Ⓔ   118 Ⓐ Ⓑ Ⓒ Ⓓ Ⓔ   163 Ⓐ Ⓑ Ⓒ Ⓓ Ⓔ
29 Ⓐ Ⓑ Ⓒ Ⓓ Ⓔ   74 Ⓐ Ⓑ Ⓒ Ⓓ Ⓔ   119 Ⓐ Ⓑ Ⓒ Ⓓ Ⓔ   164 Ⓐ Ⓑ Ⓒ Ⓓ Ⓔ
30 Ⓐ Ⓑ Ⓒ Ⓓ Ⓔ   75 Ⓐ Ⓑ Ⓒ Ⓓ Ⓔ   120 Ⓐ Ⓑ Ⓒ Ⓓ Ⓔ   165 Ⓐ Ⓑ Ⓒ Ⓓ Ⓔ

31 Ⓐ Ⓑ Ⓒ Ⓓ Ⓔ   76 Ⓐ Ⓑ Ⓒ Ⓓ Ⓔ   121 Ⓐ Ⓑ Ⓒ Ⓓ Ⓔ   166 Ⓐ Ⓑ Ⓒ Ⓓ Ⓔ
32 Ⓐ Ⓑ Ⓒ Ⓓ Ⓔ   77 Ⓐ Ⓑ Ⓒ Ⓓ Ⓔ   122 Ⓐ Ⓑ Ⓒ Ⓓ Ⓔ   167 Ⓐ Ⓑ Ⓒ Ⓓ Ⓔ
33 Ⓐ Ⓑ Ⓒ Ⓓ Ⓔ   78 Ⓐ Ⓑ Ⓒ Ⓓ Ⓔ   123 Ⓐ Ⓑ Ⓒ Ⓓ Ⓔ   168 Ⓐ Ⓑ Ⓒ Ⓓ Ⓔ
34 Ⓐ Ⓑ Ⓒ Ⓓ Ⓔ   79 Ⓐ Ⓑ Ⓒ Ⓓ Ⓔ   124 Ⓐ Ⓑ Ⓒ Ⓓ Ⓔ   169 Ⓐ Ⓑ Ⓒ Ⓓ Ⓔ
35 Ⓐ Ⓑ Ⓒ Ⓓ Ⓔ   80 Ⓐ Ⓑ Ⓒ Ⓓ Ⓔ   125 Ⓐ Ⓑ Ⓒ Ⓓ Ⓔ   170 Ⓐ Ⓑ Ⓒ Ⓓ Ⓔ

36 Ⓐ Ⓑ Ⓒ Ⓓ Ⓔ   81 Ⓐ Ⓑ Ⓒ Ⓓ Ⓔ   126 Ⓐ Ⓑ Ⓒ Ⓓ Ⓔ   171 Ⓐ Ⓑ Ⓒ Ⓓ Ⓔ
37 Ⓐ Ⓑ Ⓒ Ⓓ Ⓔ   82 Ⓐ Ⓑ Ⓒ Ⓓ Ⓔ   127 Ⓐ Ⓑ Ⓒ Ⓓ Ⓔ   172 Ⓐ Ⓑ Ⓒ Ⓓ Ⓔ
38 Ⓐ Ⓑ Ⓒ Ⓓ Ⓔ   83 Ⓐ Ⓑ Ⓒ Ⓓ Ⓔ   128 Ⓐ Ⓑ Ⓒ Ⓓ Ⓔ   173 Ⓐ Ⓑ Ⓒ Ⓓ Ⓔ
39 Ⓐ Ⓑ Ⓒ Ⓓ Ⓔ   84 Ⓐ Ⓑ Ⓒ Ⓓ Ⓔ   129 Ⓐ Ⓑ Ⓒ Ⓓ Ⓔ   174 Ⓐ Ⓑ Ⓒ Ⓓ Ⓔ
40 Ⓐ Ⓑ Ⓒ Ⓓ Ⓔ   85 Ⓐ Ⓑ Ⓒ Ⓓ Ⓔ   130 Ⓐ Ⓑ Ⓒ Ⓓ Ⓔ   175 Ⓐ Ⓑ Ⓒ Ⓓ Ⓔ

41 Ⓐ Ⓑ Ⓒ Ⓓ Ⓔ   86 Ⓐ Ⓑ Ⓒ Ⓓ Ⓔ   131 Ⓐ Ⓑ Ⓒ Ⓓ Ⓔ   176 Ⓐ Ⓑ Ⓒ Ⓓ Ⓔ
42 Ⓐ Ⓑ Ⓒ Ⓓ Ⓔ   87 Ⓐ Ⓑ Ⓒ Ⓓ Ⓔ   132 Ⓐ Ⓑ Ⓒ Ⓓ Ⓔ   177 Ⓐ Ⓑ Ⓒ Ⓓ Ⓔ
43 Ⓐ Ⓑ Ⓒ Ⓓ Ⓔ   88 Ⓐ Ⓑ Ⓒ Ⓓ Ⓔ   133 Ⓐ Ⓑ Ⓒ Ⓓ Ⓔ   178 Ⓐ Ⓑ Ⓒ Ⓓ Ⓔ
44 Ⓐ Ⓑ Ⓒ Ⓓ Ⓔ   89 Ⓐ Ⓑ Ⓒ Ⓓ Ⓔ   134 Ⓐ Ⓑ Ⓒ Ⓓ Ⓔ   179 Ⓐ Ⓑ Ⓒ Ⓓ Ⓔ
45 Ⓐ Ⓑ Ⓒ Ⓓ Ⓔ   90 Ⓐ Ⓑ Ⓒ Ⓓ Ⓔ   135 Ⓐ Ⓑ Ⓒ Ⓓ Ⓔ   180 Ⓐ Ⓑ Ⓒ Ⓓ Ⓔ